Stahl's Illustrated

# Pharmacological Treatments for Psychosis

Stephen M. Stahl
University of California, San Diego

Gabriela Alarcón
Neuroscience Education Institute

Nancy Muntner
Illustrations

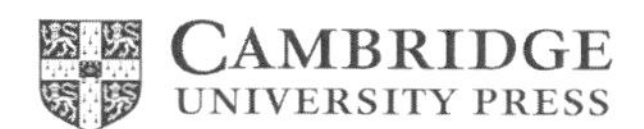
CAMBRIDGE
UNIVERSITY PRESS

COPYRIGHT

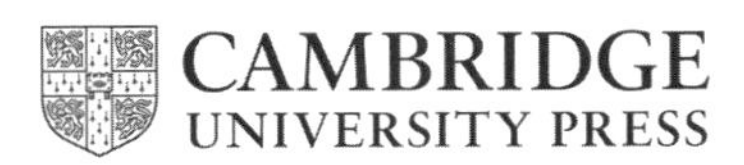

Shaftesbury Road, Cambridge CB2 8EA, United Kingdom

One Liberty Plaza, 20th Floor, New York, NY 10006, USA

477 Williamstown Road, Port Melbourne, VIC 3207, Australia

314–321, 3rd Floor, Plot 3, Splendor Forum, Jasola District Centre, New Delhi – 110025, India

103 Penang Road, #05–06/07, Visioncrest Commercial, Singapore 238467

Cambridge University Press is part of Cambridge University Press & Assessment, a department of the University of Cambridge.

We share the University's mission to contribute to society through the pursuit of education, learning and research at the highest international levels of excellence.

www.cambridge.org
Information on this title: www.cambridge.org/9781009485043

DOI: 10.1017/9781009485050



When citing this work, please include a reference to the DOI 10.1017/9781009485050

First published 2024

Printed in Mexico by Litográfica Ingramex, S.A. de C.V.

*A catalogue record for this publication is available from the British Library.*

*Library of Congress Cataloging-in-Publication Data*

ISBN 978-1-009-48504-3 Paperback

# Table of Contents

# PREFACE

These books are designed to be fun, with all concepts illustrated by full-color images and the text serving as a supplement to figures, images, and tables. The visual learner will find that this book makes psychopharmacological concepts easy to master, while the non-visual learner may enjoy a shortened text version of complex psychopharmacological concepts. Each chapter builds upon previous chapters, synthesizing information from basic biology and diagnostics to building treatment plans and dealing with complications and comorbidities.

Novices may want to approach this book by first looking through all the graphics, gaining a feel for the visual vocabulary on which our psychopharmacological concepts rely. After this once-over glance, we suggest going back through the book to incorporate the images with supporting text. Learning from visual concepts and textual supplements should reinforce one another, providing you with solid conceptual understanding at each step along the way.

Readers more familiar with these topics should find that going back and forth between images and text provides an interaction with which to vividly conceptualize complex psychopharmacology. You may find yourself using this book frequently to refresh your psychopharmacological knowledge. And you will hopefully refer your colleagues to this desk reference.

This book is intended as a conceptual overview of different topics; we provide you with a visual-based language to incorporate the rules of psychopharmacology at the expense of discussing the exceptions to these rules. The references section at the end gives you a good start for more in-depth learning about particular concepts presented here. Stahl's Essential Psychopharmacology and Stahl's Essential Psychopharmacology: The Prescriber's Guide can be helpful supplementary tools for more in-depth information on particular topics in this book. You can also search topics in psychopharmacology on the Neuroscience Education Institute's website (www.neiglobal.com) for lectures, courses, slides, and related articles.

Whether you are a novice or an experienced psychopharmacologist, this book will hopefully lead you to think critically about the complexities involved in psychiatric disorders and their treatments.

Best wishes for your educational journey into the fascinating field of psychopharmacology!

Stephen M. Stahl

# CME/CE Information

**Released:** February 1, 2024
**CME/CE credit expires:** January 31, 2027

**Target Audience:** This activity has been developed for the healthcare team or individual prescriber specializing in mental health. All other healthcare team members interested in psychopharmacology are welcome for advanced study.

**Learning Objectives:** After completing this activity, you should be better able to:

- Describe the neurobiology of psychosis and schizophrenia
- Differentiate drugs for psychosis based on their pharmacology
- Recognize how different drugs' receptor binding profiles affect symptoms of psychosis and specific side effects
- Choose the best treatment practices and switching methods when prescribing drugs for psychosis

**Accreditation:** In support of improving patient care, Neuroscience Education Institute (NEI) is jointly accredited by the Accreditation Council for Continuing Medical Education (ACCME), the Accreditation Council for Pharmacy Education (ACPE), and the American Nurses Credentialing Center (ANCC), to provide continuing education for the healthcare team.

NEI designates this enduring material for a maximum of 10.0 *AMA PRA Category 1 Credits*™. Physicians should claim only the credit commensurate with the extent of their participation in the activity.

The content in this activity pertaining to pharmacology is worth 10.0 continuing education hours of pharmacotherapeutics.

**Credit Types:** The following are being offered for this activity:

- Nurse Practitioner: ANCC contact hours
- Pharmacy: ACPE practice-based contact hours
- Physician: ACCME *AMA PRA Category 1 Credits*™
- Physician Associate: AAPA Category 1 CME credits
- Psychology: APA CE credits
- Social Work: ASWB-ACE CE credits
- Non-Physician Member of the Healthcare Team: Certificate of Participation stating the program is designated for *AMA PRA Category 1 Credits*™

**Optional Posttest and CME/CE Credit:** The optional posttest with CME/CE credits is available online for a fee (waived for NEI Members). A posttest score of 70% or higher is required to receive credit. To purchase and/or open the posttest, go to **https://nei.global/24-Stahl-illus-psychosis3**.

**Peer Review:** The content was peer reviewed by an MD specializing in forensic psychiatry to ensure the scientific accuracy and medical relevance of information presented and its independence from bias. NEI takes responsibility for the content, quality, and scientific integrity of this CME/CE activity.

**Disclosures:** All individuals in a position to influence or control content are required to disclose all relevant financial relationships. Potential conflicts were identified and mitigated prior to the activity being planned, developed, or presented.

***Authors***

**Gabriela Alarcón, PhD**
*Senior Medical Writer, Neuroscience Education Institute, Carlsbad, CA*
No financial relationships to disclose.

**Stephen M. Stahl, MD, PhD, DSc (Hon.)**
*Clinical Professor, Department of Psychiatry and Neuroscience, University of California, Riverside School of Medicine, Riverside, CA*
*Adjunct Professor, Department of Psychiatry, University of California, San Diego School of Medicine, La Jolla, CA*
*Honorary Visiting Senior Fellow, University of Cambridge, Cambridge, UK*
*Editor-in-Chief, CNS Spectrums*
*Director of Psychopharmacology Services, California Department of State Hospitals, CA*
Grant/Research: Acadia, Alkermes, Allergan/AbbVie, Arbor, AssureX, AstraZeneca, Avanir, Axovant, Biogen, Boehringer Ingelheim Braeburn, BristolMyer Squibb, Celgene, CeNeRex, Cephalon, Daiichi Sankyo-Brazil, Dey, Eisai, Forest, Genomind, GlaxoSmithKline, Harmony Biosciences, Indivior, Intra-Cellular, Ironshore, Janssen, JayMac, Jazz, Lilly, Lundbeck, Merck, Neurocrine, Neuronetics, Novartis, Otsuka, Pear, Pfizer, Reviva, Roche, Sage, Servier, Shire, Sprout, Sunovion, Supernus, Takeda, Teva, Tonix, Torrent, Vanda
Consultant/Advisor: Acadia, Adamas, Alkermes, Allergan/AbbVie, Altus, Arbor, AstraZeneca, Avanir, Axovant, Axsome, Biogen, Biomarin, Biopharma, Celgene, Cerevel, ClearView, Clexio, Concert, DepotMed, Done, EMD Serono, Eisai, Enveric, Eurolink, Fabre-Kramer, Ferring, Forest, Gedeon Richter, Genetica, Genomind, Innovative Science Solutions, Impel, Intra-Cellular, Ironshore, Janssen, Jazz, Karuna, Libbs, Lilly, Lipidio, Longboard, Lundbeck, Merck, Neos, NeuraWell, Neurocrine, NeuroPharma, Novartis, Noveida, Otsuka, Perrigo, Pfizer, Pierre Fabre, Proxymm, Recordati, Relmada, Reviva, Sage, Saniona, Servier, Shire, Sprout, Sunovion, Supernus, Takeda, Taliaz, Teva, Tonix, Tris, Trius, Vanda, Vertex, Viforpharma

Speakers Bureau: Acadia, Allergan/AbbVie, Genentech, Janssen, Lundbeck, Merck, Neurocrine, Otsuka, Servier, Sunovion, Takeda, Teva
Options Holdings: Delix, Genomind, Lipidio, NeuraWell

The **Planning Committee**, **Design Staff**, and **Peer Reviewer** have no financial relationships to disclose.

**Disclosure of Off-Label Use:** This educational activity may include discussion of unlabeled and/or investigational uses of agents that are not currently labeled for such use by the Food and Drug Administration (FDA). Please consult the product prescribing information for full disclosure of labeled uses.

**Cultural Linguistic Competencies and Implicit Bias:** A variety of resources addressing cultural and linguistic competency and strategies for understanding and reducing implicit bias can be found at: **https://nei.global/CLC-IB-handout**

**Support:** This activity is supported solely by the provider, NEI.

Stahl's Illustrated

# Introduction

Psychosis is a collection of psychological symptoms resulting in the loss of touch with reality. It is a common feature to many psychiatric disorders, particularly schizophrenia and other conditions in the schizophrenia spectrum, as well as mood disorders (bipolar disorder and major depression with psychotic features). Psychosis may also manifest due to an underlying medical disease or substance use. Approximately 1.5 to 3.5% of people will meet diagnostic criteria for a psychotic disorder. The presence of psychosis generally indicates a serious mental illness, which often requires early intervention and long-term treatment to achieve favorable outcomes (Calabrese & Al Khalili, 2023).

So-called antipsychotics (serotonin/dopamine antagonists) are the gold-standard treatment for psychotic episodes and disorders. However, advancements in our understanding of the neurobiology of psychosis, particularly schizophrenia, may soon expand our treatment options. This expansion also challenges our conceptualization of the "antipsychotic." Antipsychotics are synonymous with dopamine D2 antagonism, but newer medications in development do not directly target this receptor. Furthermore, D2 antagonists are used to successfully treat non-psychotic symptoms like depression. Therefore, throughout this book we use the neuroscience-based nomenclature, which is based on mechanism of action and not therapeutic indication, wherever possible when referring to drugs for psychosis.

In the following pages, we describe the symptoms of psychosis, the neurocircuitry that underlies those symptoms, and the evidence-based therapeutic targets for the treatment of those symptoms. Chapters 1–2 describe the neurobiological models and neurocircuitry that underlie psychosis and how malfunctioning circuits are connected to symptoms. An emphasis is placed on schizophrenia as the prototypical psychotic disorder; however, Parkinson's disease psychosis and dementia-related psychosis are also discussed. Chapter 3 addresses additional receptor actions that lead to common side effects of serotonin/dopamine antagonists. Chapters 4–5 review pharmacological properties of dopamine receptor blocking agents and strategies for switching medications. Finally, Chapter 6 describes advancements in the development of novel pharmacological treatments for psychosis that do not directly target the dopamine D2 receptor.

Stahl's Illustrated

Chapter 1

# Schizophrenia as the Prototypical Psychotic Disorder

Schizophrenia is the prototypical psychotic disorder since it is the most common and best known and expresses prototypical psychotic symptoms. Delusions and hallucinations are the hallmarks of schizophrenia and are often called the "positive symptoms" of psychosis. Delusions are fixed beliefs—often bizarre—that have an inadequate rational basis and can't be changed by rational arguments or evidence to the contrary. Hallucinations are perceptual experiences of any sensory modality—especially auditory—that occur without a real external stimulus yet are vivid and clear, just like normal perceptions, but not under voluntary control. Schizophrenia can also include other symptoms like disorganized speech and behavior and the so-called "negative symptoms" of psychosis, including diminished emotional expression and decreased motivation (American Psychiatric Association, 2022).

Both disease pathophysiology and novel treatments are pivoting from the postsynaptic dopamine D2 receptor to the presynaptic dopamine terminals of overly-active dopamine fibers that drive positive symptoms. High levels of dopamine in presynaptic terminals of psychotic unmedicated patients have been documented and replicated with in-vivo human neuroimaging (Brugger et al., 2020; Weinstein et al., 2017). Emerging genetic research shows this is likely due to aberrant presynaptic D2 receptors being inadequately sensitive and thus unable to turn off dopamine release (Benjamin et al., 2023). Mechanisms whereby upstream modulation of dopamine by various neurotransmitters may treat symptoms of psychosis are presented.

# Schizophrenia Phenotype: Positive and Negative Symptoms

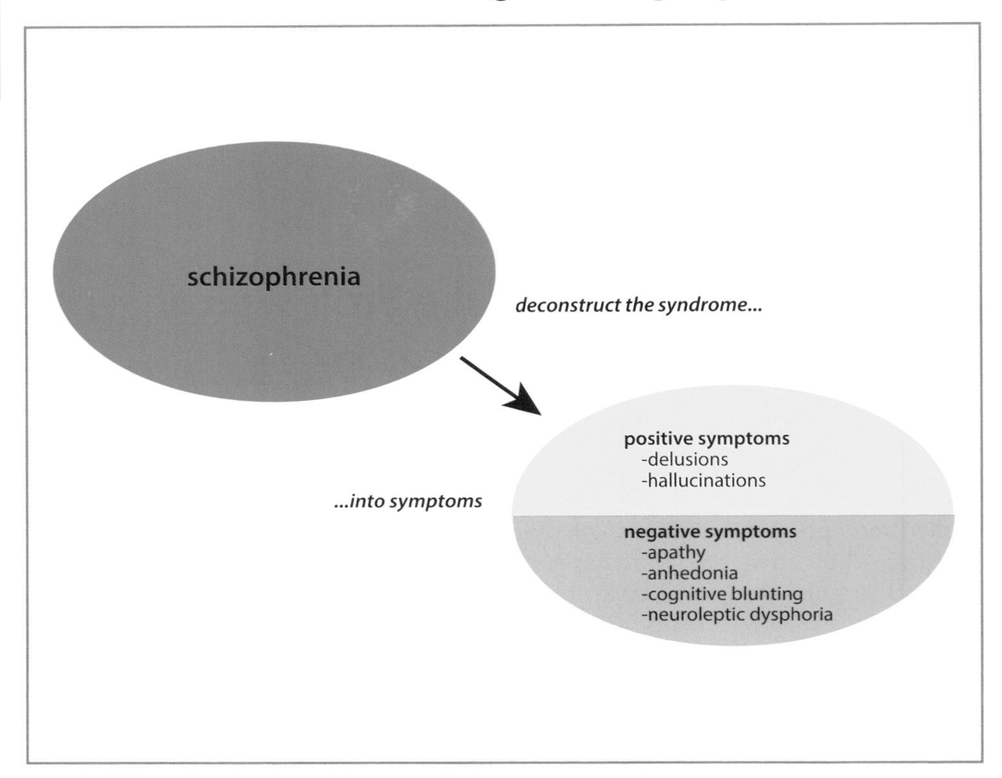


**FIGURE 1.1.** The syndrome of schizophrenia consists of a mixture of symptoms that are commonly divided into two major categories, positive and negative. Positive symptoms, such as delusions and hallucinations, reflect the development of the symptoms of psychosis; they can be dramatic and may reflect loss of touch with reality. Negative symptoms reflect the loss of normal functions and feelings, such as losing interest in things and not being able to experience pleasure (Stahl, 2021).

# Localization of Symptom Domains

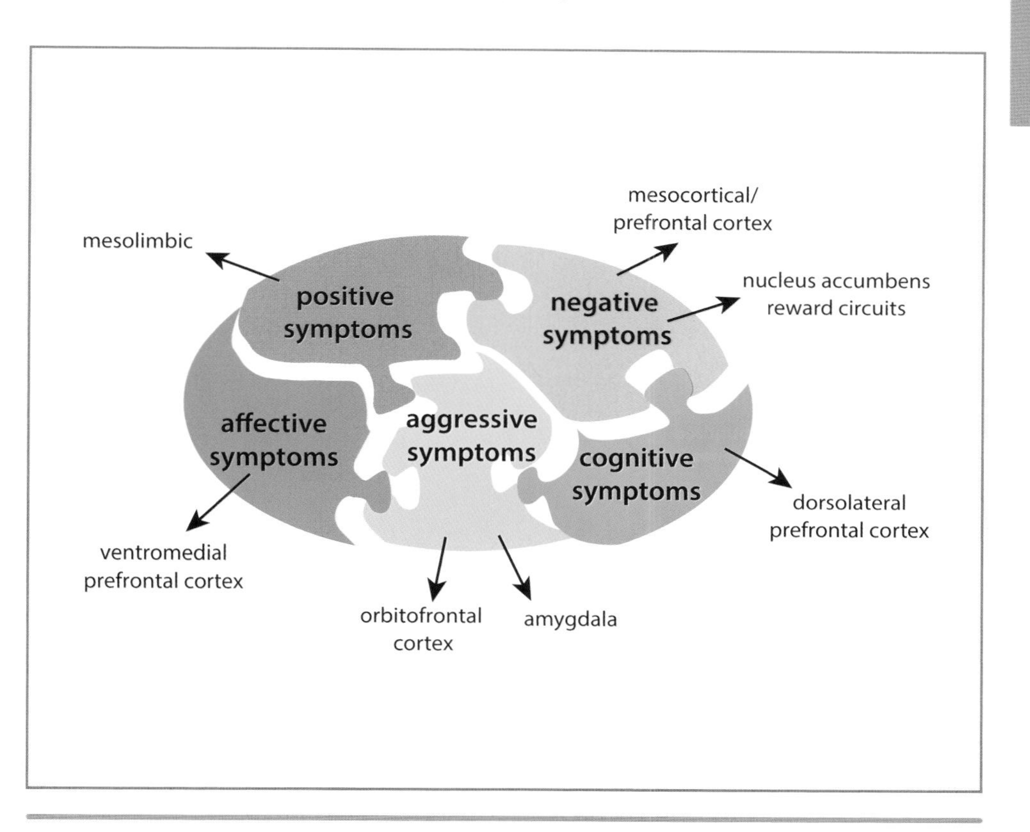


**FIGURE 1.2.** Although not recognized formally as part of the diagnostic criteria for schizophrenia, numerous studies subcategorize the symptoms of this illness into five dimensions: positive, negative, cognitive, affective, and aggressive. Each of these symptom domains may hypothetically be mediated by unique brain regions (Stahl, 2021).

# The Nature and Nurture of Schizophrenia

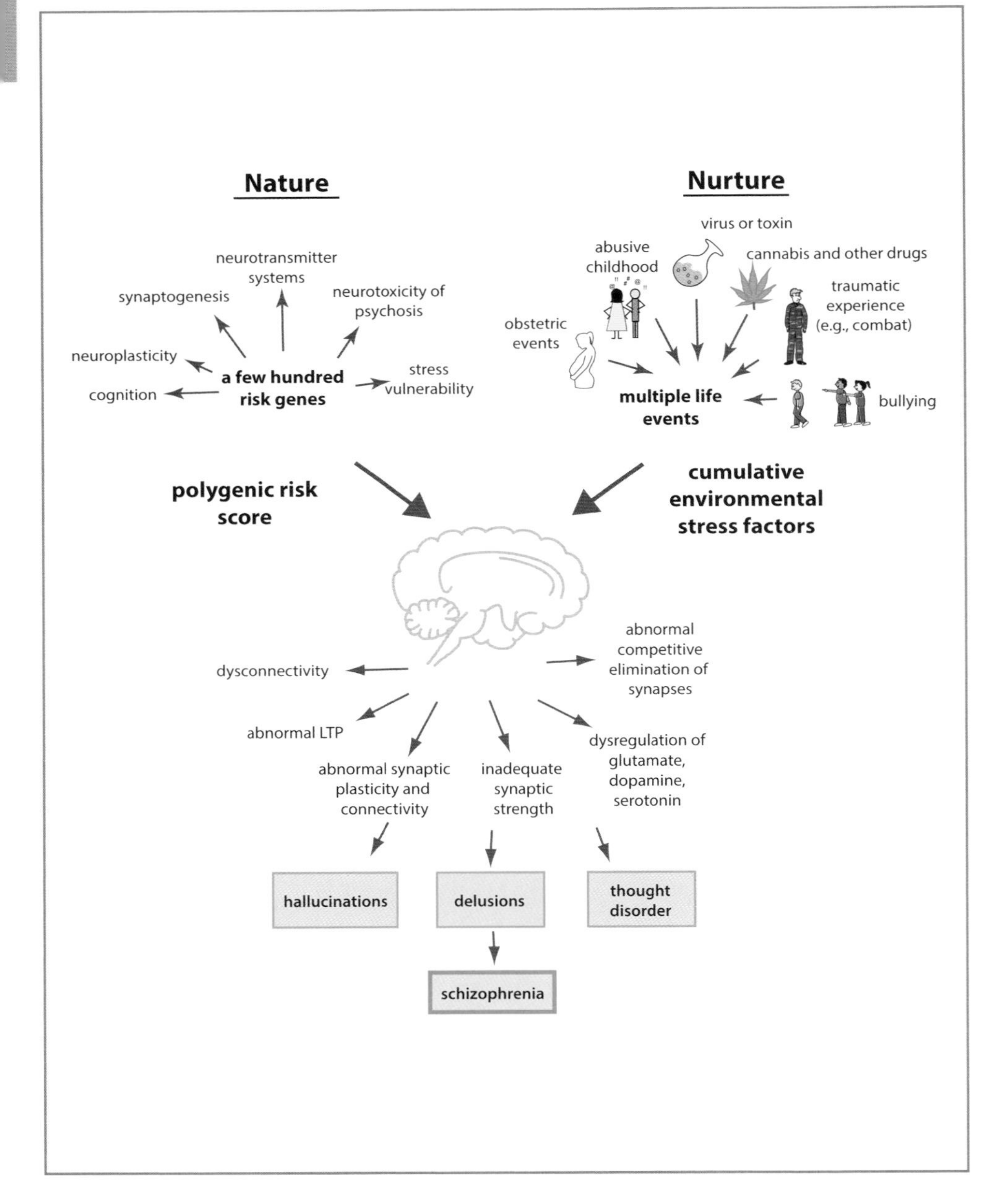

# The Nature and Nurture of Schizophrenia

**FIGURE 1.3.** Schizophrenia may occur as the result of both genetic (nature) and epigenetic (nurture) factors. That is, an individual with multiple genetic risk factors, combined with multiple stressors causing epigenetic changes, may have abnormal information processing in the form of dysconnectivity, abnormal long-term potentiation (LTP), reduced synaptic plasticity, inadequate synapse strength, dysregulated neurotransmission, and abnormal competitive elimination of synapses. The result may be psychiatric symptoms such as hallucinations, delusions, and thought disorder (Stahl, 2021; St Clair & Lang, 2021; Wahbeh & Avrampolous, 2021).

# Neurodevelopmental Hypothesis of Schizophrenia: Abnormal Synaptogenesis

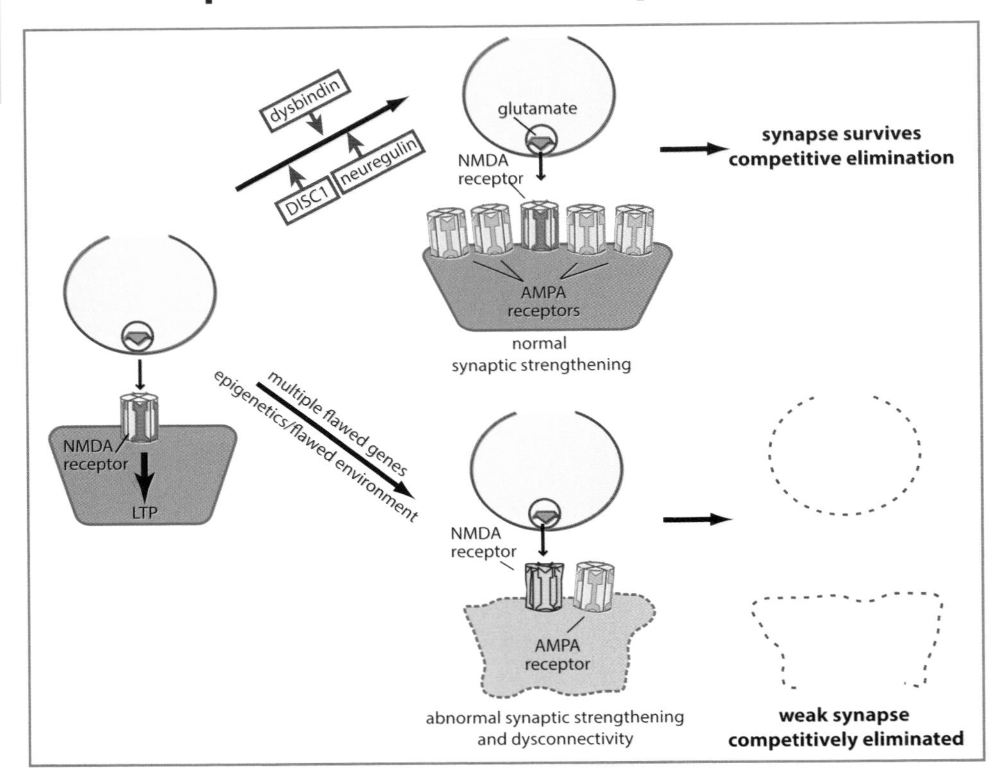

# Neurodevelopmental Hypothesis of Schizophrenia: Abnormal Synaptogenesis

**FIGURE 1.4.** Dysbindin, DISC1 (disrupted in schizophrenia-1), and neuregulin are proteins involved in "strengthening" of glutamate synapses. Under normal circumstances, N-methyl-D-aspartate (NMDA) receptors in active glutamate synapses trigger long-term potentiation (LTP), which leads to structural and functional changes of the synapse to make it more efficient, or "strengthened." This process leads to an increased number of α-amino-3-hydroxy-5 methyl-4-isoxazolepropionic acid (AMPA) receptors, which are important for mediating glutamatergic neurotransmission. Normal synaptic strengthening means that the synapse will survive during competitive elimination. If the genes that regulate strengthening of glutamate synapses are abnormal, combined with environmental insults, then this could cause hypofunctioning of NMDA receptors with a resultant decrease in LTP and fewer AMPA receptors. This abnormal synaptic strengthening and dysconnectivity would lead to weak synapses that would not survive competitive elimination. This would theoretically lead to increased risk of developing schizophrenia, and these abnormal synapses could mediate the symptoms of schizophrenia (Bubeníková-Valesová et al., 2008; Stahl, 2021).

# Elevated DA Synthesis and Release in Schizophrenia

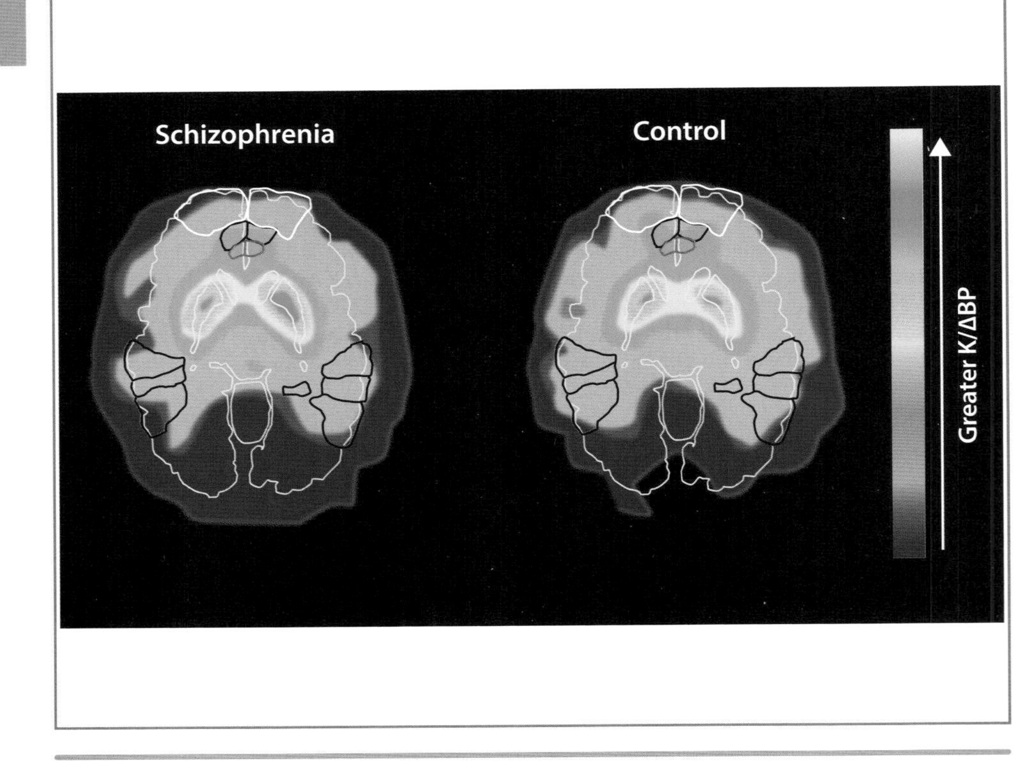


**FIGURE 1.5.** Molecular imaging studies indicate that individuals with schizophrenia have elevated presynaptic striatal dopamine (DA) synthesis and release capacities compared to healthy controls. Dopamine synthesis is measured by the uptake of radiolabeled L-DOPA tracer (K), while dopamine release capacity is measured by a change in tracer binding to the postsynaptic dopamine receptor following a psychostimulant challenge (ΔBP) (Brugger et al., 2020; Howes et al., 2011; Lindström et al., 1999; Weinstein et al., 2017).

# D2 Receptor Short Isoform Is a Risk Factor for Schizophrenia

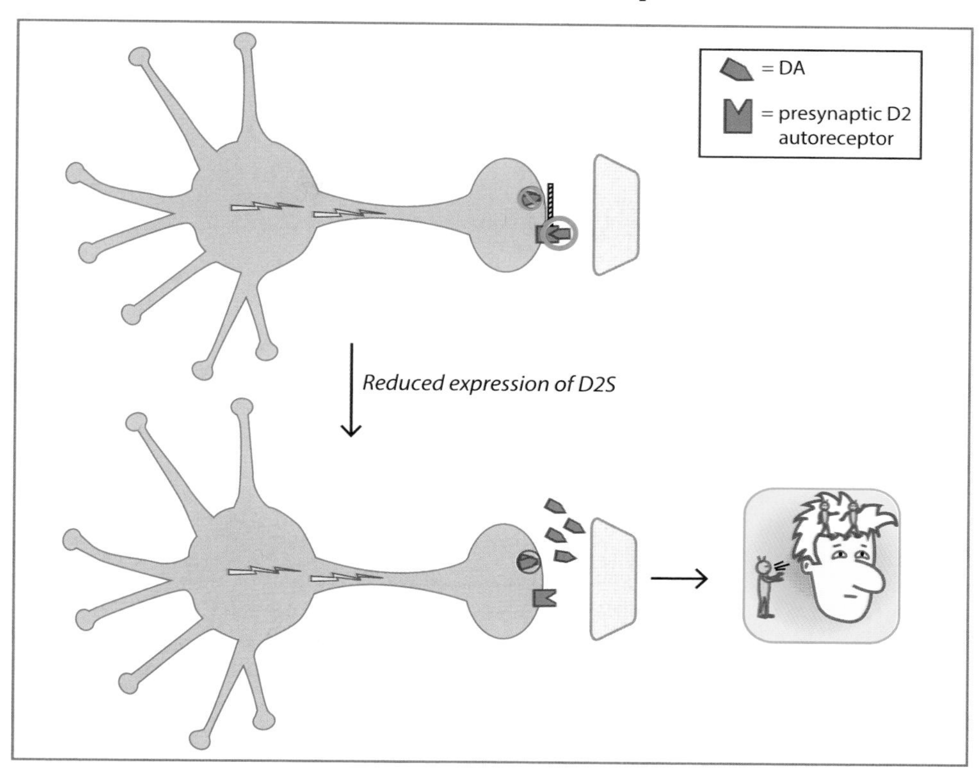


**FIGURE 1.6.** Presynaptic D2 autoreceptors can be located on the axon terminal. When dopamine builds up in the synapse it is available to bind to the autoreceptor, which then inhibits dopamine release. The *DRD2* gene generates two principal receptor dopamine D2 isoforms, D2L (long) and D2S (short). D2L functions as a postsynaptic dopamine receptor, while D2S functions as a presynaptic autoreceptor. Genetic analyses of postmortem brain tissue show reduced expression of D2S isoforms in the caudate nucleus of people with schizophrenia. Consequently, this compromised presynaptic autoregulation leads to increased synaptic dopamine in the striatum that putatively places individuals at risk for schizophrenia (Benjamin et al., 2022).

# The Psychosis Circuit: Upstream Cholinergic Modulation of DA

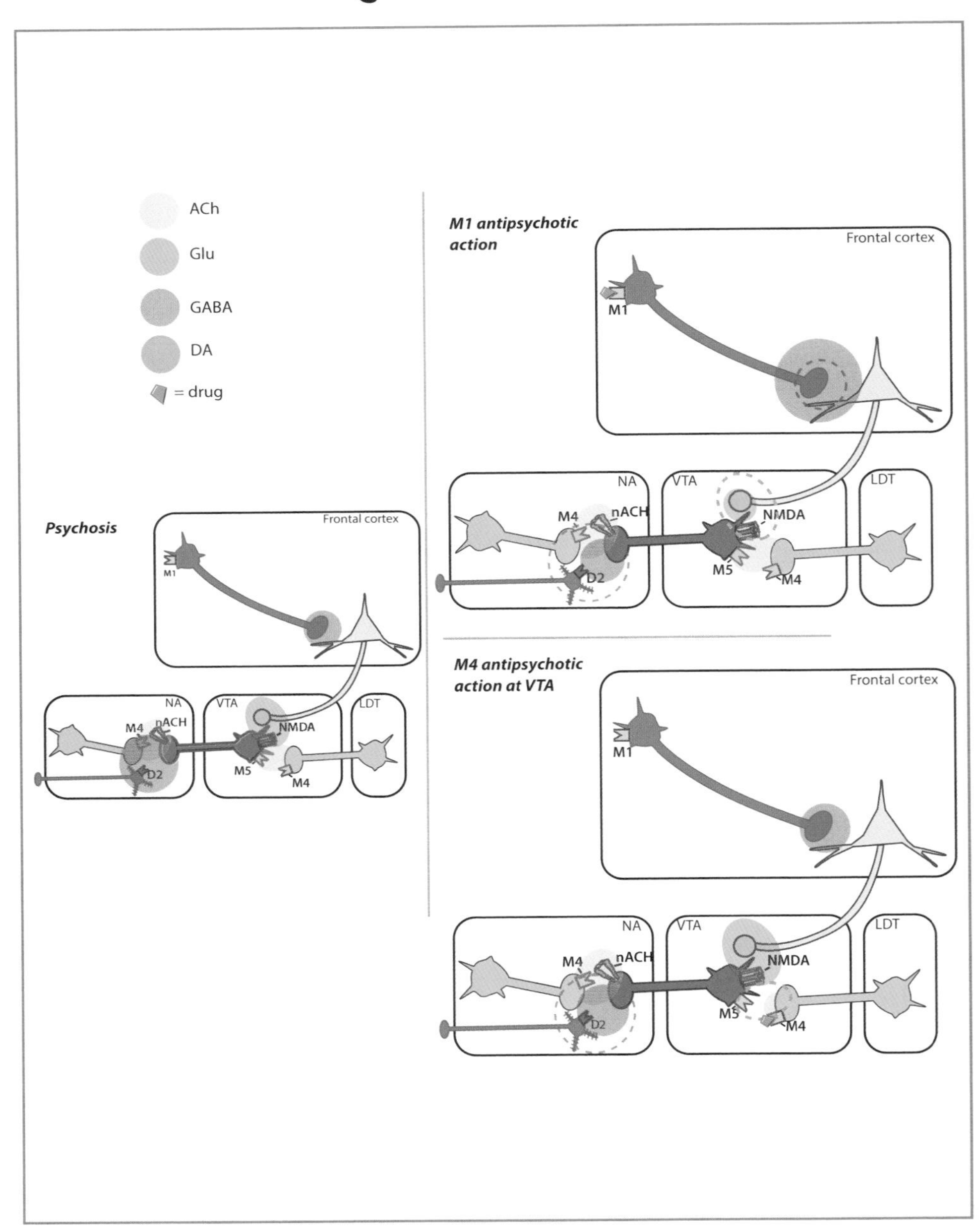

# The Psychosis Circuit: Upstream Cholinergic Modulation of DA

**FIGURE 1.7.** Muscarinic M1 and M4 receptors modulate dopamine (DA) release upstream in psychosis circuits. In a state of psychosis, low γ-aminobutyric acid (GABA) interneuron activity in the frontal cortex leads to increased neuronal excitability from the ventral tegmental area (VTA), which in turn leads to excess dopamine in the nucleus accumbens (NA) (left). In the frontal cortex, activation of M1 receptors on GABA interneurons leads to a reduction of excitatory glutamate (Glu) release in the VTA. This reduction in Glu decreases the activity of DA neurons via N-methyl-D-aspartate (NMDA) receptors, resulting in a decrease in DA release and a hypothetical decrease in the positive symptoms of psychosis (top right). In addition, M4 receptors on cholinergic projections from the laterodorsal tegmental nucleus (LDT) in the hindbrain act as autoreceptors and turn off acetylcholine (ACh) release from these projections when activated. This reduction in ACh leads to decreased activation of muscarinic M5 receptors located on DA cell bodies, decreased neuronal excitability in the VTA, and hypothethically decreased positive symptoms of psychosis (bottom right) (Paul et al., 2022; Yohn et al., 2022).

# The Psychosis Circuit: Upstream Trace Amine Modulation of DA

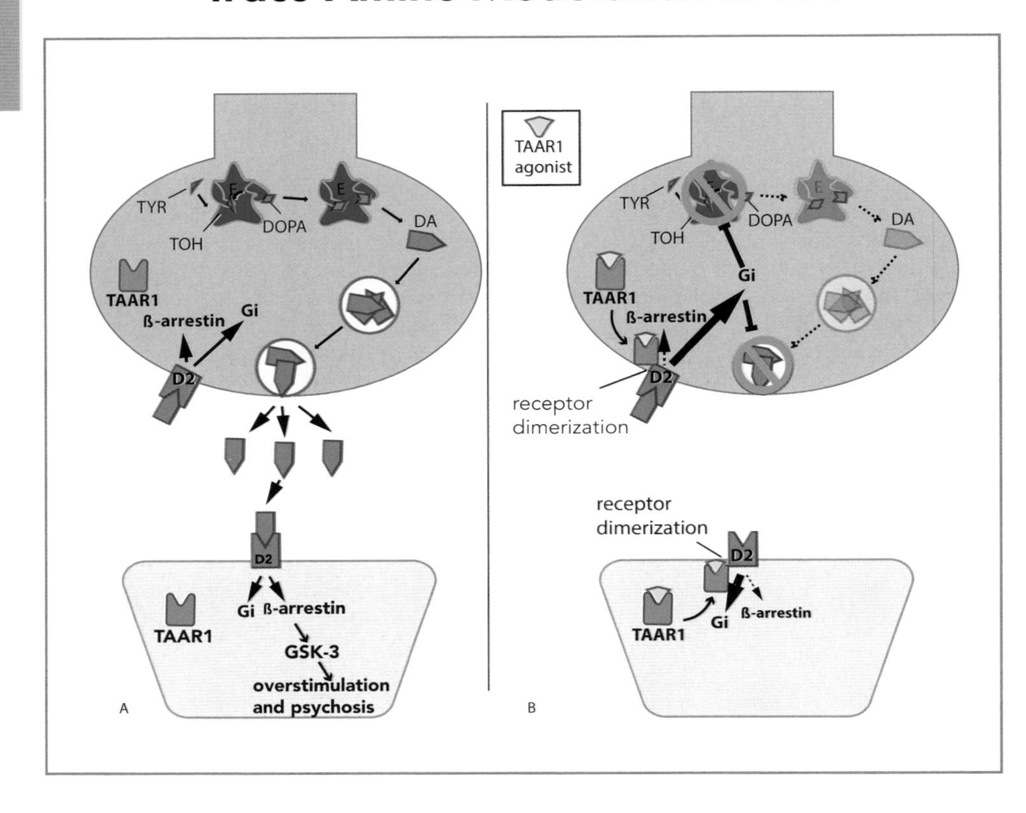

# The Psychosis Circuit: Upstream Trace Amine Modulation of DA

**FIGURE 1.8.** Trace amines are formed from amino acids when either the tyrosine hydroxylase (TYR) step or the tryptophan hydroxylase (TOH) step is omitted during production of dopamine or serotonin, respectively. (A) Dopamine is produced and packaged into synaptic vesicles, then released into the synapse. Dopamine binding at both pre- and postsynaptic D2 receptors can either trigger the inhibitory G (Gi) protein signal transduction cascade or the β-arrestin 2 signal transduction cascade. The β-arrestin 2 cascade leads to production of glycogen synthase kinase 3 (GSK-3); too much GSK-3 activation may be associated with psychosis. (B) When TAAR1 receptors are bound by an agonist, they translocate to the synaptic membrane and couple with D2 receptors (heterodimerization). This biases the D2 receptor toward activating the Gi signal transduction cascade instead of the β-arrestin cascade. Presynaptically, amplification of the Gi pathway leads to inhibition of the synthesis and release of dopamine, which would be beneficial in cases of psychosis. Postsynaptically, amplification of the Gi pathway can lead to reduced production of GSK-3 (Pei et al., 2016; Stahl, 2021).

# The Psychosis Circuit: Upstream Glutamate Modulation of DA

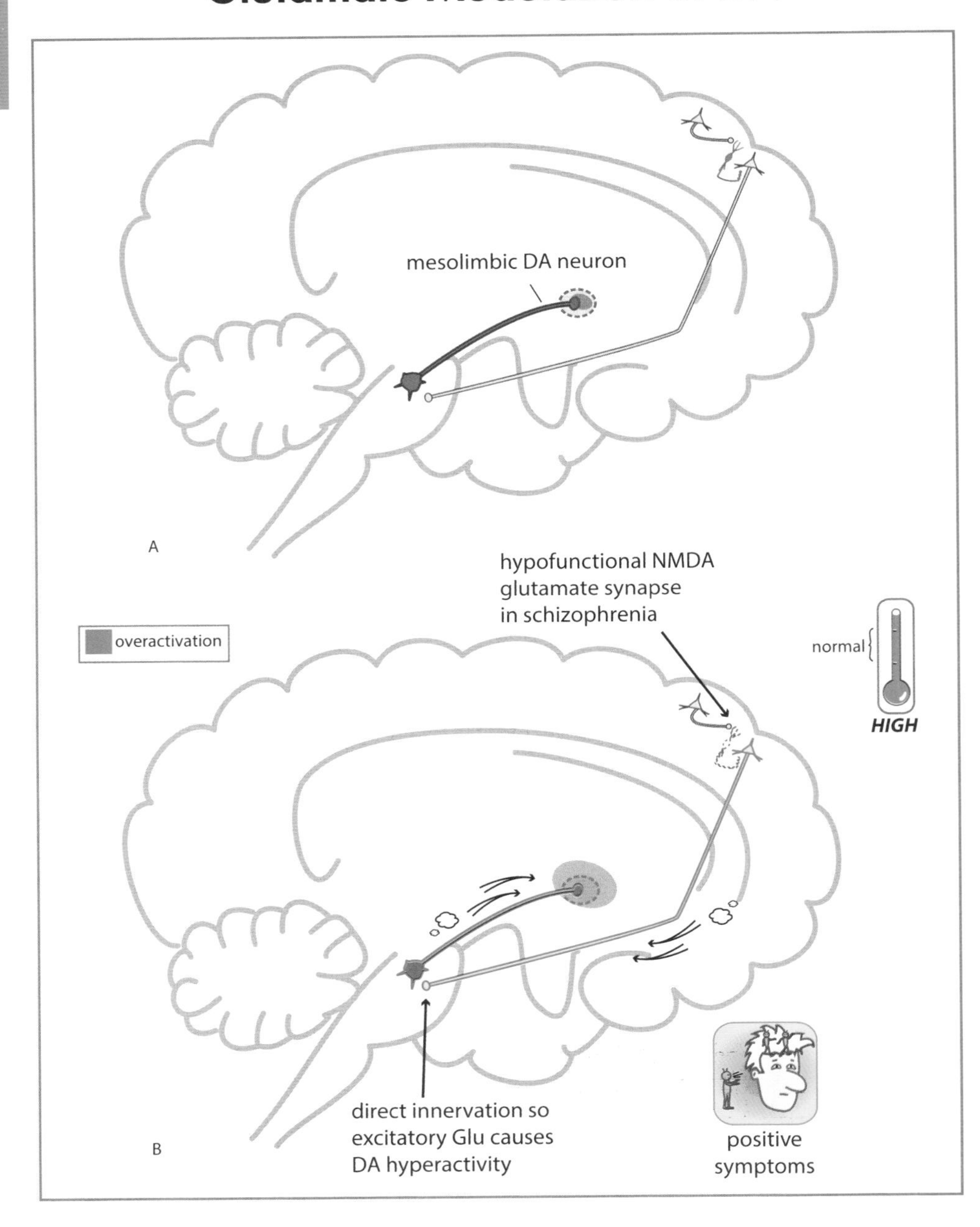

# The Psychosis Circuit: Upstream Glutamate Modulation of DA

**FIGURE 1.9.** (A) The cortical brainstem glutamate projection communicates with the mesolimbic dopamine pathway in the ventral tegmental area (VTA) to regulate dopamine release in the nucleus accumbens. (B) If NMDA receptors on cortical GABA interneurons are hypoactive, then GABA release is inhibited and the cortical brainstem pathway to the VTA will be overactivated, leading to excessive release of glutamate in the VTA. This will lead to excessive stimulation of the mesolimbic dopamine pathway and thus excessive dopamine release in the nucleus accumbens. This is the theoretical biological basis for the mesolimbic dopamine hyperactivity thought to be associated with the positive symptoms of psychosis (de Bartolomeis et al., 2005; Paz et al., 2008; Stahl, 2018; Stahl, 2021).

# The Psychosis Circuit: Upstream Serotonin Modulation of DA

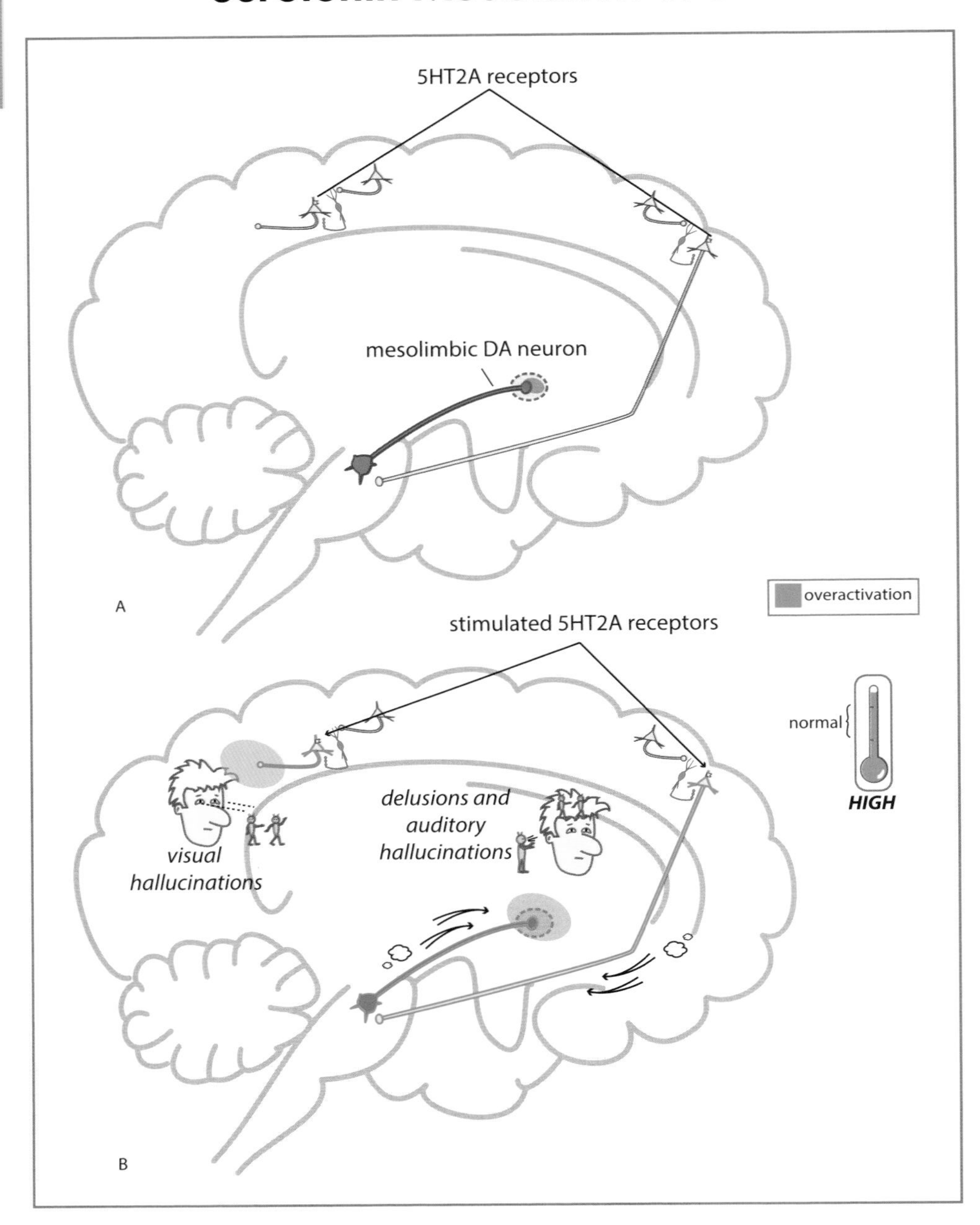

# The Psychosis Circuit: Upstream Serotonin Modulation of DA

**FIGURE 1.10.** (A) Shown here is a cortico-brainstem glutamatergic pathway projecting from the prefrontal cortex to the ventral tegmental area (VTA), and an indirect cortico-cortical glutamatergic pathway in the visual cortex. Activity of both pathways is regulated by serotonergic neurons that project from the raphe nucleus as well as by GABA interneurons in the prefrontal cortex. At baseline, normal stimulation of excitatory 5HT2A receptors on the glutamate neurons is balanced by tonic stimulation of GABA receptors on the same neurons; the net effect is thus normal activation of the glutamatergic neurons. (B) When 5HT2A agonists stimulate 5HT2A receptors on glutamatergic pyramidal neurons in the prefrontal cortex, this causes overactivation of the glutamate neurons. Excessive glutamate release into the VTA causes hyperactivity of the mesolimbic dopamine (DA) pathway, resulting in delusions and auditory hallucinations. Excessive glutamate release in the visual cortex can cause visual hallucinations (Alex et al., 2007; Gellings et al., 2012; Stahl, 2018; Stahl, 2021).

# Course of Illness in Schizophrenia

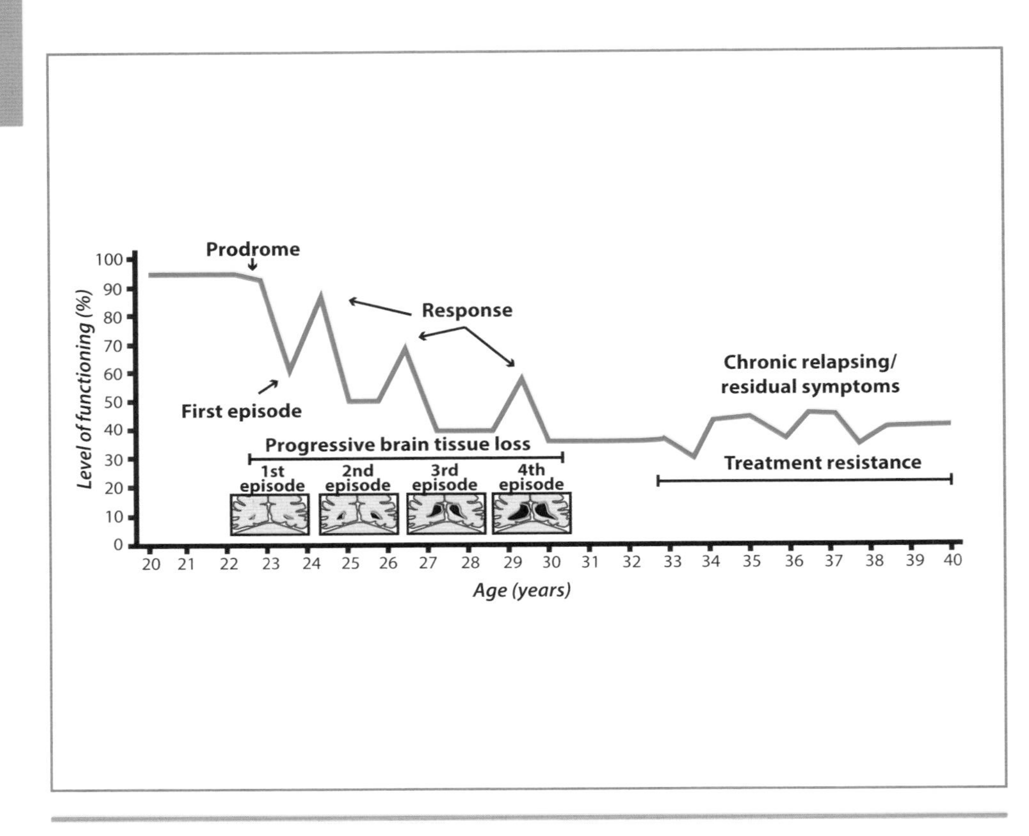


**FIGURE 1.11.** Although schizophrenia may begin as a neurodevelopmental disorder, its progressive nature suggests that it may also be a neurodegenerative disorder. Strengthening and weakening of synapses occurs throughout the lifetime. In schizophrenia, it is possible that abnormal synaptogenesis prevents normal synapses from strengthening even if they are being "used" and/or allows the "wrong" synapses to strengthen and be retained. There is evidence that recurrent episodes of psychotic breaks are associated with progressive loss of brain tissue in schizophrenia and loss of treatment responsiveness (Arango et al., 2012; Goff et al., 2018; Reckziegel et al., 2022; Stahl, 2021).

# Other Disorders With Psychosis

| Disorders in which psychosis is a defining feature |
|---|
| Substance/medication-induced psychotic disorders |
| Schizophreniform disorder |
| Schizoaffective disorder |
| Delusional disorder |
| Brief psychotic disorder |
| Shared psychotic disorder |
| Psychotic disorder due to another medical condition |
| Childhood psychotic disorder |

| Disorders in which psychosis is an associated feature |
|---|
| Mania |
| Depression |
| Cognitive disorders |
| Alzheimer's disease and other dementias |
| Parkinson's disease |

**TABLE 1.1.**

Stahl's Illustrated | Chapter 2

# Three Neurotransmitter Networks Linked to Psychosis

Psychosis has been theoretically linked to three major neurotransmitter pathways. The longstanding dopamine (DA) theory centers around the concept of hyperactive dopamine 2 (D2) receptors in the mesolimbic pathway (projection from ventral tegmental area to ventral striatum). Although recent neuroimaging data indicate that a better conception of this pathway is as the mesostriatal pathway (projection from substantia nigra to associative striatum), this book will continue to refer to the classic mesolimbic pathway as the body of evidence grows. The glutamate theory proposes that N-methyl D-aspartate (NMDA) receptors are hypoactive at critical synapses in the prefrontal cortex, which could lead to downstream hyperactivity in the mesolimbic dopamine pathway. The serotonin theory posits that there is serotonergic hyperactivity particularly at serotonin 2A (5HT2A) receptors in the cortex, which also could result in hyperactivity in the mesolimbic dopamine pathway. It is likely that one or more of these three pathways is involved in the development of psychosis, not only schizophrenia, but psychoses associated with Parkinson's disease, with various forms of dementia, and with numerous psychotomimetic drugs (psychostimulants, dissociative anesthetics, psychedelics).

# SECTION 1
# Classic Dopamine (DA) Pathways

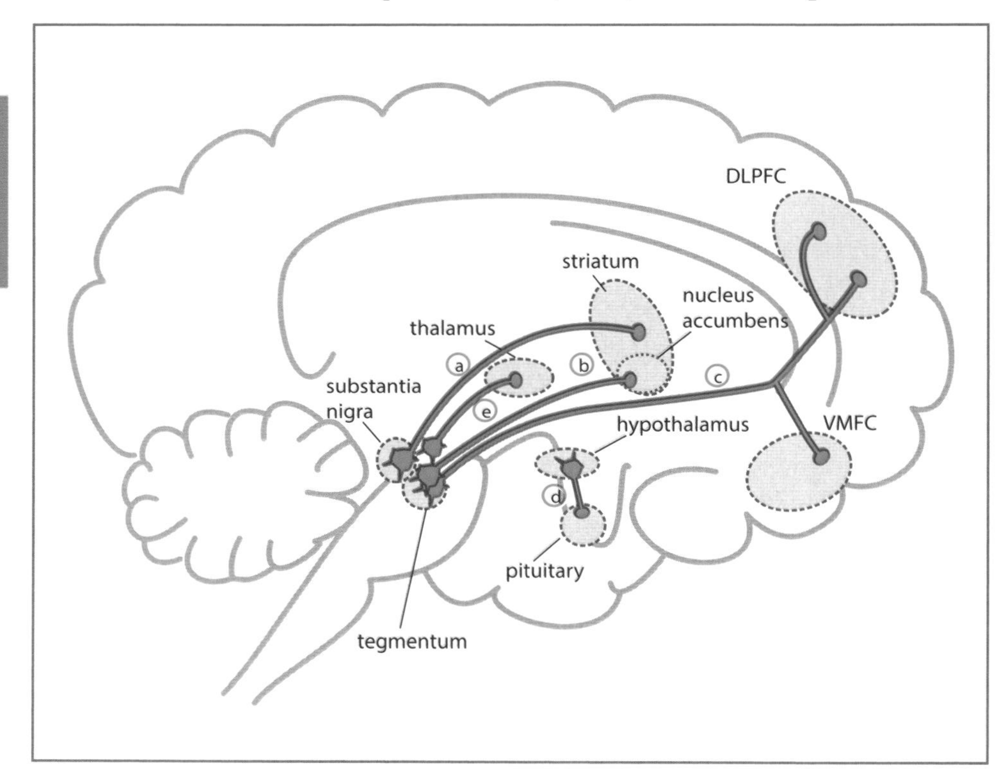


**FIGURE 2.1.** (a) The nigrostriatal dopamine pathway, which projects from the substantia nigra to the basal ganglia or striatum, is part of the extrapyramidal nervous system and controls motor function and movement. (b) The mesolimbic dopamine pathway projects from the midbrain ventral tegmental area (VTA) to the nucleus accumbens, a part of the limbic system of the brain thought to be involved in many behaviors such as pleasurable sensations, the powerful euphoria of drugs of abuse, and delusions and hallucinations of psychosis. (c) The mesocortical dopamine pathway also projects from the midbrain VTA but sends its axons to areas of the prefrontal cortex, where they may have a role in mediating cognitive symptoms (dorsolateral prefrontal cortex or DLPFC) and affective symptoms (ventromedial prefrontal cortex or VMPFC) of schizophrenia. (d) The tuberoinfundibular dopamine pathway projects from the hypothalamus to the anterior pituitary gland and controls prolactin secretion. (e) The fifth dopamine pathway arises from multiple sites, including the periaqueductal gray, ventral mesencephalon, hypothalamic nuclei, and lateral parabrachial nucleus, and projects to the thalamus. Its function is not currently well known (Stahl, 2021).

# Dopamine Synthesis

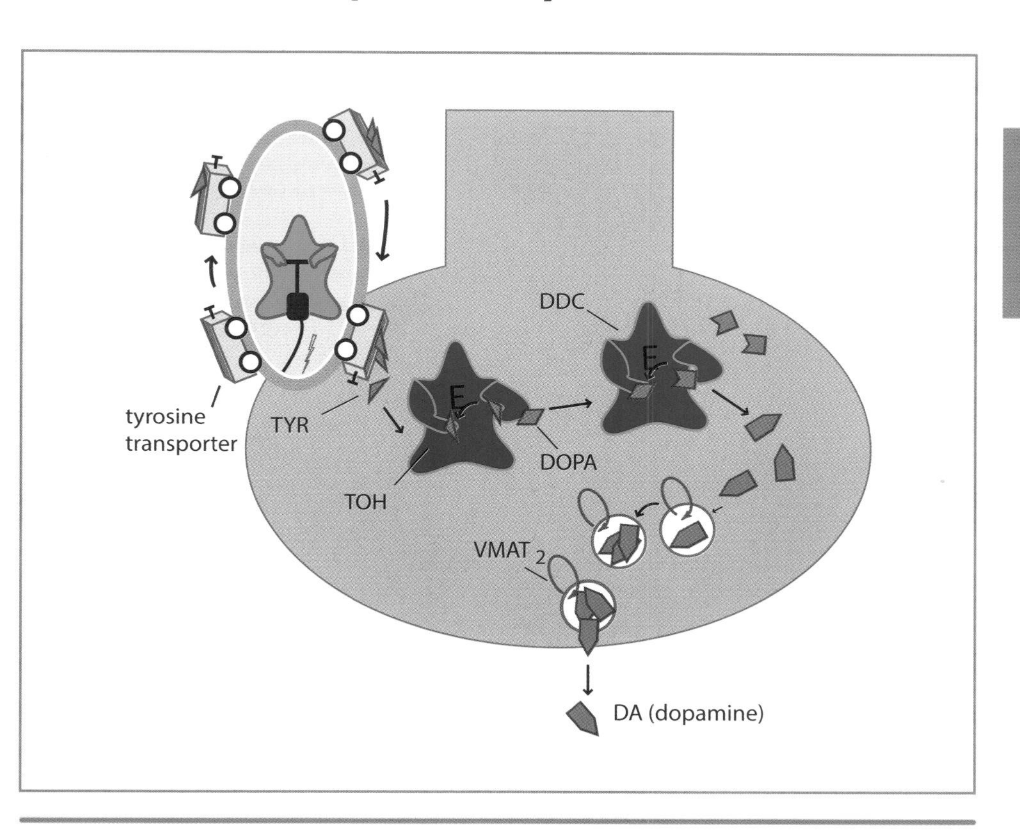


**FIGURE 2.2.** Tyrosine (TYR), a precursor to DA, is taken up into DA nerve terminals via a tyrosine transporter and converted into DOPA by the enzyme tyrosine hydroxylase (TOH). DOPA is then converted into DA by the enzyme DOPA decarboxylase (DDC). After synthesis, DA is packaged into synaptic vesicles via the vesicular monoamine transporter (VMAT2) and stored there until its release into the synapse during neurotransmission (Stahl, 2021).

# Dopamine Termination

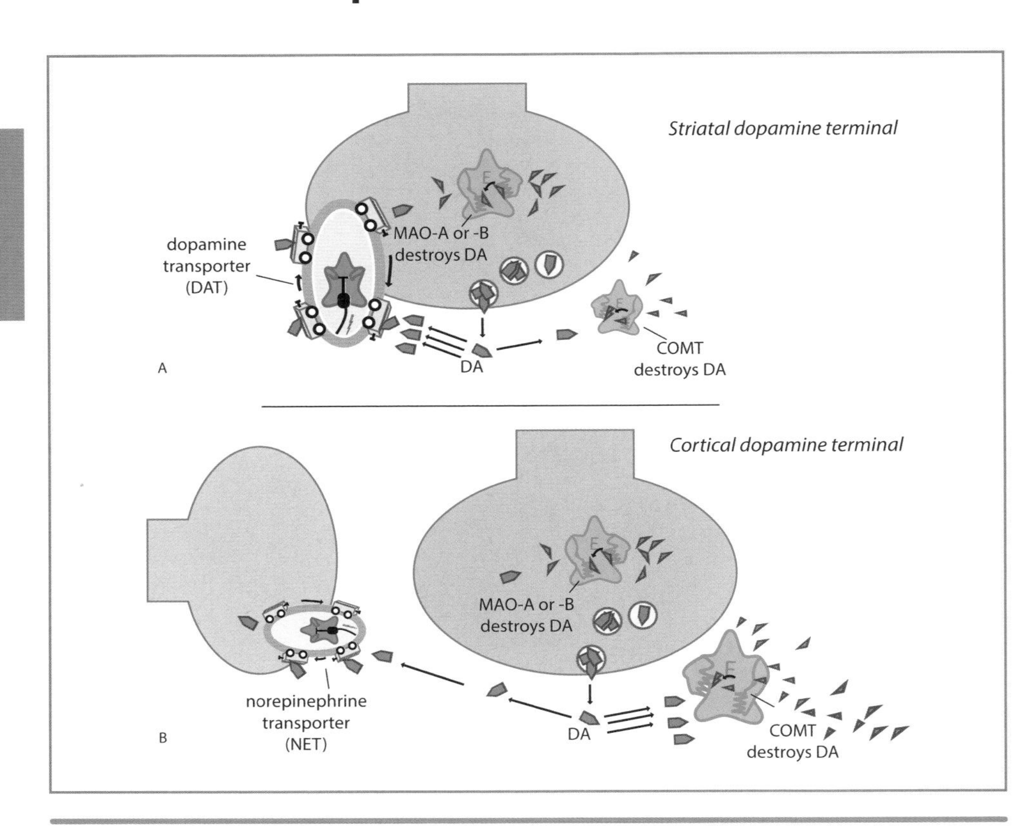


**FIGURE 2.3.** DA can be transported out of the synaptic cleft and back into the presynaptic neuron via the dopamine transporter (DAT). Alternatively, DA may be broken down extracellularly via the enzyme catechol O-methyltransferase (COMT). Other enzymes that break down DA are monoamine oxidase A (MAO-A) and monoamine oxidase B (MAO-B) (A). In the prefrontal cortex, the predominant method of DA inactivation is via MAO-A or MAO-B intracellularly, and COMT extracellularly. DA can also diffuse away from the synapses and be taken up by the norepinephrine transporter (NET) at nearby neurons (B) (Stahl, 2021).

# Postsynaptic DA Receptors

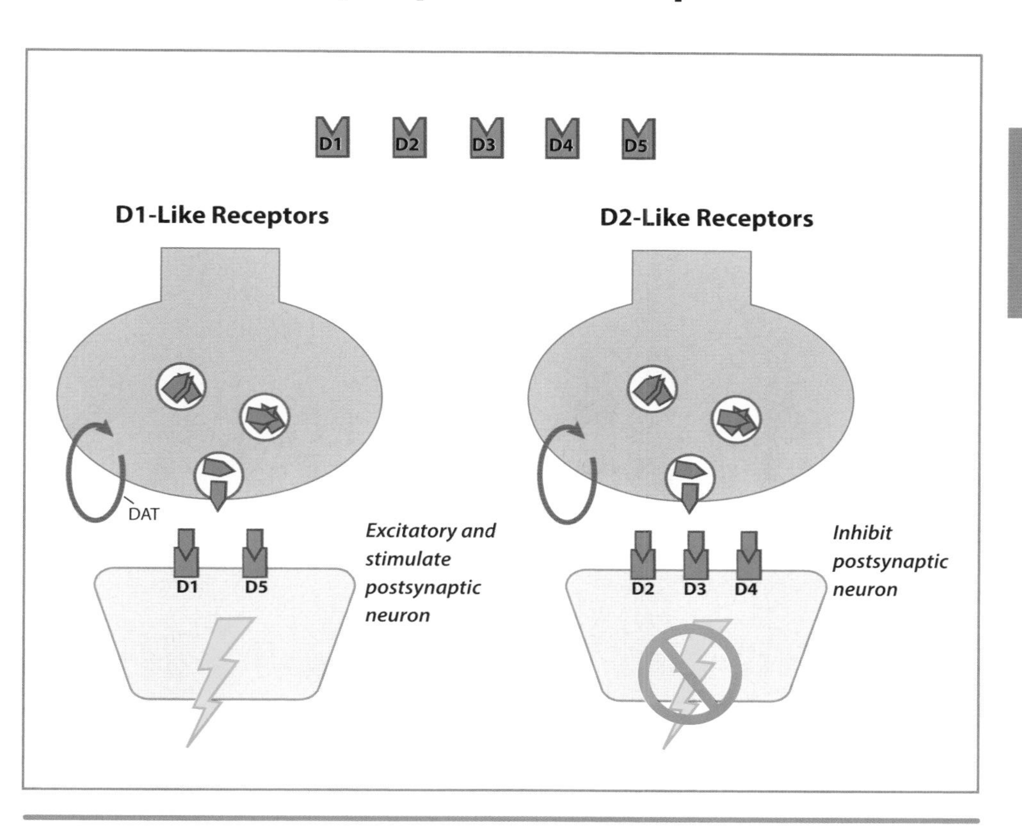


**FIGURE 2.4.** There are two groups of postsynaptic DA receptors. D1-like receptors, which include both D1 and D5 receptors, are excitatory and thus stimulate the postsynaptic neuron. D2-like receptors, which include D2, D3, and D4, are inhibitory and thus inhibit the postsynaptic neuron (Beaulieu & Gainetdinov, 2011; Stahl, 2017; Stahl, 2021).

# Presynaptic DA Receptors

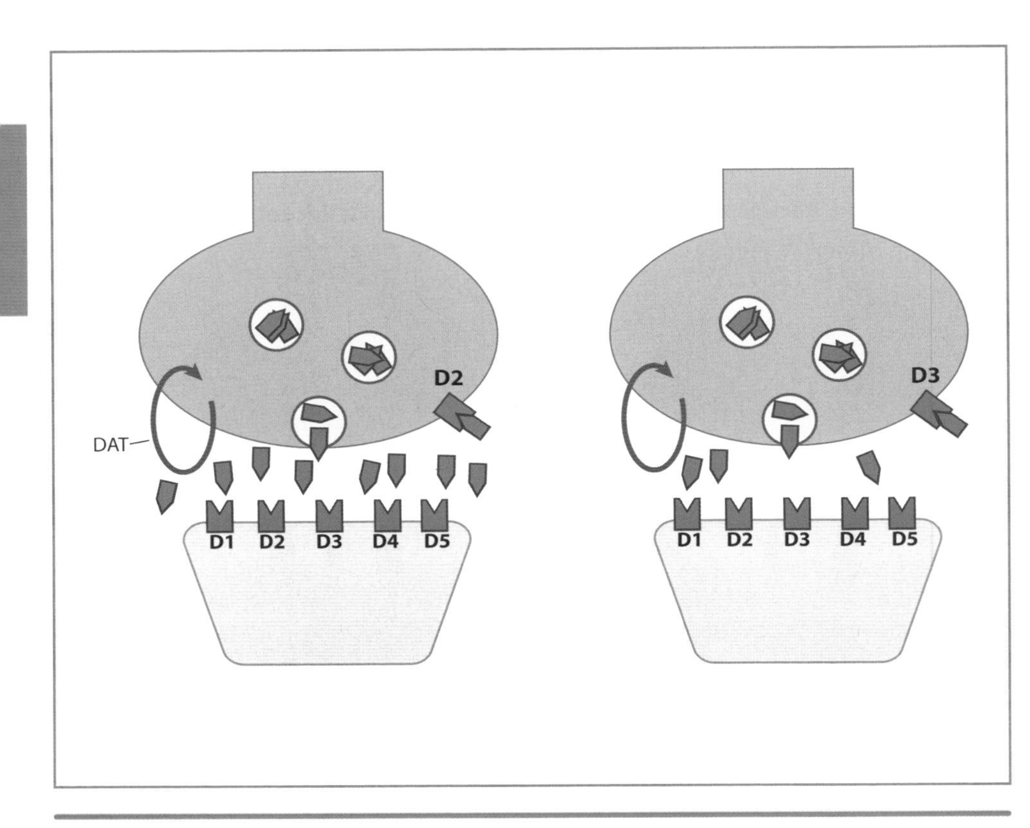


**FIGURE 2.5.** Dopamine (DA) D2 and D3 receptors are also located presynaptically, where, due to their inhibitory actions, they act as autoreceptors to inhibit further dopamine release. The D2 autoreceptor is less sensitive to DA than the D3 autoreceptor and thus it takes a higher concentration of synaptic DA for the D2 autoreceptor to become activated (left) than it does for the D3 autoreceptor to become activated (right) (Beaulieu & Gainetdinov, 2011; Stahl, 2017; Stahl, 2021).

Presynaptic D2 and D3 autoreceptors can also be found in the somatodendritic area, where DA binding shuts off neuronal impulse flow in the DA neuron and further DA release (Beaulieu & Gainetdinov, 2011; Stahl, 2017; Stahl, 2021).

# Nigrostriatal DA Pathway Controls Movement Via CSTC Loop

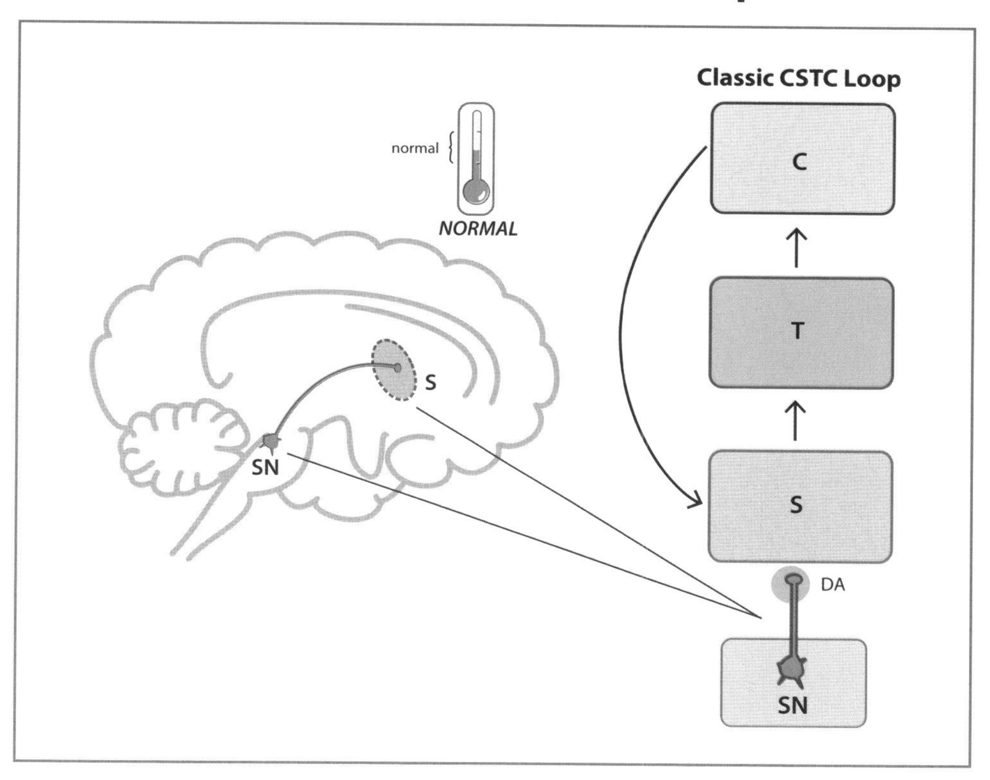


**FIGURE 2.6.** The nigrostriatal dopamine pathway projects from the substantia nigra (SN) to the basal ganglia or striatum (S). It is part of the extrapyramidal nervous system and plays a key role in regulating movements. When DA is deficient, it can cause parkinsonism with tremor, rigidity, and akinesia/bradykinesia. When DA is in excess, it can cause hyperkinetic movements such as tics and dyskinesias. In untreated schizophrenia, activation of this pathway is believed to be "normal." The nigrostriatal DA pathway is considered to control motor movements via its connections with the thalamus (T) and cortex (C) in a circuit known as the cortico-striato-thalamo-cortical (CSTC) loop (Calabresi et al., 2014; DeLong & Wichmann, 2007; Stahl, 2021).

# DA Regulates CSTC Loop

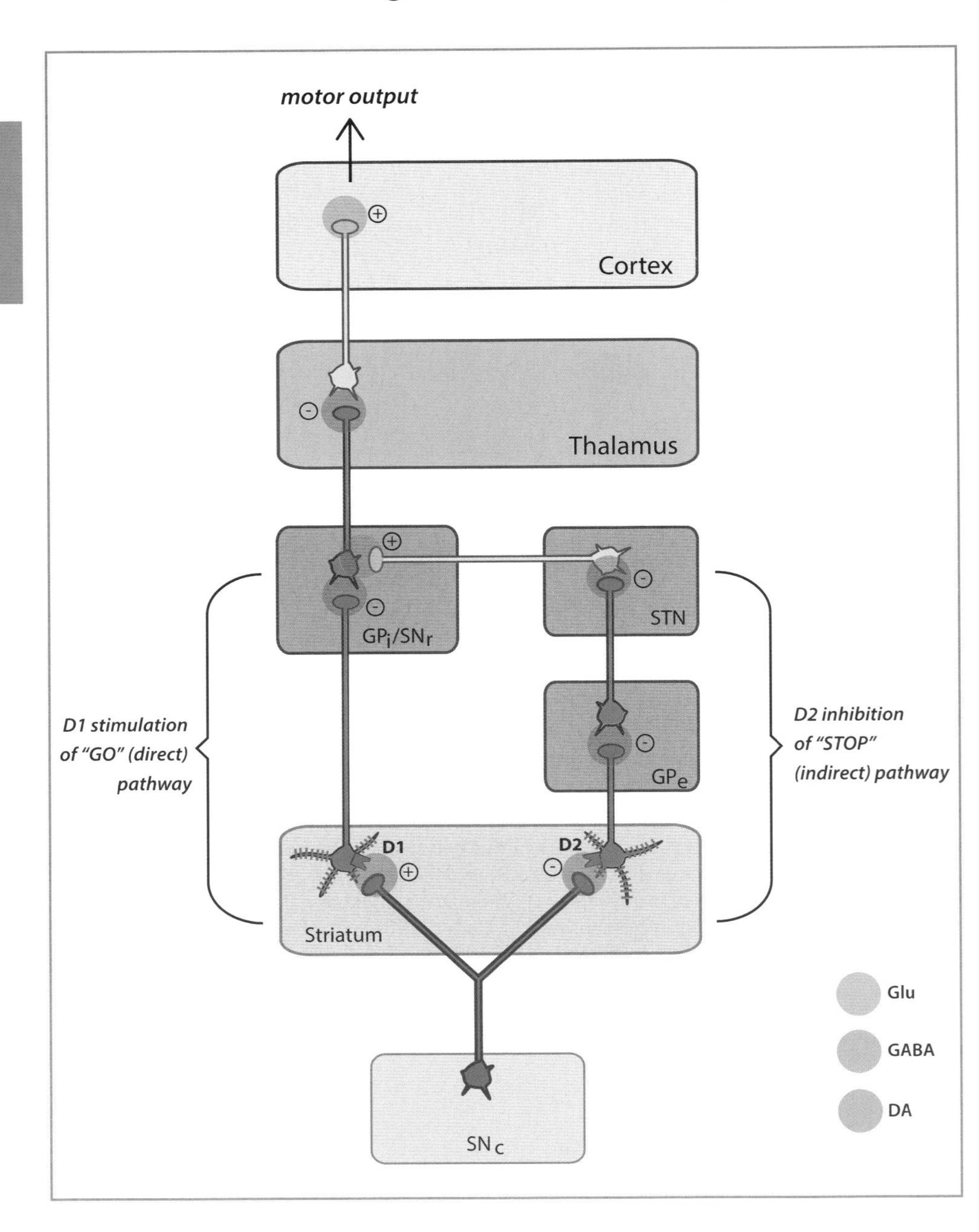

# DA Regulates CSTC Loop

**FIGURE 2.7.** Populated with excitatory D1 receptors, the direct pathway for dopamine regulation of motor movements (left) projects from the striatum to the globus pallidus interna and results in the stimulation of movement. The indirect pathway for dopamine regulation of motor movements (right) projects to the globus pallidus interna via the globus pallidus externa and subthalamic nuclei. This pathway is populated with inhibitory D2 receptors and normally blocks motor movements (Calabresi et al., 2014; DeLong & Wichmann, 2007; Stahl, 2021). CSTC: cortico-striato-thalamo-cortical; D1: dopamine 1 receptor; D2: dopamine 2 receptor; DA: dopamine; GABA: gamma-aminobutyric acid; Glu: glutamate; GPe: globus pallidus externa; GPi: globus pallidus interna; SNc: substantia nigra compacta; SNr: substantia nigra reticulata; STN: subthalamic nucleus.

# The DA Hypothesis of Psychosis: Classic Mesolimbic Pathway

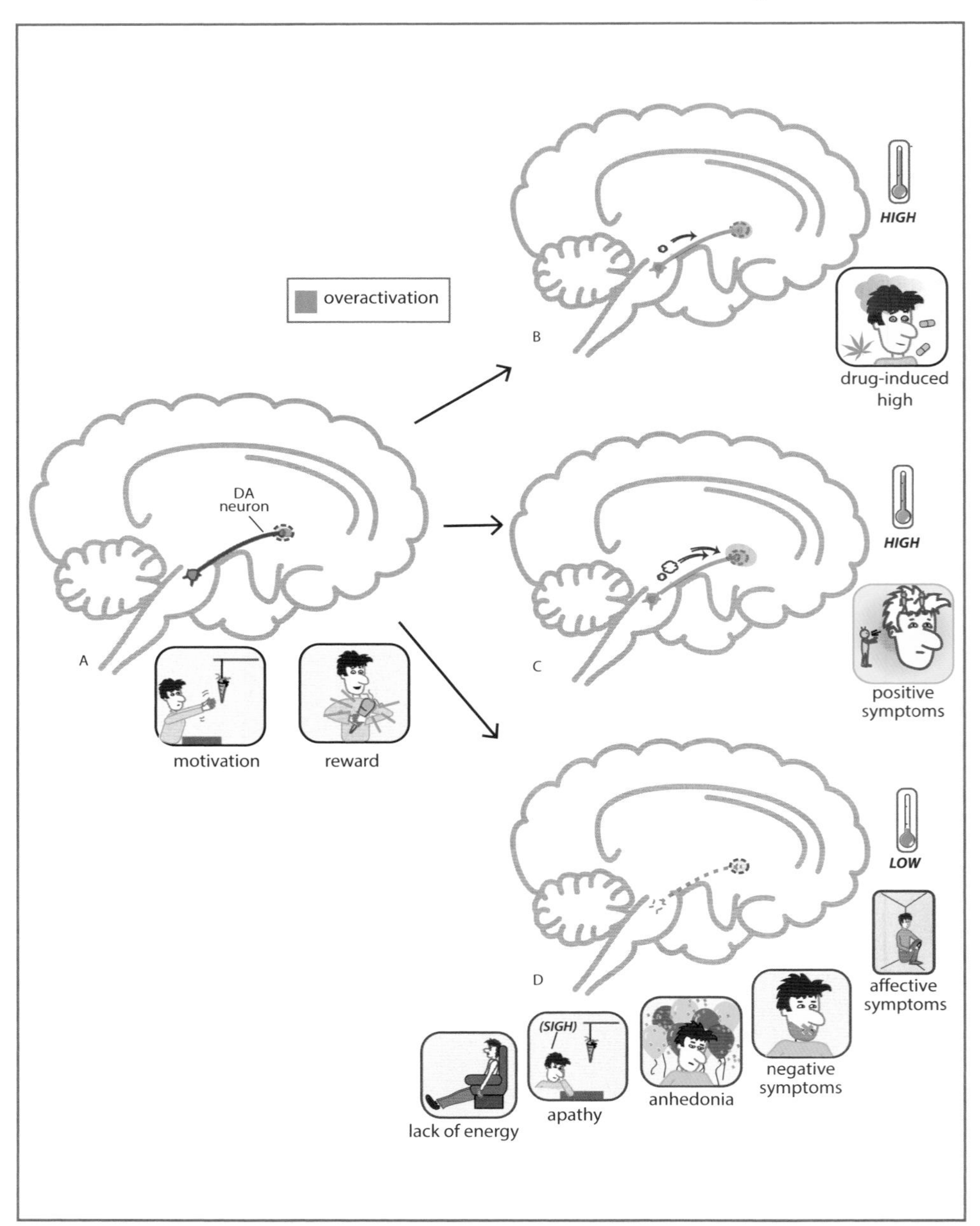

# The DA Hypothesis of Psychosis: Classic Mesolimbic Pathway

**FIGURE 2.8.** (A) The mesolimbic dopamine pathway, which projects from the ventral tegmental area (VTA) in the brainstem to the nucleus accumbens in the ventral striatum, is involved in regulation of motivation and reward. Classically, hyperactivity of this pathway is associated with drug-induced highs (B) and is believed to account for the positive symptoms of psychosis (C). The mesolimbic dopamine hypothesis states that hyperactivity of the dopamine neurons in the mesolimbic dopamine pathway mediates the positive symptoms of psychosis, such as delusions and hallucinations. Mesolimbic overactivity may also be associated with impulsivity, agitation, violence/aggression, and hostility. By contrast, hypoactivity of this pathway is associated with symptoms of anhedonia, apathy, and lack of energy as well as with the negative symptoms of schizophrenia (D) (Gellings et al., 2012; Stahl, 2018; Stahl, 2021).

Neuroimaging data in unmedicated patients with schizophrenia suggest that dopaminergic activity may be unaltered in the ventral striatum, but may instead be overactive in an intermediate part of the striatum called the associative striatum, which receives input from the substantia nigra rather than the VTA. Rather than separate nigrostriatal and mesolimbic projections, a better conception may be that of a mesostriatal pathway (McCutcheon et al., 2019; Stahl, 2021).

# The DA Hypothesis of Psychosis: Classic Mesocortical Pathway

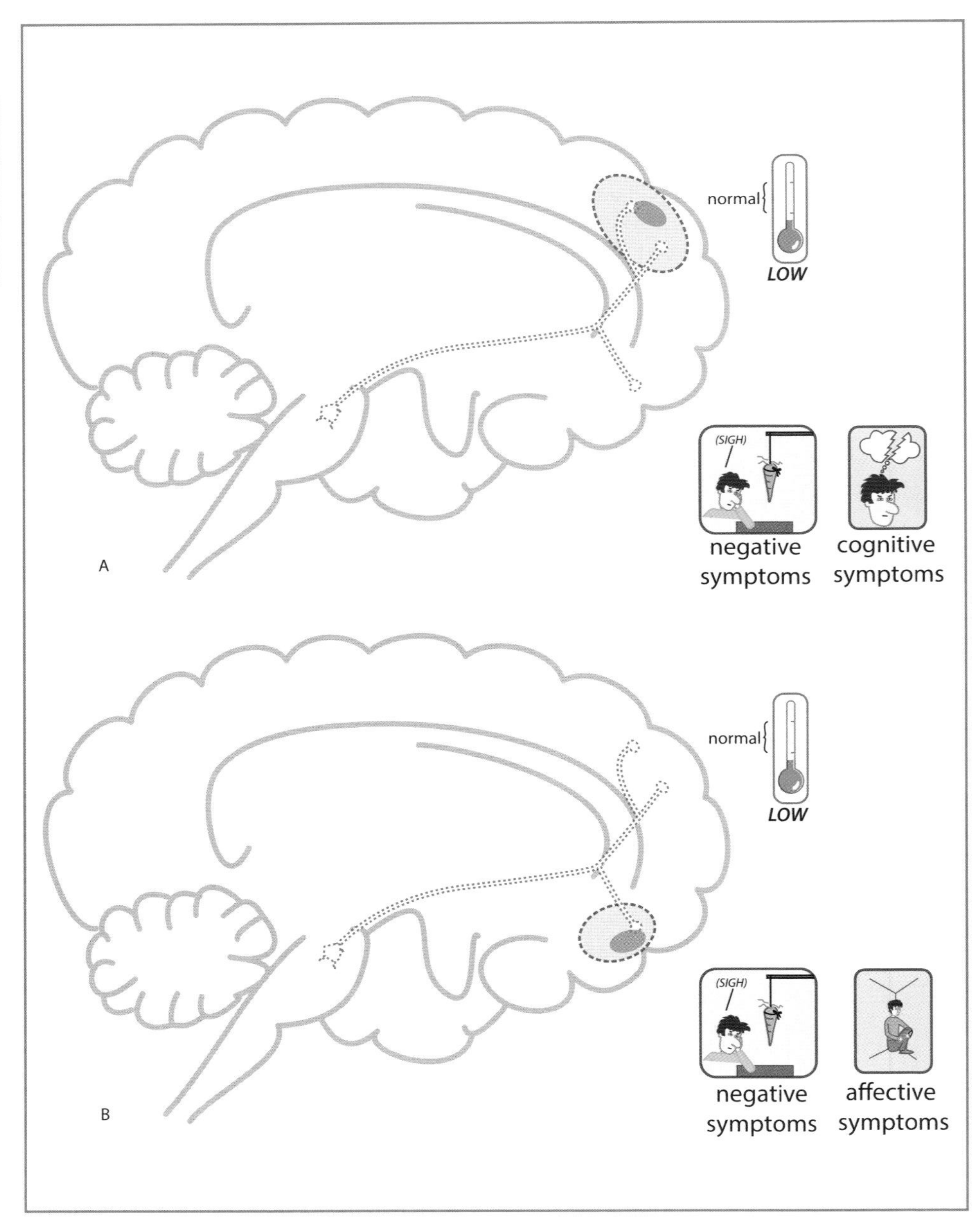

# The DA Hypothesis of Psychosis: Classic Mesocortical Pathway

**FIGURE 2.9.** The mesocortical dopamine pathway projects from the ventral tegmental area (VTA) to the prefrontal cortex. Projections specifically to the dorsolateral prefrontal cortex are associated with cognitive and executive functioning, with hypoactivity of the dopamine neurons in this pathway classically believed to be involved in the cognitive and some negative symptoms of schizophrenia (A). Projections specifically to the ventromedial prefrontal cortex are associated with emotions and affect, with hypoactivity of the dopamine neurons in this pathway classically believed to be involved in the negative and affective symptoms of schizophrenia (B) (Stahl, 2021).

# Key Glutamate Pathways

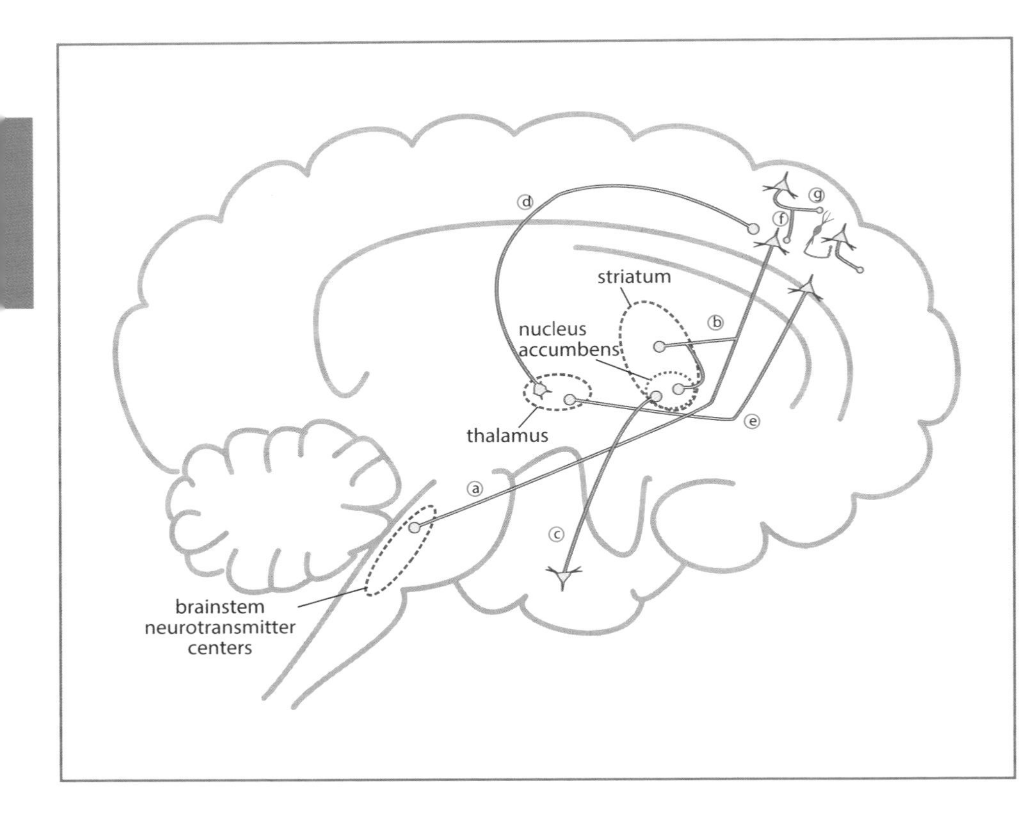

# Key Glutamate Pathways

**FIGURE 2.10.** Although glutamate can have actions at virtually all neurons in the brain, there are key glutamate pathways particularly relevant to schizophrenia. (a) The cortico-brainstem glutamate projection is a descending pathway that projects from cortical pyramidal neurons in the prefrontal cortex to brainstem neurotransmitter centers (raphe nucleus, locus coeruleus, ventral tegmental area, substantia nigra) and regulates neurotransmitter release. (b) Another descending glutamatergic pathway projects from the prefrontal cortex to the striatal complex (cortico-striatal glutamate pathway). (c) There is also a glutamatergic projection from the ventral hippocampus to the nucleus accumbens. (d) Thalamo-cortical glutamate pathways ascend from the thalamus and innervate pyramidal neurons in the cortex. (e) Cortico-thalamic glutamate pathways descend from the prefrontal cortex to the thalamus. (f) Intracortical pyramidal neurons can communicate directly with each other via the neurotransmitter glutamate; these pathways are known as direct cortico-cortical glutamatergic pathways and are excitatory. (g) Intracortical pyramidal neurons can also communicate via GABAergic interneurons; these indirect cortico-cortical glutamate pathways are therefore inhibitory (Stahl, 2021).

# Glutamate Is Recycled and Regenerated

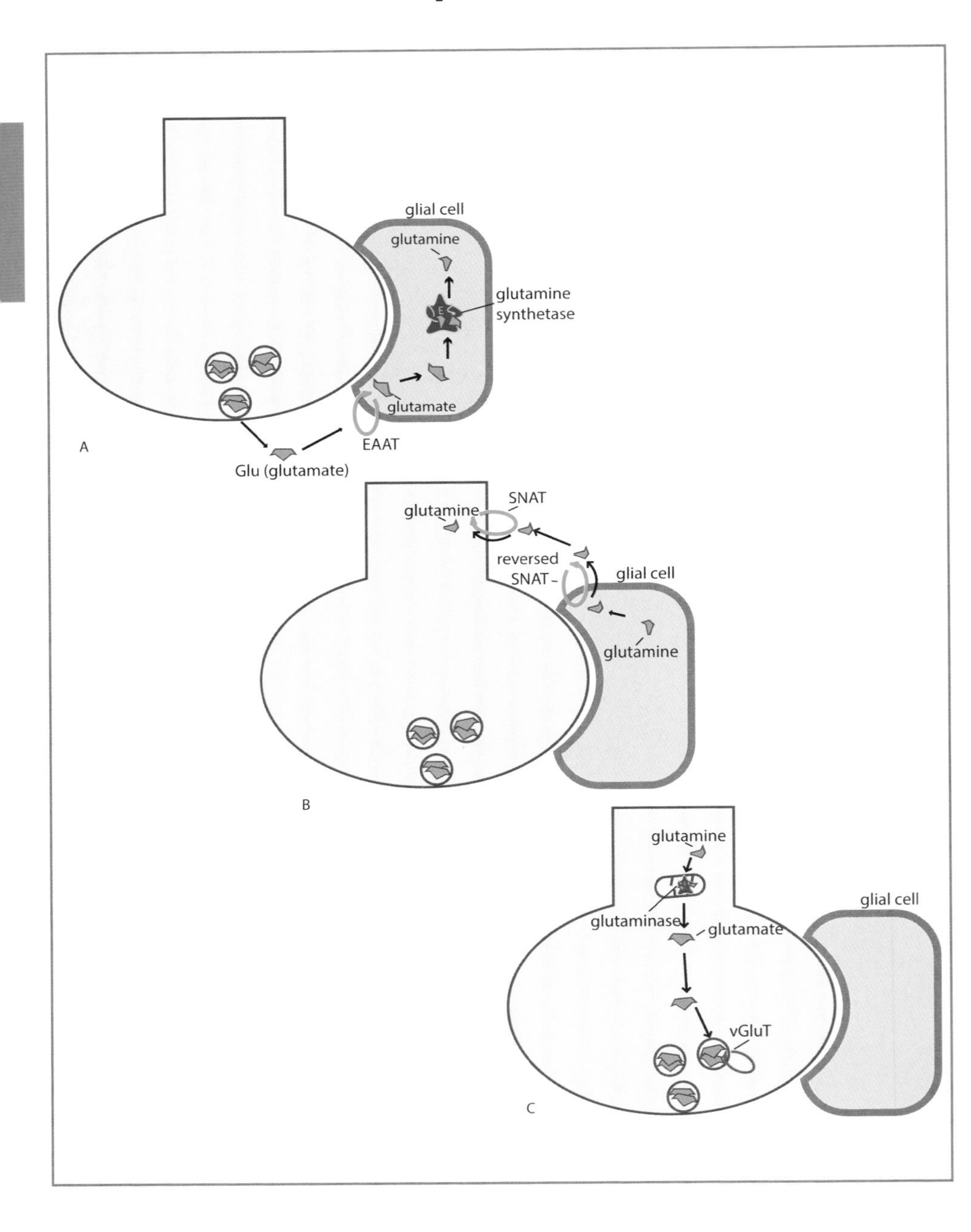

# Glutamate Is Recycled and Regenerated

**FIGURE 2.11.** After release of glutamate from the presynaptic neuron, it is taken up into glial cells via the excitatory amino acid transporter (EAAT). Once inside the glial cell, glutamate is converted into glutamine by the enzyme glutamine synthetase (A). Glutamine is released from glial cells by a specific glial neutral amino acid transporter (SNAT) through the process of reverse transport, and then taken up by SNATs on glutamate neurons (B). Glutamine is converted into glutamate within the presynaptic glutamate neuron by the enzyme glutaminase and taken up into synaptic vesicles by the vesicular glutamate transporter (vGluT), where it is stored for future release (C) (Stahl, 2021).

# Glutamate Receptors

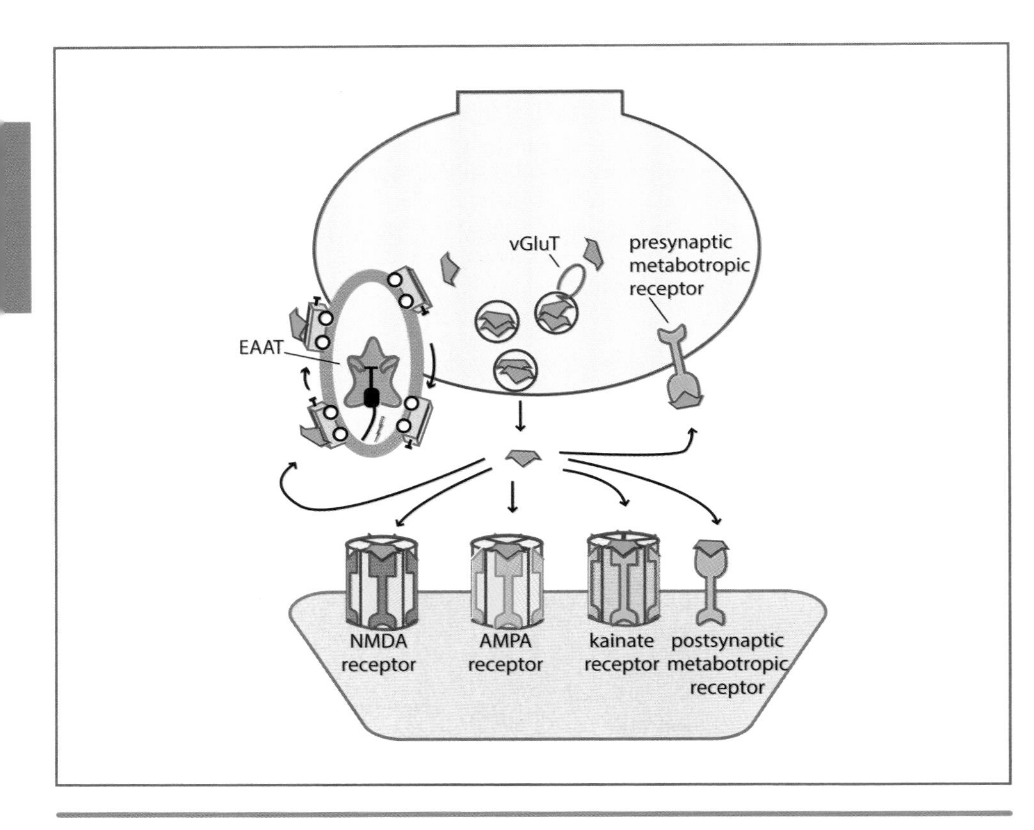


**FIGURE 2.12.** The excitatory amino acid transporter (EAAT) exists presynaptically and is responsible for clearing excess glutamate out of the synapse. The vesicular transporter for glutamate (vGluT) transports glutamate into synaptic vesicles, where it is stored until used in a future neurotransmission. Metabotropic glutamate receptors (linked to G proteins) can occur either pre- or postsynaptically. Three types of postsynaptic glutamate receptors are linked to ion channels and are known as ligand-gated ion channels: N-methyl-D-aspartate (NMDA) receptors, α-amino-3-hydroxy-5-methyl-4-isoxazole-propionic acid (AMPA) receptors, and kainate receptors, all named for the agonists that bind to them (Scheefhals & MacGillavry, 2018; Stahl, 2021).

# Metabotropic Glutamate Autoreceptors

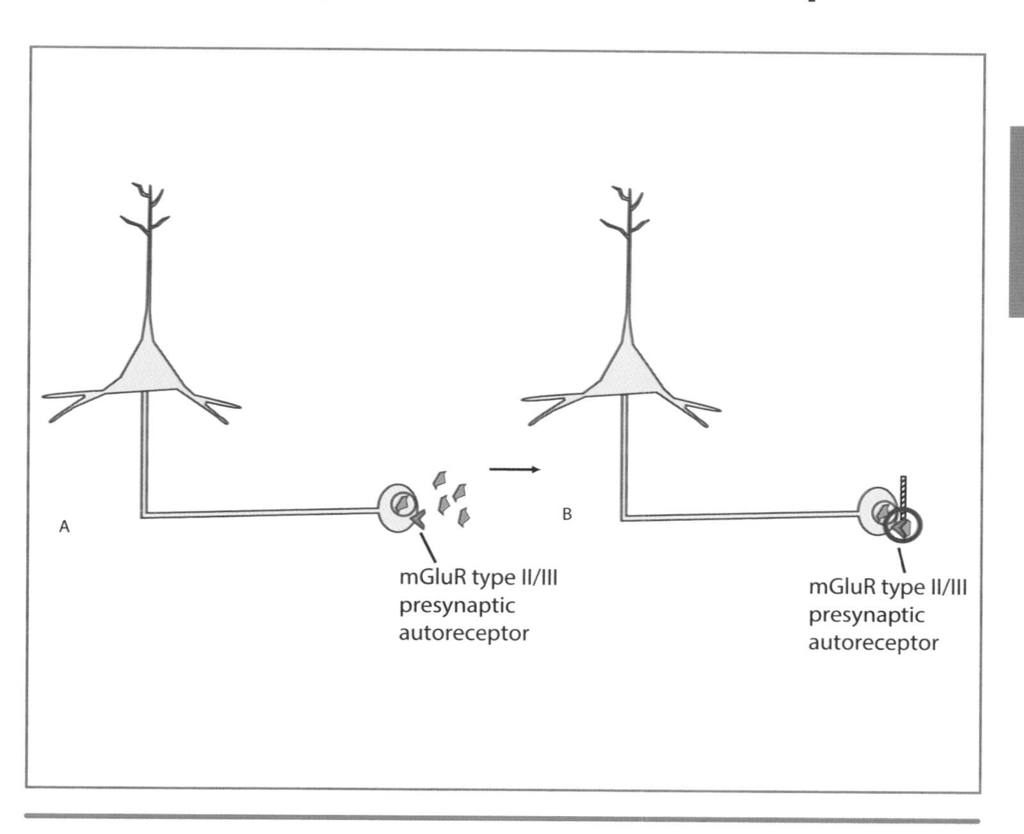


**FIGURE 2.13.** Groups II and III metabotropic glutamate receptors can exist presynaptically as autoreceptors to regulate the release of glutamate. When glutamate builds up in the synapse (A), it is available to bind to the autoreceptor, which then inhibits glutamate release (B) (Stahl, 2021).

# Ionotropic Glutamate Receptors: AMPA & Kainate

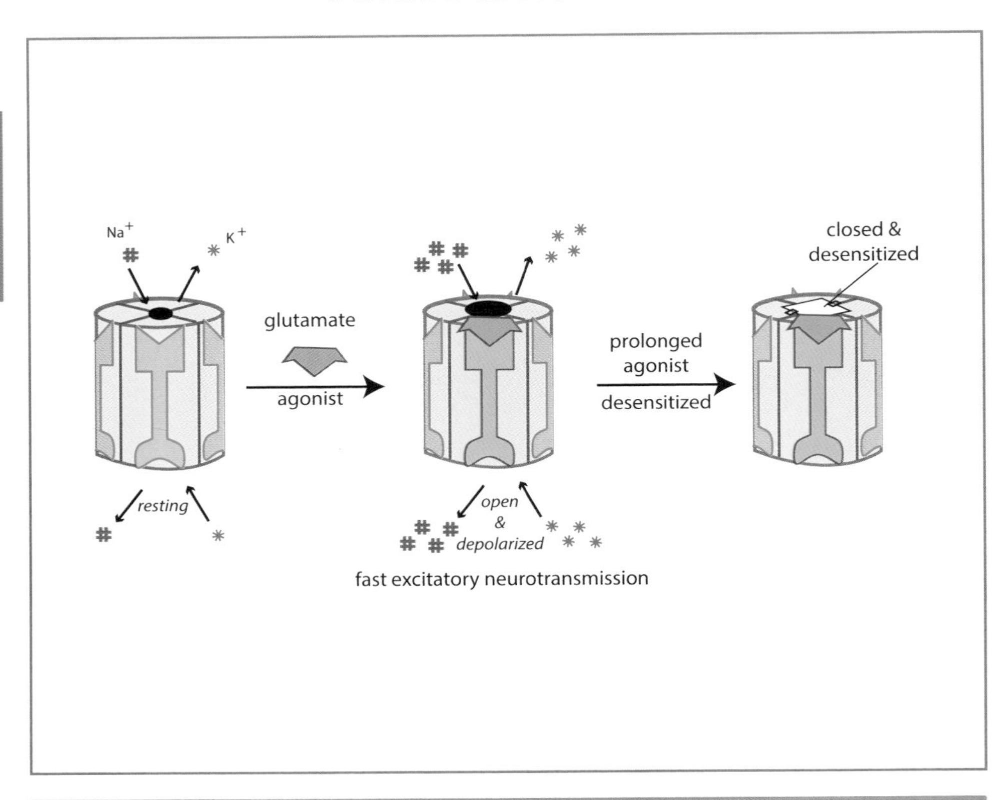


**FIGURE 2.14.** When glutamate binds to AMPA and kainate receptors, this leads to fast excitatory neurotransmission and membrane depolarization. Sustained binding of the agonist glutamate will lead to receptor desensitization, causing the channel to close and be transiently unresponsive to agonist (Stahl, 2021).

# Ionotropic Glutamate Receptors: NMDA

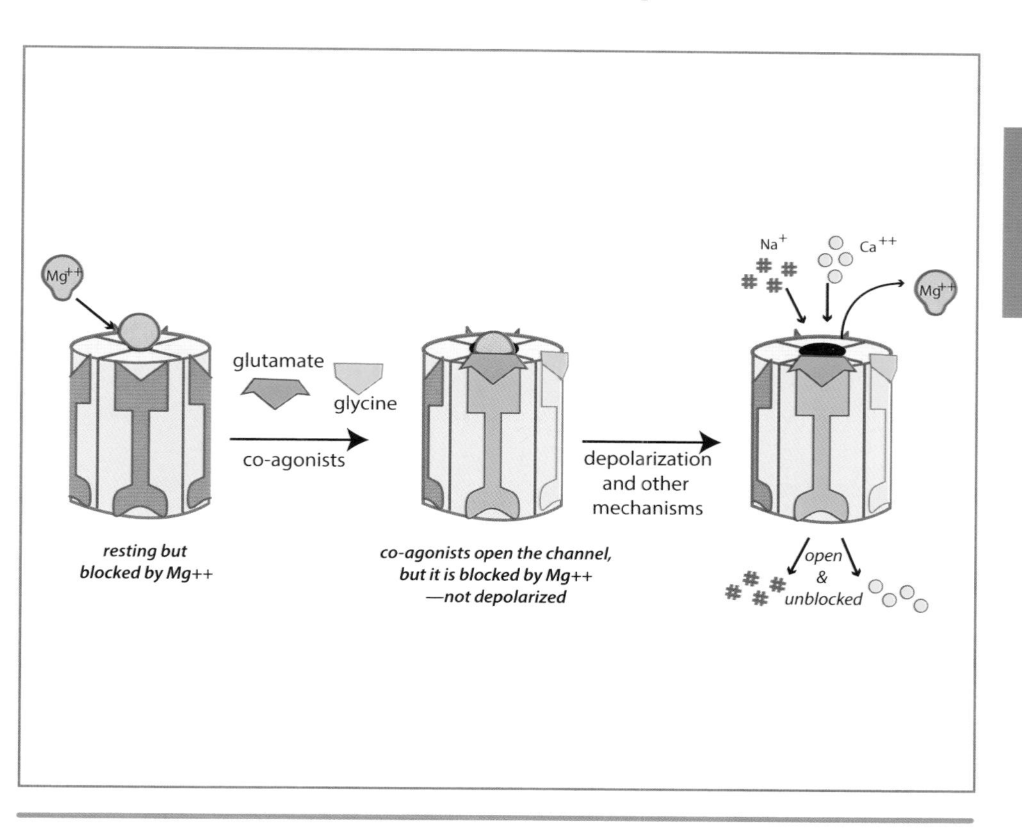


**FIGURE 2.15.** Magnesium is a negative allosteric modulator at NMDA glutamate receptors. Opening of NMDA glutamate receptors requires the presence of both glutamate and glycine, each of which bind to a different site on the receptor. When magnesium is also bound and the membrane is not depolarized, it prevents the effects of glutamate and glycine and thus does not allow the ion channel to open. For the channel to open, depolarization must remove magnesium while both glutamate and glycine are bound to their sites on the ligand-gated ion channel complex (Hansen et al., 2018; Paoletti et al., 2007; Stahl, 2021).

# Hypothetical Site of Glutamate Dysfunction in Psychosis

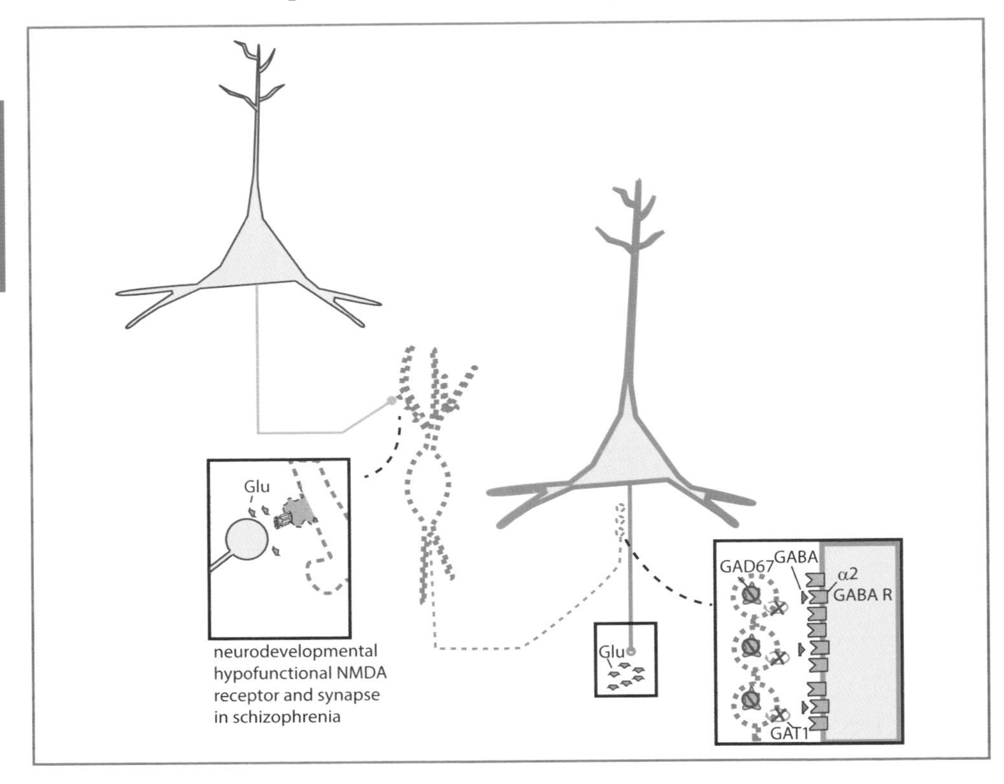


**FIGURE 2.16.** Shown here is a close-up of intracortical pyramidal neurons communicating via GABAergic interneurons in the presence of hypofunctional NMDA receptors. Glutamate is released from an intracortical pyramidal neuron. However, the NMDA receptor that it would normally bind to is hypofunctional due to neurodevelopmental abnormalities, preventing glutamate from exerting its effects at the receptor. This prevents GABA release from the interneuron; thus, stimulation of α2 GABA receptors on the axon of another glutamate neuron does not occur. When GABA does not bind to the α2 GABA receptors on its axon, the pyramidal neuron is no longer inhibited. Instead, it is disinhibited and overactive, releasing excessive glutamate into the cortex (Homayoun & Moghaddam, 2007; Stahl, 2018; Stahl, 2021).

# Hypothetical Site of Glutamate Dysfunction in Psychosis Related to Dementia

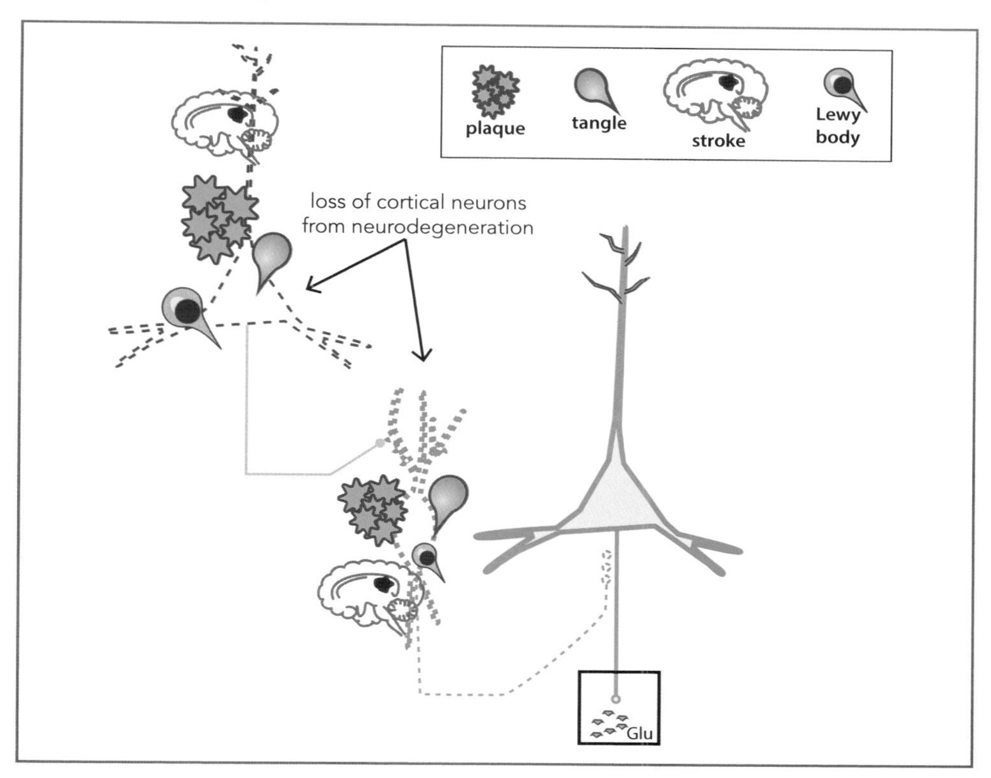


**FIGURE 2.17.** Shown here is a close-up of intracortical pyramidal neurons communicating via GABAergic interneurons in the presence of neurodegeneration associated with dementia. Not all patients with dementia develop symptoms of psychosis. It may be that in those that do, the neurodegeneration associated with the accumulation of amyloid plaques, tau tangles, and/or Lewy bodies, as well as the damage caused by strokes, may destroy some glutamatergic pyramidal neurons and GABAergic interneurons while leaving others intact, at least temporarily. The end result may be excessive glutamate activity in the cortex, as in schizophrenia or in ketamine abuse (Stahl, 2021).

# NMDA Receptor Hypofunction and Psychosis in Schizophrenia

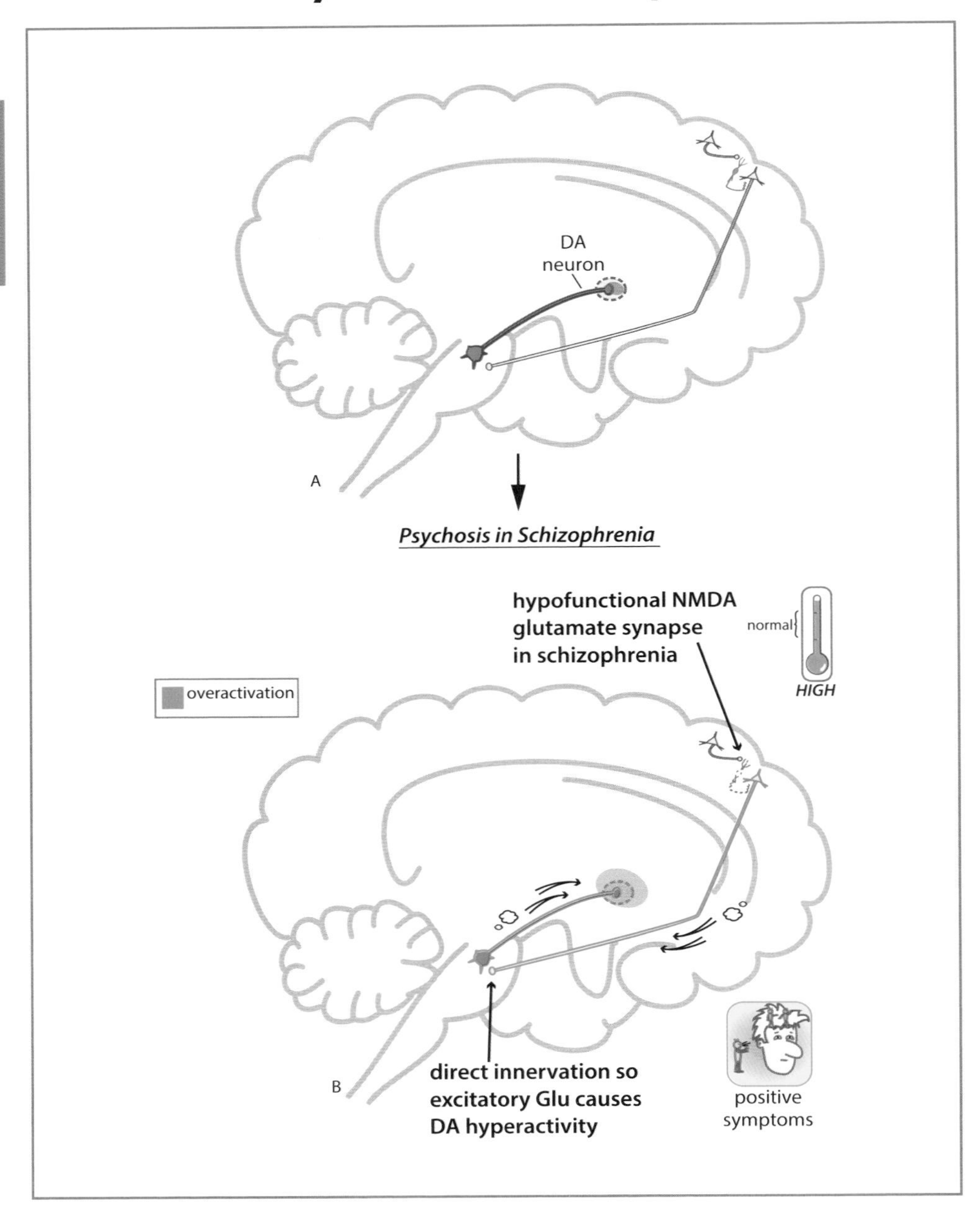

# NMDA Receptor Hypofunction and Psychosis in Schizophrenia

**FIGURE 2.18.** (A) The cortical glutamate projection communicates with the mesolimbic dopamine pathway in the ventral tegmental area (VTA) to regulate dopamine release in the nucleus accumbens. (B) If NMDA receptors on cortical GABA interneurons are hypoactive, then GABA release is inhibited and the cortical brainstem pathway to the VTA will be overactivated, leading to excessive release of glutamate in the VTA. This will lead to excessive stimulation of the mesolimbic dopamine pathway and thus excessive dopamine release in the nucleus accumbens. This is the theoretical biological basis for the mesolimbic dopamine hyperactivity thought to be associated with the positive symptoms of psychosis (Homayoun & Moghaddam, 2007; Stahl, 2018; Stahl, 2021).

# Neurodegeneration and Psychosis in Dementia

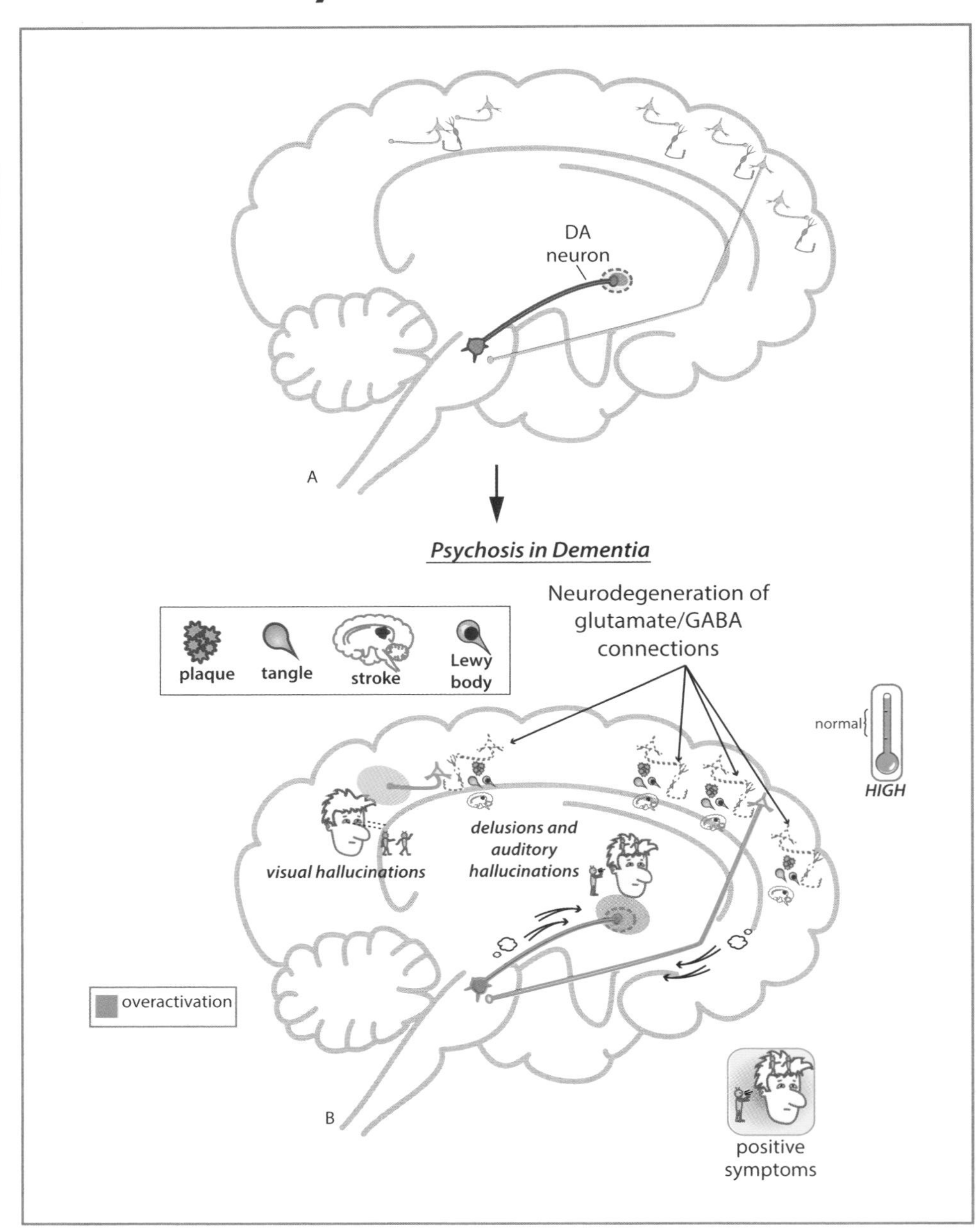

# Neurodegeneration and Psychosis in Dementia

**FIGURE 2.19.** (A) The cortical brainstem glutamate projection communicates with the mesolimbic dopamine pathway in the ventral tegmental area (VTA) to regulate dopamine release in the nucleus accumbens. (B) If neurodegeneration leads to the destruction of some glutamatergic neurons and some GABAergic interneurons, but not others, then this could lead to excessive release of glutamate in various brain regions. In the VTA, this could lead to excessive stimulation of the mesolimbic dopamine pathway and thus excessive dopamine release in the nucleus accumbens, resulting in delusions and auditory hallucinations. In the visual cortex, excessive glutamatergic activity could result in visual hallucinations (Cummings et al., 2022; Stahl, 2021).

# NMDA Receptor Hypofunction and Negative Symptoms of Schizophrenia

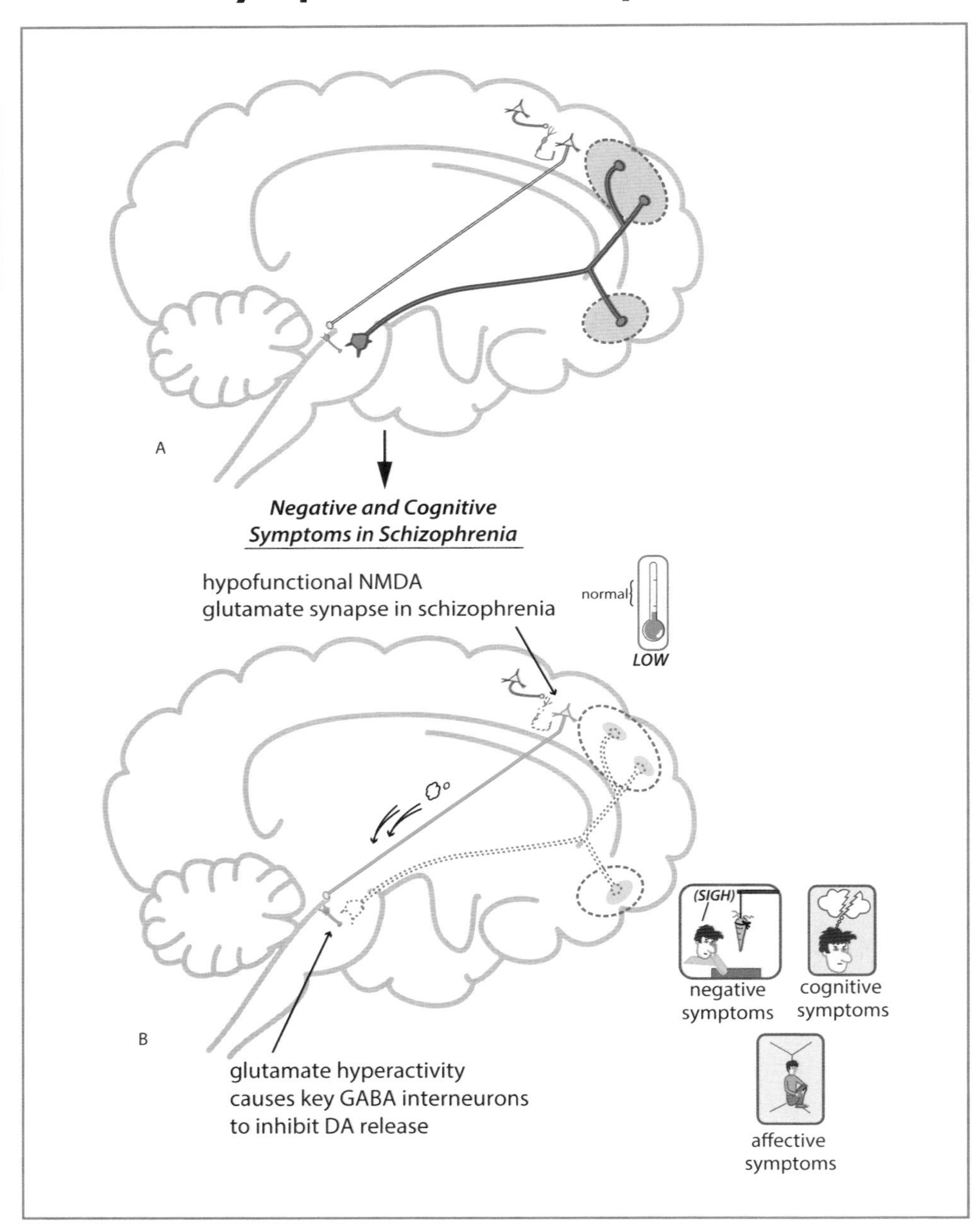

# NMDA Receptor Hypofunction and Negative Symptoms of Schizophrenia

**FIGURE 2.20.** (A) The cortical brainstem glutamate projection communicates with the mesocortical dopamine pathway in the ventral tegmental area (VTA) via GABAergic interneurons, thus regulating dopamine release in the prefrontal cortex. (B) If NMDA receptors on cortical GABA interneurons are hypoactive, then the cortical brainstem pathway to the VTA will be overactivated, leading to excessive release of glutamate in the VTA. This will lead to excessive stimulation of the brainstem GABA interneurons, which in turn leads to inhibition of mesocortical dopamine neurons. This reduces dopamine release in the prefrontal cortex and is the theoretical biological basis for the negative symptoms of psychosis (Homayoun & Moghaddam, 2007; Stahl, 2021).

# SECTION 3
# Key Serotonin Pathways

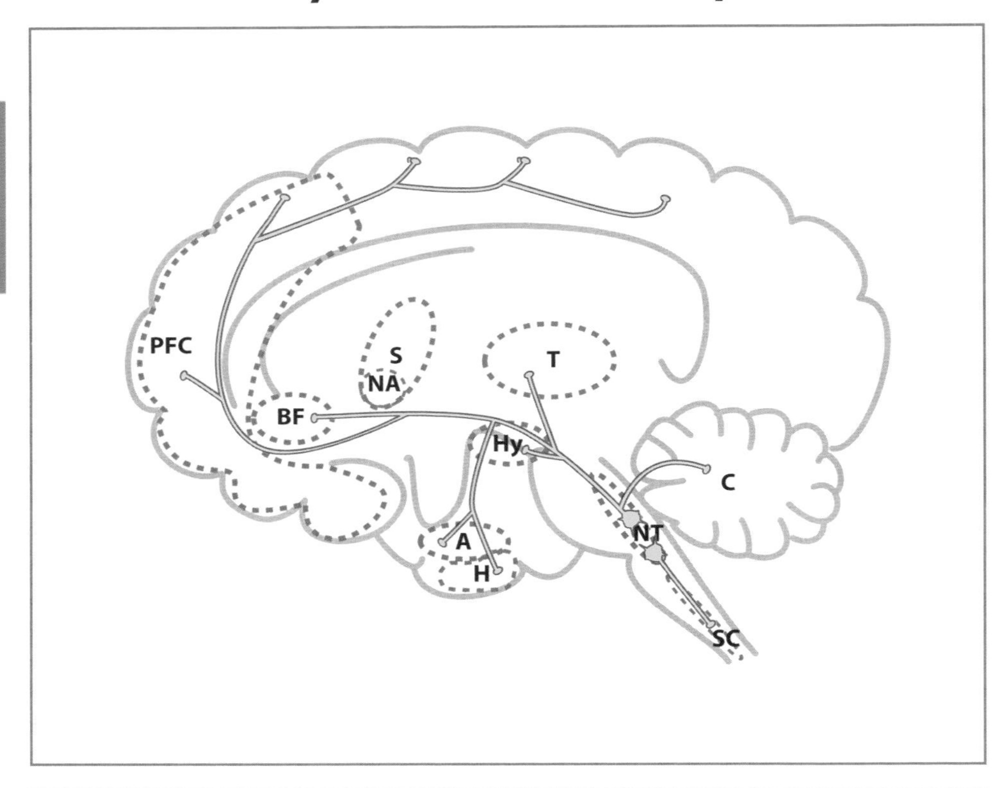


**FIGURE 2.21.** In order to fully understand the properties of pharmacological treatments for psychosis, it is imperative to examine the serotonin (5HT) pathways throughout the brain and how they modulate DA and glutamate circuits. Ascending 5HT projections originate in the raphe nucleus in the brainstem and extend to many of the same regions as noradrenergic projections, with additional projections to the striatum and nucleus accumbens. These ascending projections may regulate mood, anxiety, sleep, and other functions. Descending 5HT projections extend down the brainstem and through the spinal cord and may regulate pain (Stahl, 2021). A: amygdala; BF: basal forebrain; C: cerebellum; H: hippocampus; Hy: hypothalamus; NA: nucleus accumbens; NT: brainstem neurotransmitter centers; PFC: prefrontal cortex; S: striatum; SC: spinal cord; T: thalamus.

# Serotonin Synthesis

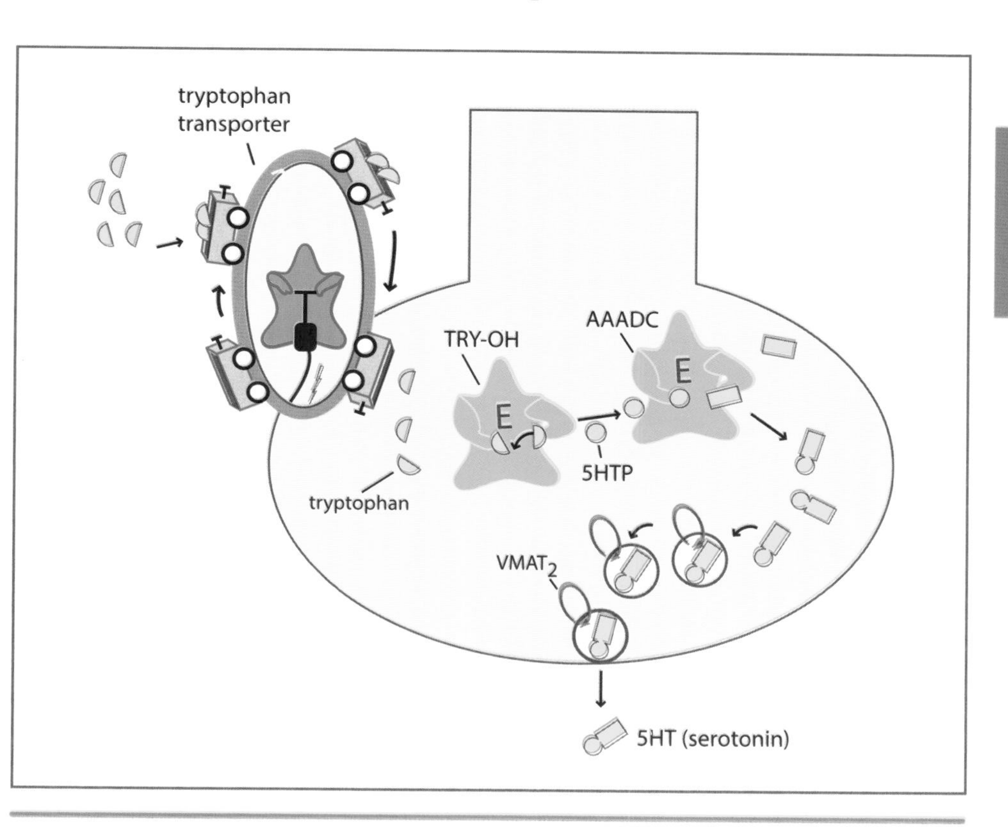


**FIGURE 2.22.** Serotonin (5-hydroxytryptamine [5HT]) is produced from enzymes after the amino acid precursor tryptophan is transported into the serotonin neuron. Once transported into the serotonin neuron, tryptophan is converted by the enzyme tryptophan hydroxylase (TRY-OH) into 5-hydroxytryptophan (5HTP), which is then converted into 5HT by the enzyme aromatic amino acid decarboxylase (AAADC). Serotonin is then taken up into synaptic vesicles via the vesicular monoamine transporter (VMAT2), where it stays until released by a neuronal impulse (Stahl, 2021).

# Serotonin Termination

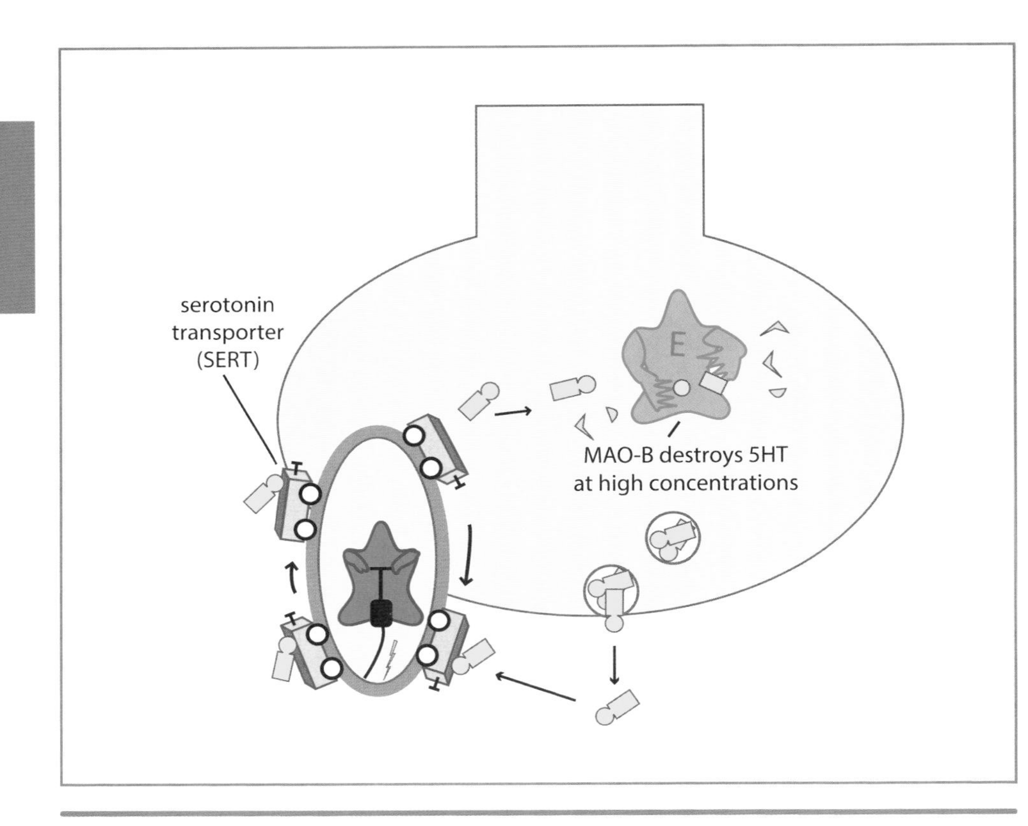


**FIGURE 2.23.** Serotonin's (5HT) action is terminated enzymatically by monoamine oxidase B (MAO-B) within the neuron when it is present in high concentrations. These enzymes convert serotonin into an inactive metabolite. There is also a presynaptic transport pump selective for serotonin, called the serotonin transporter (SERT), which clears serotonin out of the synapse and back into the presynaptic neuron (Stahl, 2021).

# Serotonin Receptor Subtypes

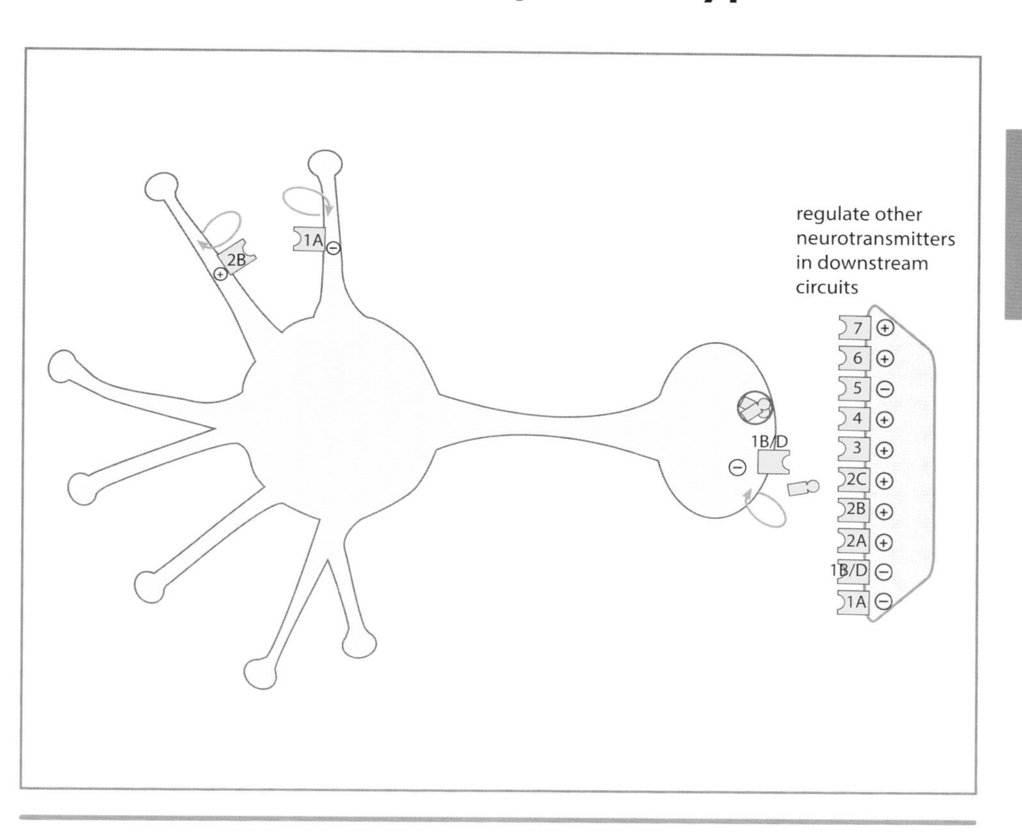


**FIGURE 2.24.** Presynaptic serotonin (5HT) receptors include 5HT1A, 5HT1B/D, and 5HT2B, all of which act as autoreceptors. There are also numerous postsynaptic serotonin receptors, which regulate other neurotransmitters in downstream circuits (Stahl, 2021).

Presynaptic 5HT1A autoreceptors are located on the cell body and dendrites and are therefore called somatodendritic autoreceptors. When 5HT is released somatodendritically, it binds to these 5HT1A receptors and causes a shutdown of 5HT neuronal impulse flow and a reduction in the release of 5HT from the synapse. Presynaptic 5HT2B autoreceptors are located on the cell body and dendrites and are therefore called somatodendritic autoreceptors. When 5HT is released somatodendritically, it binds to these 5HT2B receptors and causes increased 5HT neuronal impulse flow and increased release of 5HT from the synapse. Presynaptic 5HT1B/D autoreceptors are located on the presynaptic axon terminal. They act by detecting the presence of 5HT in the synapse and causing a shutdown of further 5HT release. When 5HT builds up in the synapse, it is available to bind to the autoreceptor, which then inhibits 5HT release (Stahl, 2021).

# Serotonin Regulates All Major Neurotransmitter Systems

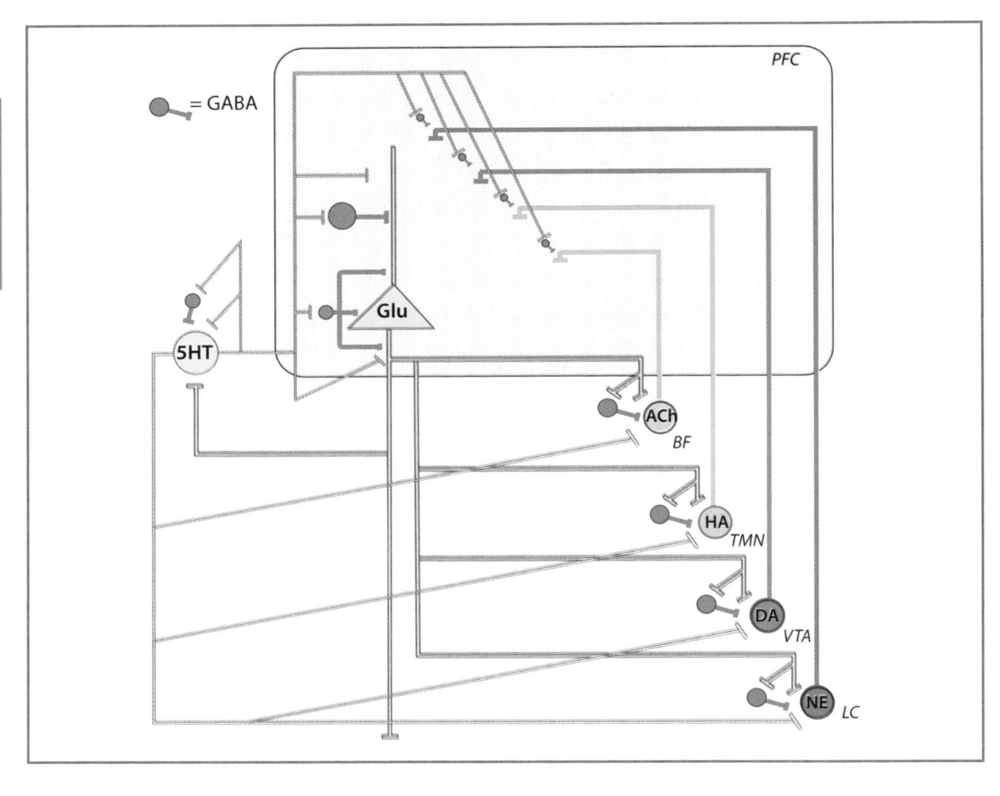

# Serotonin Regulates All Major Neurotransmitter Systems

**FIGURE 2.25.** 5HT circuits arise from discrete brainstem nuclei, including the dorsal and median raphe nuclei. These circuits project to a wide range of cortical and subcortical brain areas, including the prefrontal cortex (PFC) and the loci for the cell bodies of neurons of other neurotransmitters, such as the locus coeruleus (LC) for norepinephrine, the ventral tegmental area (VTA) for dopamine, the tuberomammillary nucleus of the hypothalamus (TMN) for histamine, and the basal forebrain (BF) for acetylcholine. Through these connections, the 5HT network may both modulate itself and directly and indirectly influence virtually all other neurotransmitter networks. Thus, it is not surprising that the 5HT network is thought to regulate a variety of behaviors, including mood, sleep, and appetite, or that dysregulation of the 5HT network has been implicated in many psychiatric disorders (Fink & Göthert, 2007; Stahl, 2021).

# Serotonin 5HT2A Receptors and Hallucinogen Psychosis

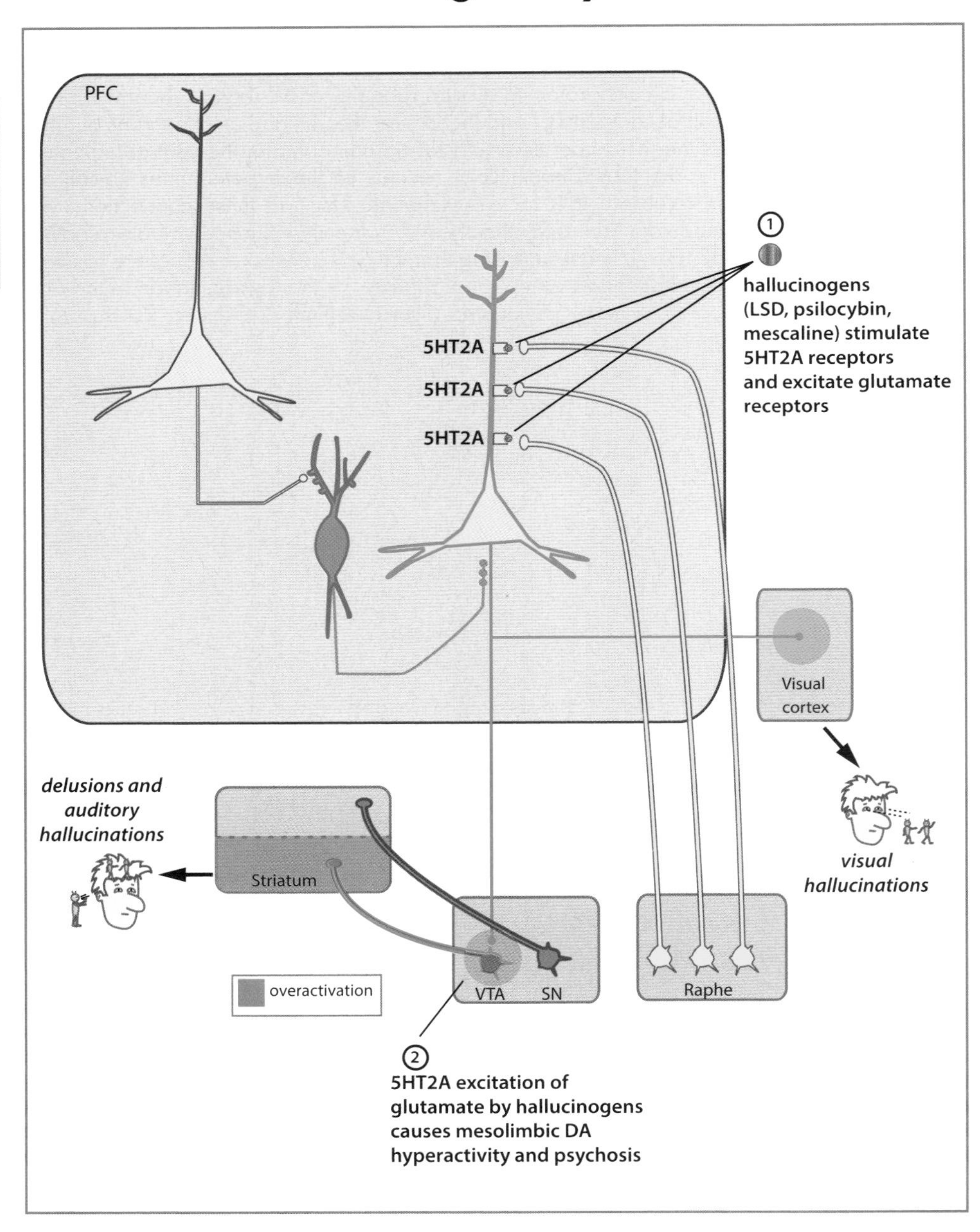

# Serotonin 5HT2A Receptors and Hallucinogen Psychosis

**FIGURE 2.26.** Hallucinogens such as LSD, psilocybin, and mescaline are 5HT2A agonists. (1) When these agents stimulate 5HT2A receptors on glutamatergic pyramidal neurons in the prefrontal cortex (PFC), this causes overactivation of the glutamate neuron. (2) The resultant release of glutamate into the ventral tegmental area (VTA) causes hyperactivity of the mesolimbic dopamine (DA) pathway, resulting in delusions and auditory hallucinations. Excessive glutamate release in the visual cortex can cause visual hallucinations (Amargós-Bosch et al., 2004; Gellings et al., 2012; Stahl, 2021).

# Serotonin 5HT2A Receptors and Parkinson's Disease Psychosis

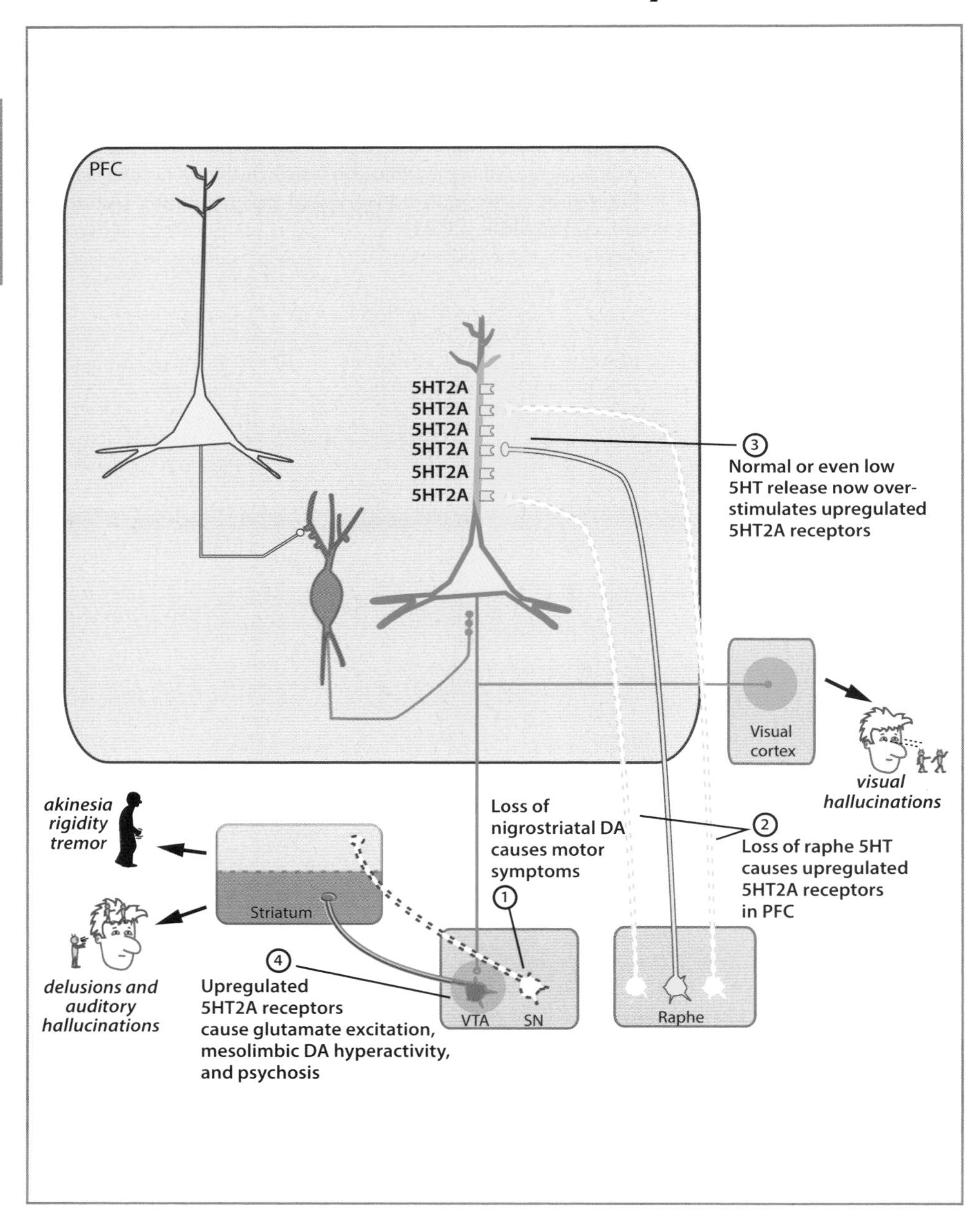

# Serotonin 5HT2A Receptors and Parkinson's Disease Psychosis

**FIGURE 2.27.** (1) Loss of nigrostriatal DA neurons causes the motor symptoms of Parkinson's disease, such as akinesia, rigidity, and tremor. (2) Parkinson's disease also causes loss of serotonergic neurons that project from the raphe to the prefrontal cortex (PFC). (3) This leads to upregulation of 5HT2A receptors, in which case normal or even low 5HT release can overstimulate these receptors, causing overactivation of the glutamatergic pyramidal neuron. (4) Excessive Glu release into the ventral tegmental area (VTA) causes hyperactivity of the mesolimbic DA pathway, resulting in delusions and auditory hallucinations. Excessive Glu release in the visual cortex can cause visual hallucinations (Stahl, 2021).

# Serotonin 5HT2A Receptors and Psychosis in Dementia

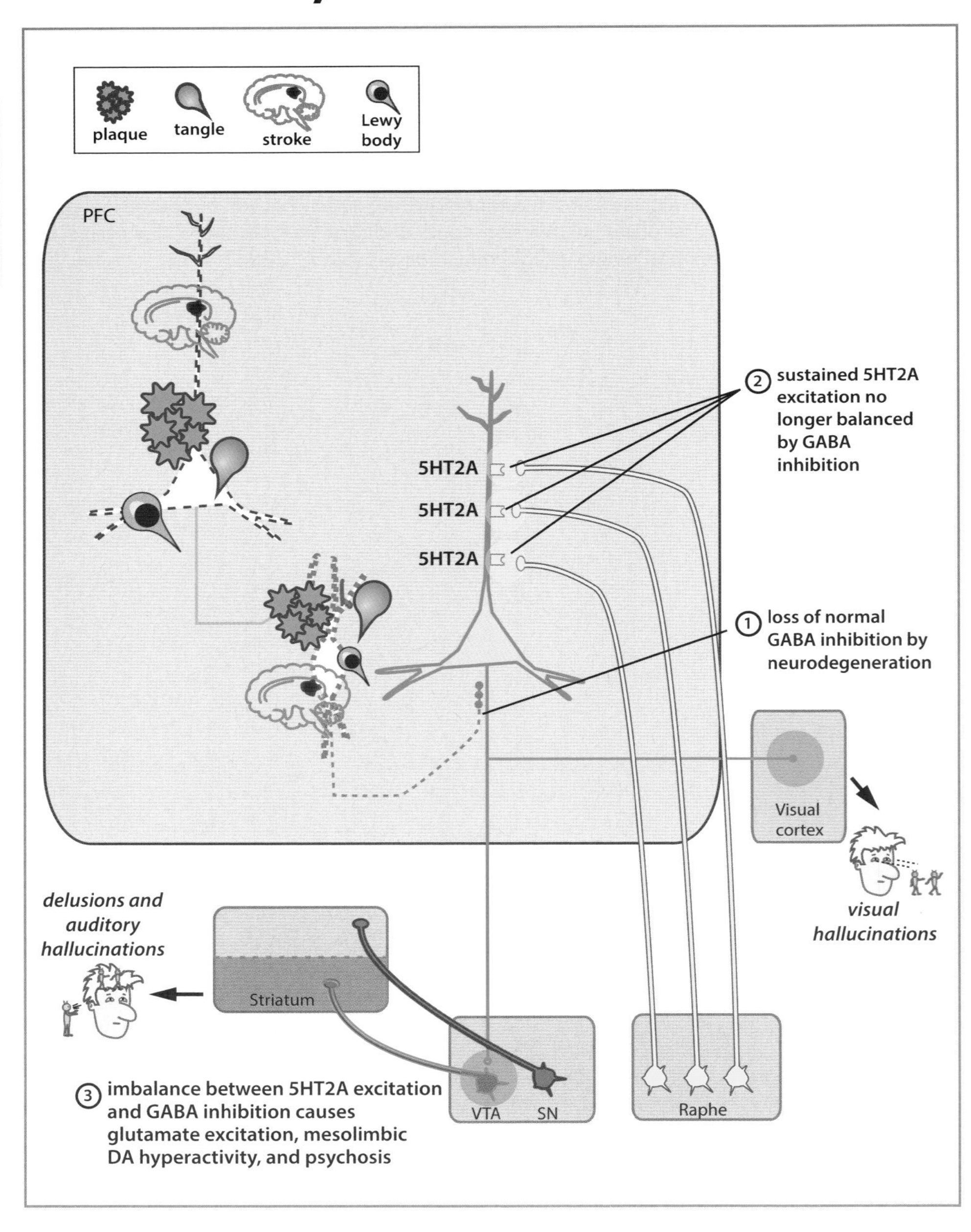

# Serotonin 5HT2A Receptors and Psychosis in Dementia

**FIGURE 2.28.** (1) Accumulation of amyloid plaques, tau tangles, and/or Lewy bodies, as well as the damage caused by strokes, may destroy some glutamatergic pyramidal neurons and GABAergic interneurons while leaving others intact. The loss of GABA inhibition upsets the balance of control over glutamatergic pyramidal neurons. (2) When the effects of stimulation of excitatory 5HT2A receptors are not countered by GABA inhibition, there is a net increase in glutamatergic neurotransmission. (3) Excessive Glu release into the ventral tegmental area (VTA) causes hyperactivity of the mesolimbic DA pathway, resulting in delusions and auditory hallucinations. Excessive Glu release in the visual cortex can cause visual hallucinations (Cummings et al., 2022; Stahl, 2021).

# Hallucinogen Psychosis

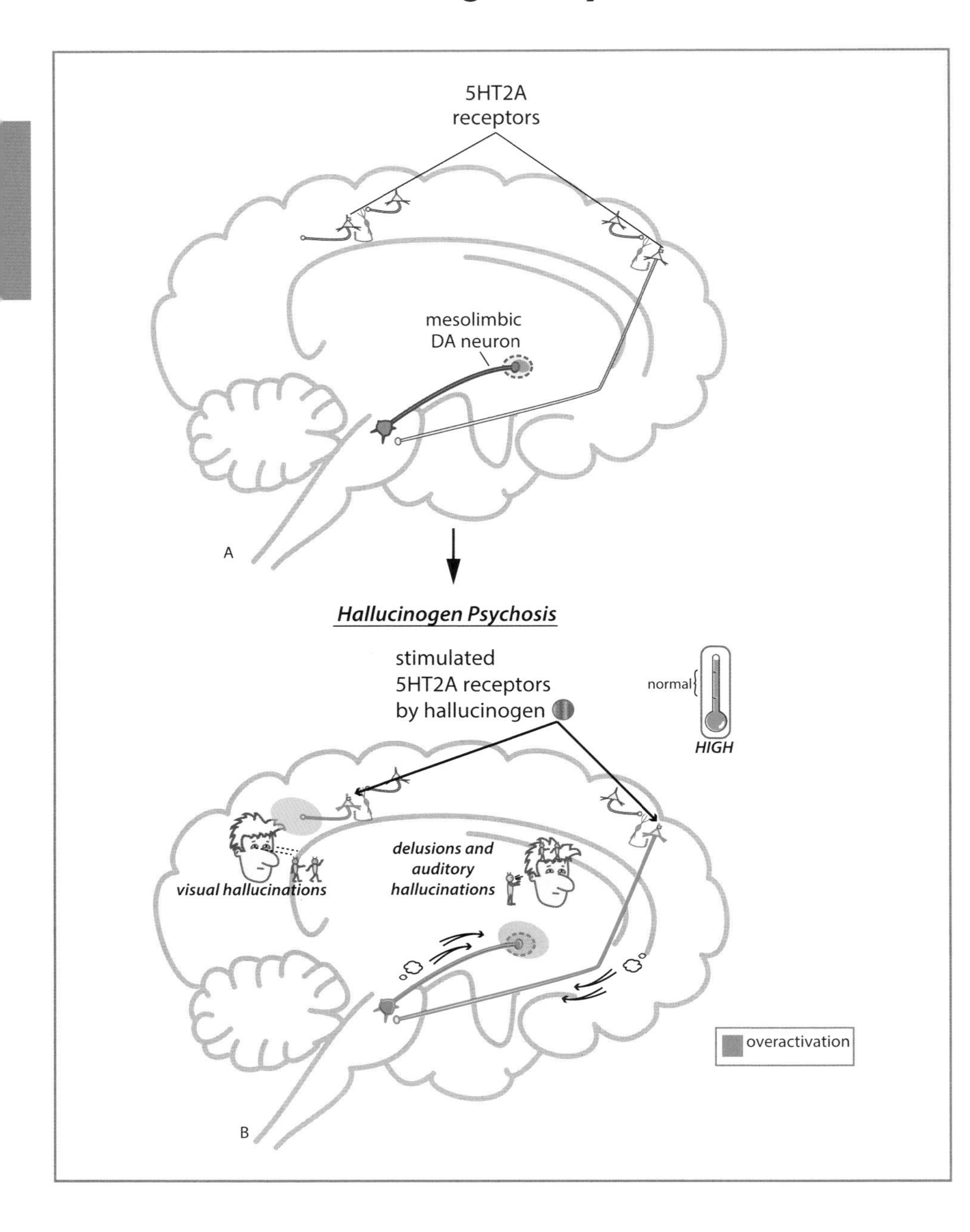

# Hallucinogen Psychosis

**FIGURE 2.29.** (A) Shown here is a cortico-brainstem glutamatergic pathway projecting from the prefrontal cortex to the ventral tegmental area (VTA), and an indirect cortico-cortical glutamatergic pathway in the visual cortex. Activity of both pathways is regulated by serotonergic neurons that project from the raphe nucleus as well as by GABA interneurons in the prefrontal cortex. At baseline, normal stimulation of excitatory 5HT2A receptors on the Glu neurons is balanced by tonic stimulation of GABA receptors on the same neurons; the net effect is thus normal activation of the glutamatergic neurons. (B) Hallucinogens such as LSD, psilocybin, and mescaline are 5HT2A agonists. When these agents stimulate 5HT2A receptors on glutamatergic pyramidal neurons in the prefrontal cortex, this causes overactivation of the Glu neurons. Excessive Glu release into the VTA causes hyperactivity of the mesolimbic DA pathway, resulting in delusions and auditory hallucinations. Excessive Glu release in the visual cortex can cause visual hallucinations (Amargós-Bosch et al., 2004; Gellings et al., 2012; Stahl, 2021).

# Psychosis in Parkinson's Disease

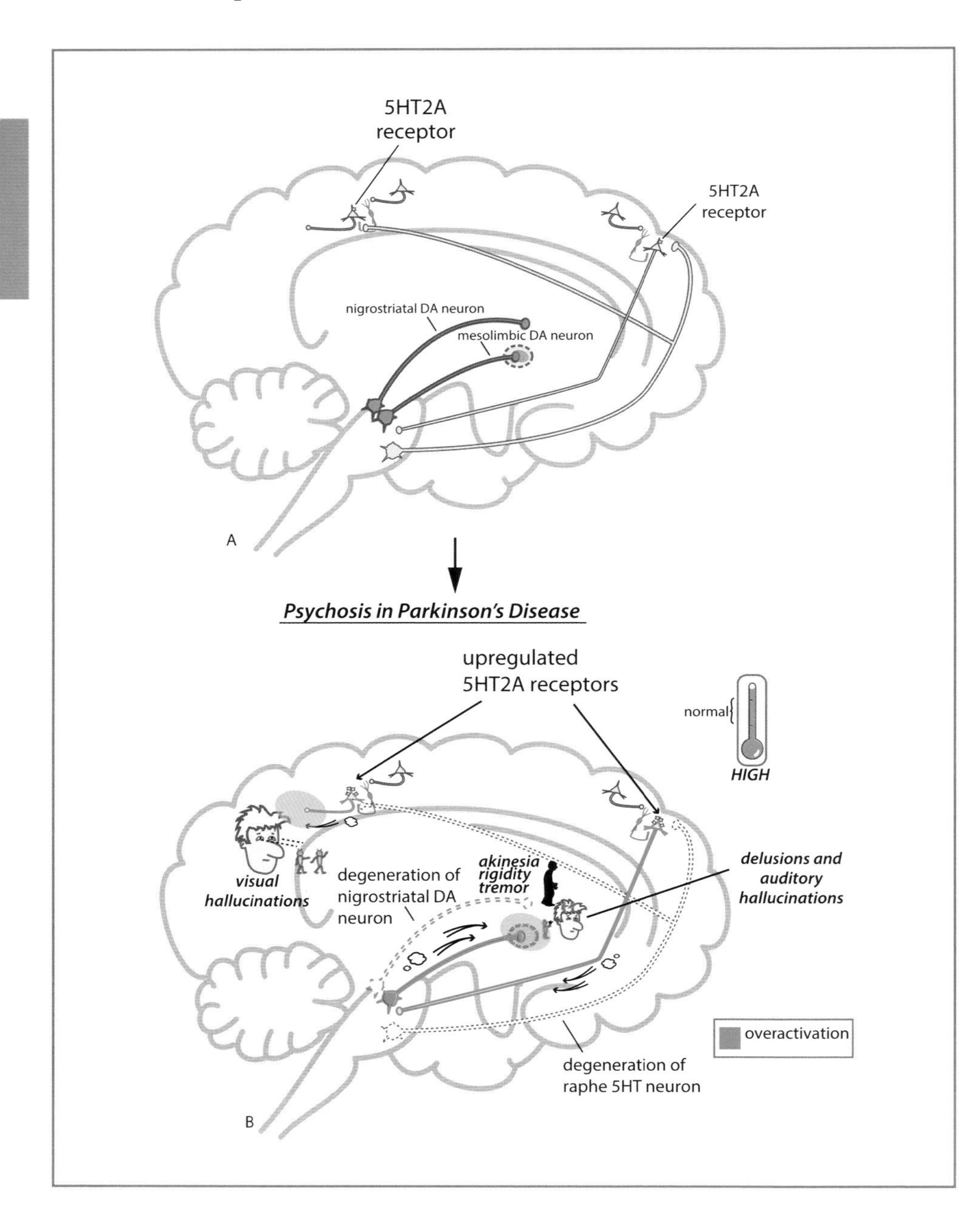

# Psychosis in Parkinson's Disease

**FIGURE 2.30.** (A) Shown here is a cortico-brainstem glutamatergic pathway projecting from the prefrontal cortex to the ventral tegmental area (VTA), and an indirect cortico-cortical glutamatergic pathway in the visual cortex. Activity of both pathways is regulated by serotonergic neurons that project from the raphe nucleus as well as by GABA interneurons in the prefrontal cortex. At baseline, normal stimulation of excitatory 5HT2A receptors on the Glu neurons is balanced by tonic stimulation of GABA receptors on the same neurons; the net effect is thus normal activation of the glutamatergic neurons. (B) Loss of nigrostriatal dopamine neurons causes the motor symptoms of Parkinson's disease, such as akinesia, rigidity, and tremor. Parkinson's disease also causes loss of serotonergic neurons that project from the raphe to the prefrontal cortex and to the visual cortex. This leads to upregulation of 5HT2A receptors on glutamatergic pyramidal neurons in the prefrontal cortex, in which case normal or even low 5HT release can overstimulate these receptors. Excessive glutamate release into the VTA causes hyperactivity of the mesolimbic DA pathway, resulting in delusions and auditory hallucinations. Excessive Glu release in the visual cortex can cause visual hallucinations (Stahl, 2016; Stahl, 2021).

# Psychosis in Dementia

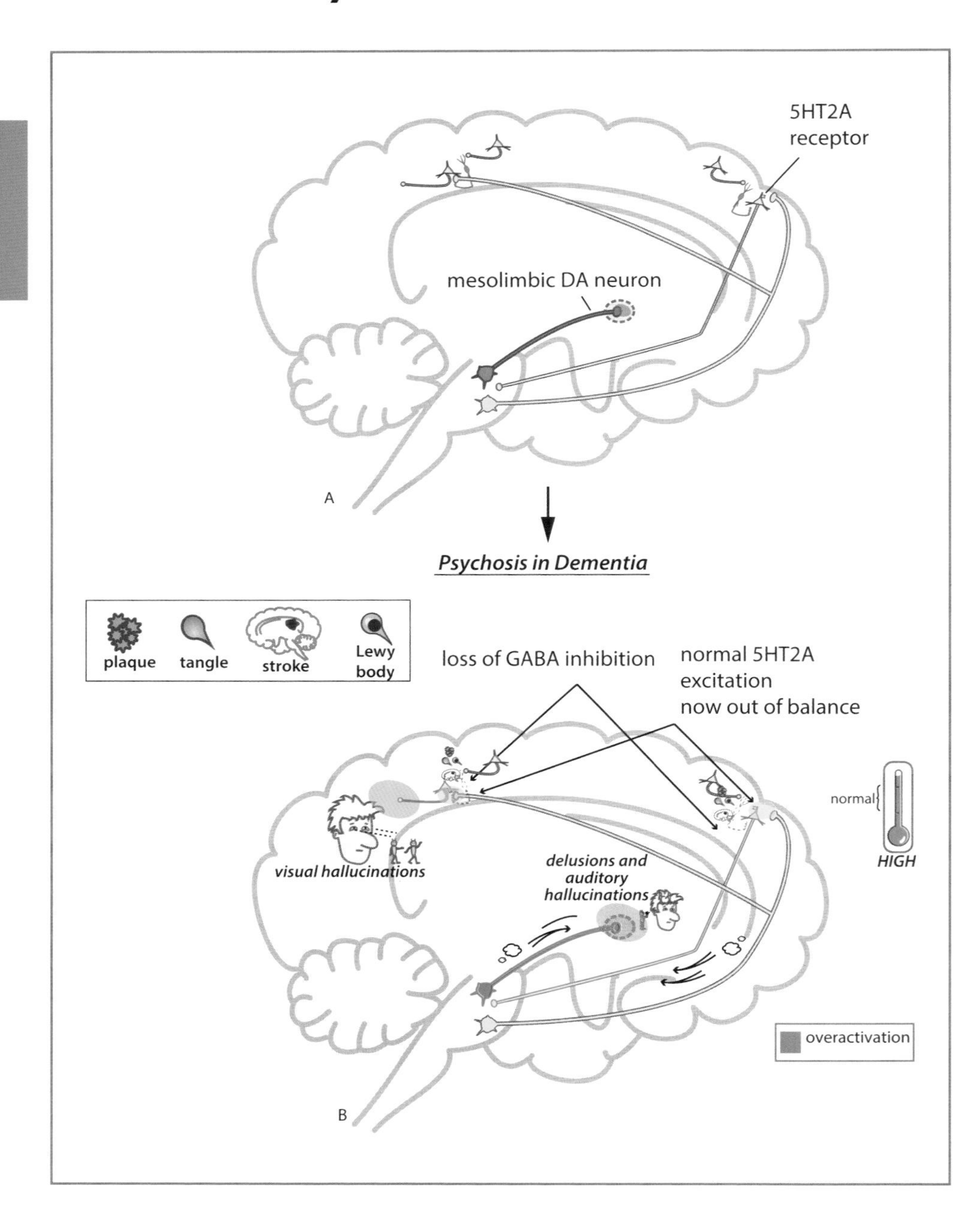

# Psychosis in Dementia

**FIGURE 2.31.** (A) Shown here is a cortico-brainstem glutamatergic pathway projecting from the prefrontal cortex to the ventral tegmental area (VTA), and an indirect cortico-cortical glutamatergic pathway in the visual cortex. Activity of both pathways is regulated by serotonergic neurons that project from the raphe nucleus as well as by GABA interneurons in the prefrontal cortex. At baseline, normal stimulation of excitatory 5HT2A receptors on the Glu neurons is balanced by tonic stimulation of GABA receptors on the same neurons; the net effect is thus normal activation of the glutamatergic neurons. (B) Accumulation of amyloid plaques, tau tangles, and/or Lewy bodies, as well as the damage caused by strokes, may destroy some glutamatergic pyramidal neurons and GABA interneurons while leaving others intact. When the effects of stimulation of excitatory 5HT2A receptors are not countered by GABA inhibition, there is a net increase in glutamatergic neurotransmission. Excessive Glu release into the VTA causes hyperactivity of the mesolimbic DA pathway, resulting in delusions and auditory hallucinations. Excessive Glu release in the visual cortex can cause visual hallucinations (Cummings et al., 2022; Stahl, 2021).

Stahl's Illustrated | Chapter 3

# Circuits to Mechanisms of Treatments for Psychosis and Side Effects

Currently available drugs for psychosis are associated with an array of side effects. Many of these side effects are hypothetically linked to interactions at dopamine D2, serotonin 5HT2A, and serotonin 5HT1A receptors. Binding at additional receptors (e.g., muscarinic M1, α1 adrenergic, histamine H1, serotonin 5HT2C, and others) may lead to other notable side effects. This chapter reviews how binding at these receptors in dopamine pathways and beyond can lead to side effects like tardive dyskinesia, hyperprolactinemia, weight gain, and others. This chapter will also explain how an informed psychopharmacologist can ensure side effects are minimized and, in certain cases, optimally treated.

# Therapeutic Mechanisms of Drugs for Psychosis

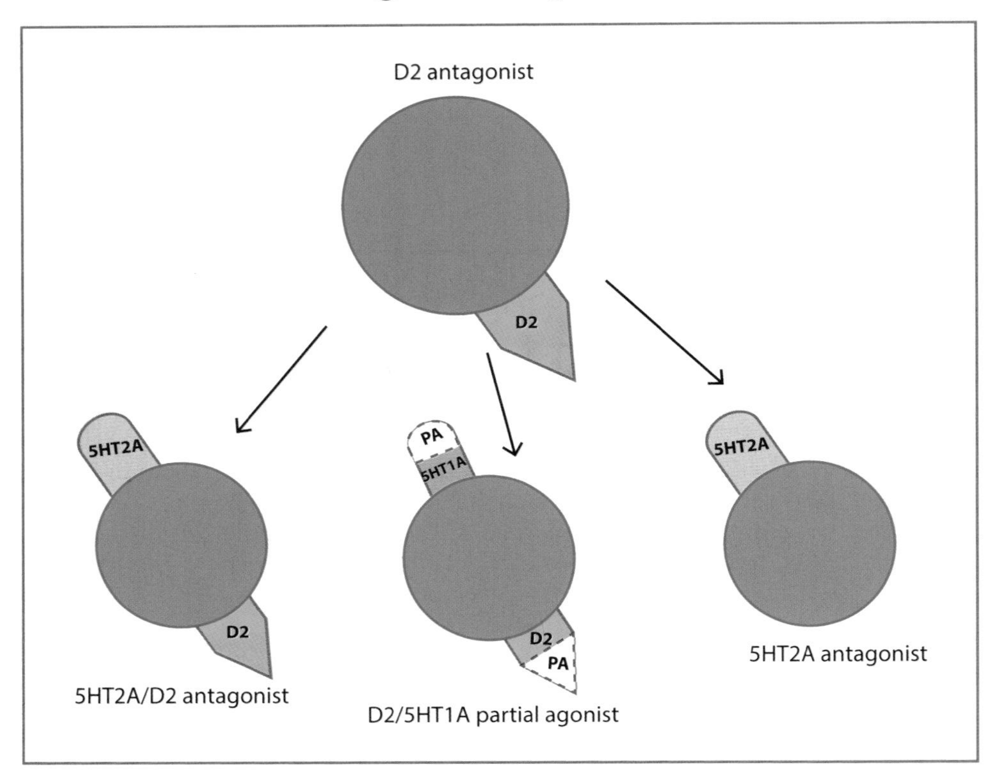


**FIGURE 3.1.** The first mechanism identified to treat psychosis was dopamine 2 (D2) antagonism, and for several decades all available medications to treat psychosis were D2 antagonists. Today, there are many agents available with additional mechanisms, including D2 antagonism combined with serotonin (5HT) 2A (5HT2A) antagonism, D2 partial agonism (PA) combined with serotonin 1A (5HT1A) partial agonism, and 5HT2A antagonism alone (Stahl, 2021).

# Mesolimbic DA Pathway and D2 Antagonist/Partial Agonist

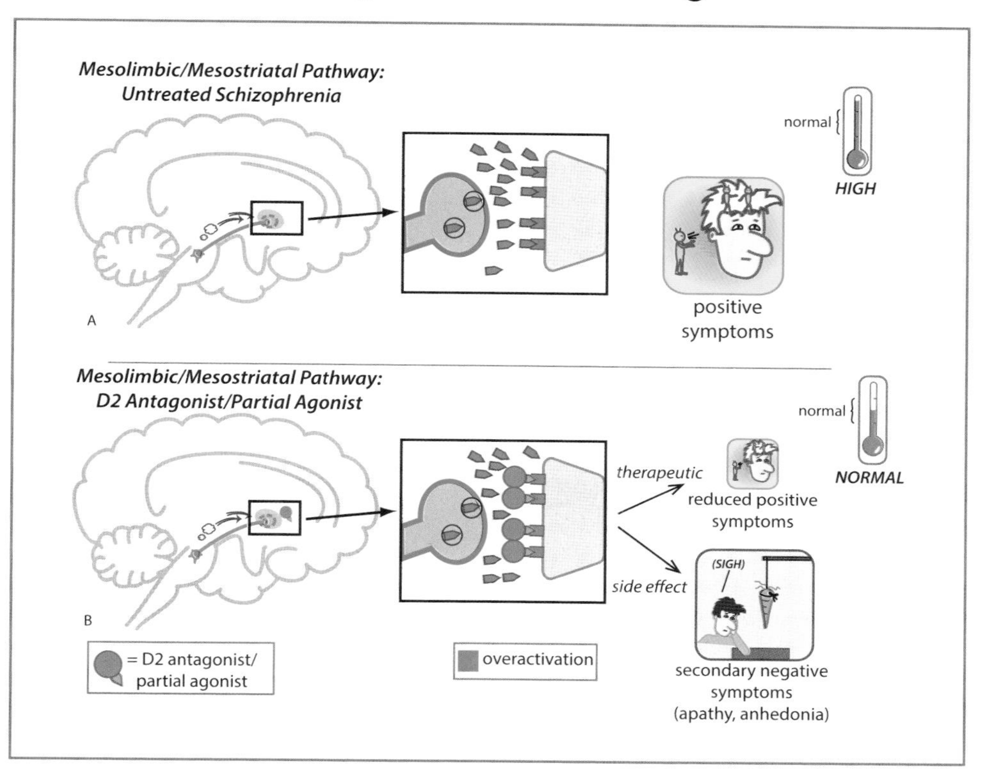


**FIGURE 3.2.** (A) In untreated schizophrenia, the mesolimbic/mesostriatal DA pathway is hypothesized to be hyperactive, indicated here by the pathway appearing red as well as by the excess dopamine in the synapse. This leads to positive symptoms such as delusions and hallucinations. (B) Administration of a D2 antagonist or partial agonist blocks DA from binding to the D2 receptor, which reduces hyperactivity in this pathway and thereby reduces positive symptoms as well. However, because the mesolimbic/mesostriatal DA pathway also plays a role in regulating motivation and reward, blockade of D2 receptors can cause secondary negative symptoms such as apathy and anhedonia (Stahl, 2021).

# Mesocortical DA Pathway in Untreated Schizophrenia

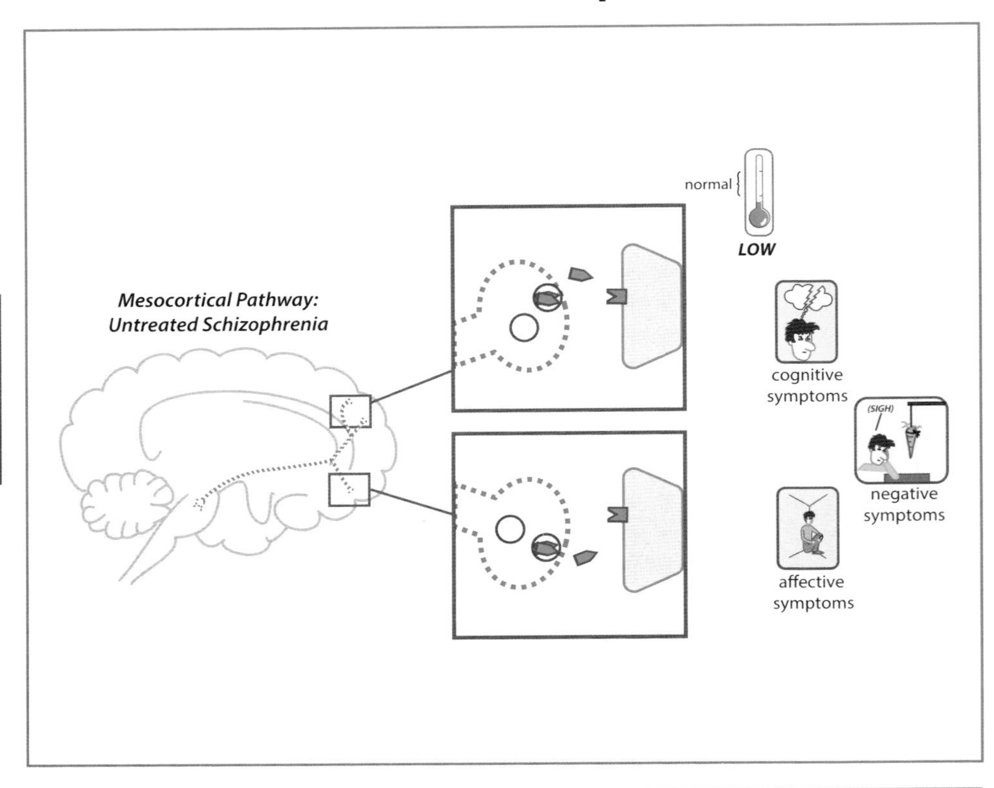


**FIGURE 3.3.** In untreated schizophrenia, the mesocortical DA pathways to the dorsolateral prefrontal cortex (DLPFC) and to the ventromedial prefrontal cortex (VMPFC) are hypothesized to be hypoactive, indicated here by the dotted outlines of the pathway. This hypoactivity is related to cognitive symptoms (in the DLPFC), negative symptoms (in the DLPFC and VMPFC), and affective symptoms of schizophrenia (in the VMPFC) (Stahl, 2021).

# Mesocortical DA Pathway With D2 Antagonist/Partial Agonist

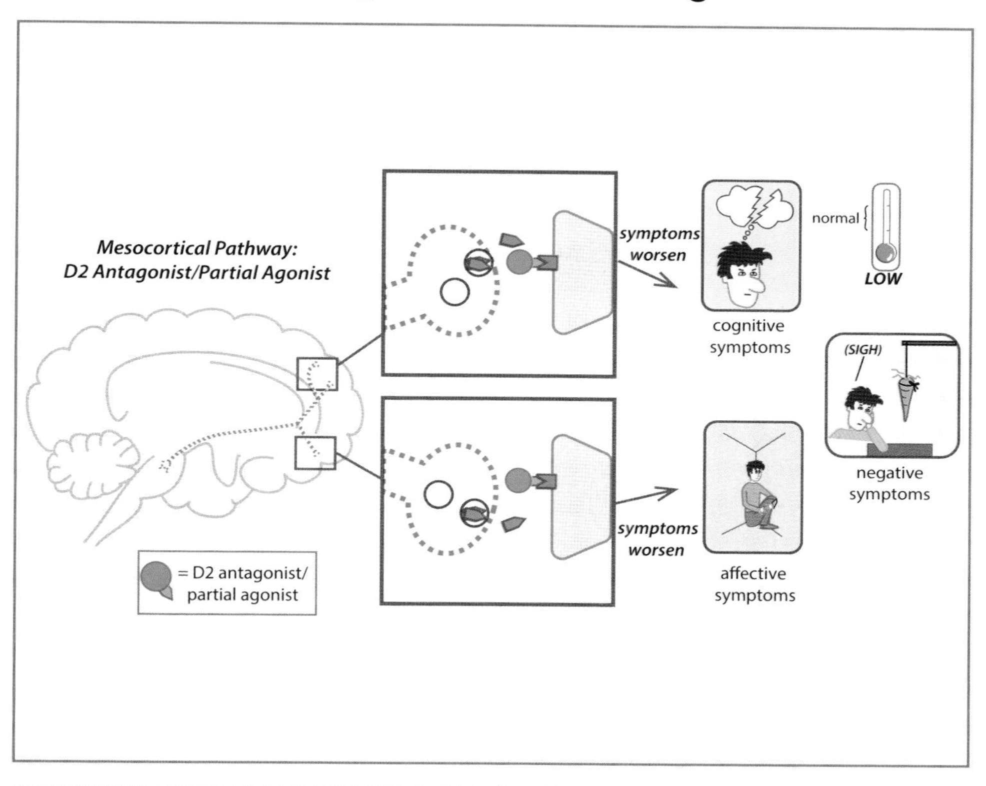


**FIGURE 3.4.** Administration of a D2 antagonist or partial agonist could further reduce activity in this pathway and thus potentially worsen these symptoms (Stahl, 2021).

# Tuberoinfundibular DA Pathway and D2 Antagonist

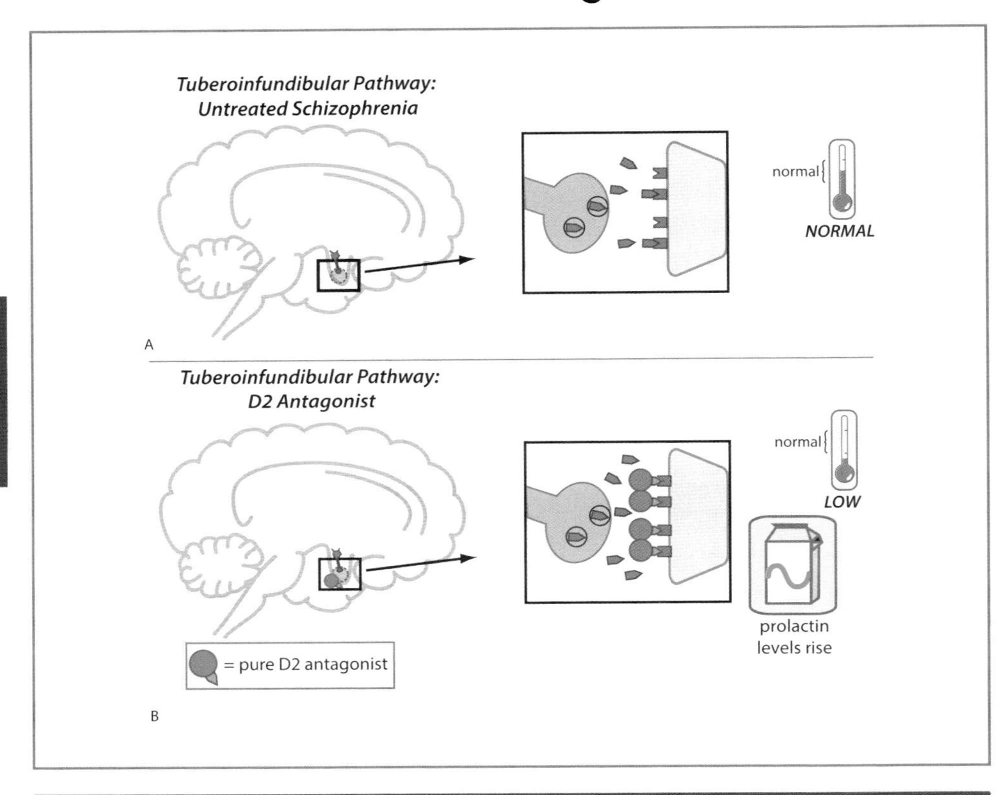


**FIGURE 3.5.** (A) The tuberoinfundibular DA pathway, which projects from the hypothalamus to the pituitary gland, is theoretically "normal" in untreated schizophrenia. (B) D2 antagonists reduce activity in this pathway by preventing DA from binding to D2 receptors. This causes prolactin levels to rise, which is associated with side effects such as galactorrhea (breast secretions) and amenorrhea (irregular menstrual periods) (Stahl, 2021).

# Nigrostriatal DA Pathway and D2 Antagonist/Partial Agonist

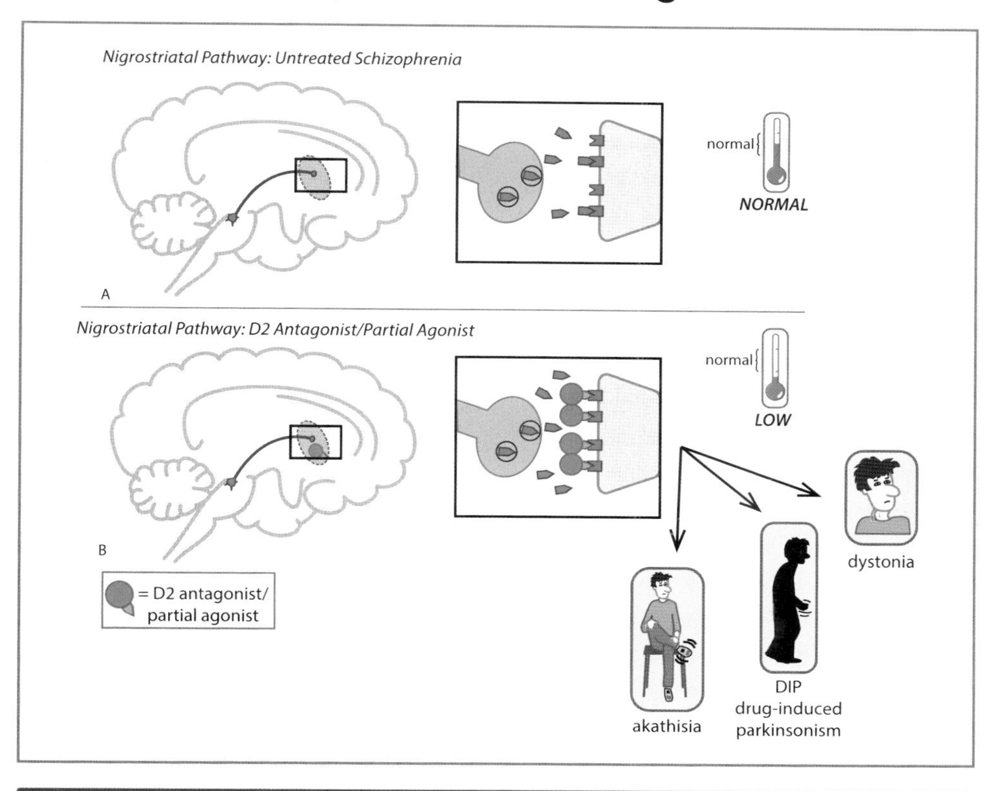


**FIGURE 3.6.** (A) The nigrostriatal DA pathway is theoretically unaffected in untreated schizophrenia. (B) Blockade of D2 receptors prevents DA from binding there and can cause motor side effects such as drug-induced parkinsonism (tremor, muscle rigidity, slowing or loss of movement), akathisia (motor restlessness), and dystonia (involuntary twisting and contractions) (Stahl, 2021).

# Tardive Dyskinesia

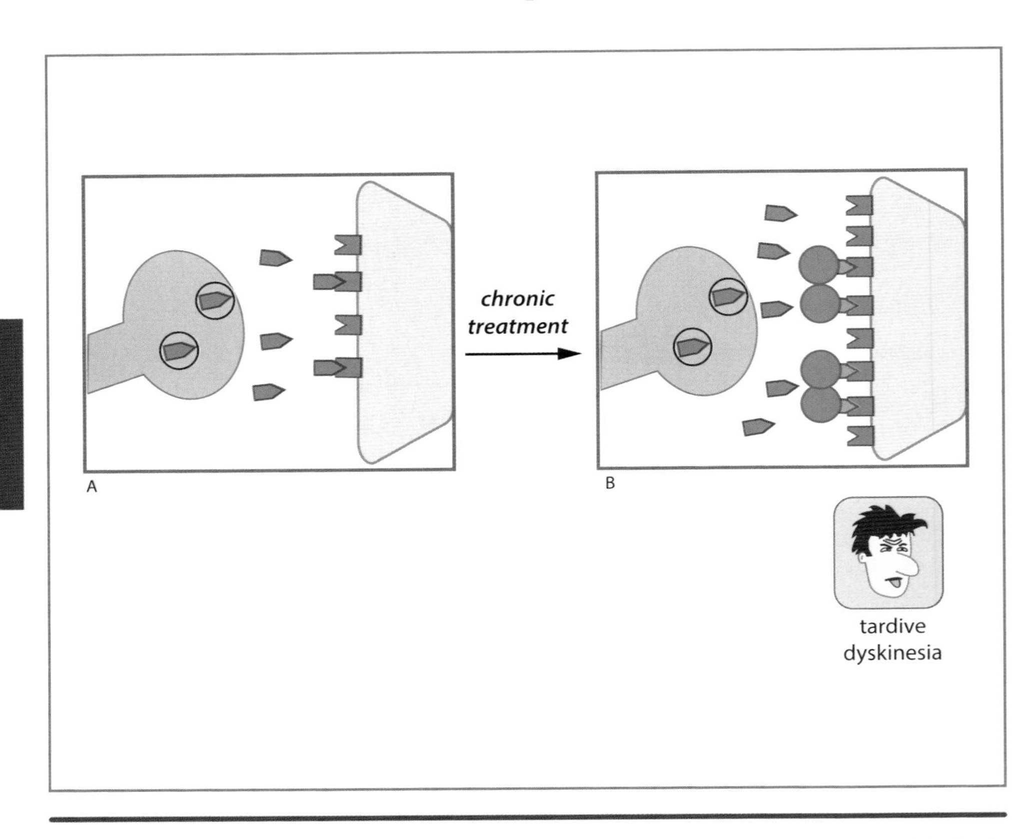


**FIGURE 3.7.** (A) DA binds to D2 receptors in the nigrostriatal pathway. (B) Chronic blockade of D2 receptors in the nigrostriatal DA pathway can cause upregulation of those receptors, which can lead to a hyperkinetic motor condition known as tardive dyskinesia, characterized by facial and tongue movements (e.g., tongue protrusions, facial grimaces, chewing) as well as quick, jerky limb movements (Stahl, 2017; Stahl, 2021).

# Reciprocal Relationship of DA and ACh

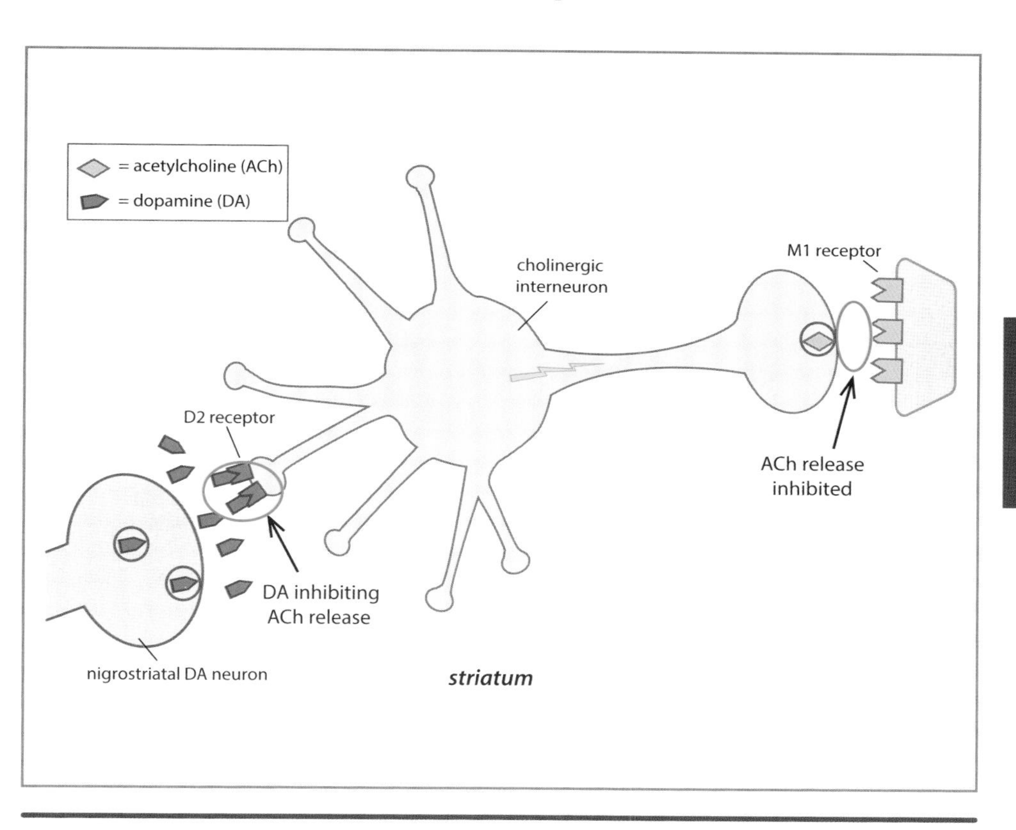


**FIGURE 3.8.** DA and ACh have a reciprocal relationship in the nigrostriatal DA pathway. DA neurons here make postsynaptic connections with the dendrite of a cholinergic neuron. Normally, DA binding at D2 receptors suppresses ACh activity (no ACh being released from the cholinergic axon on the right) (Stahl, 2021).

# DA, ACh, and D2 Antagonism

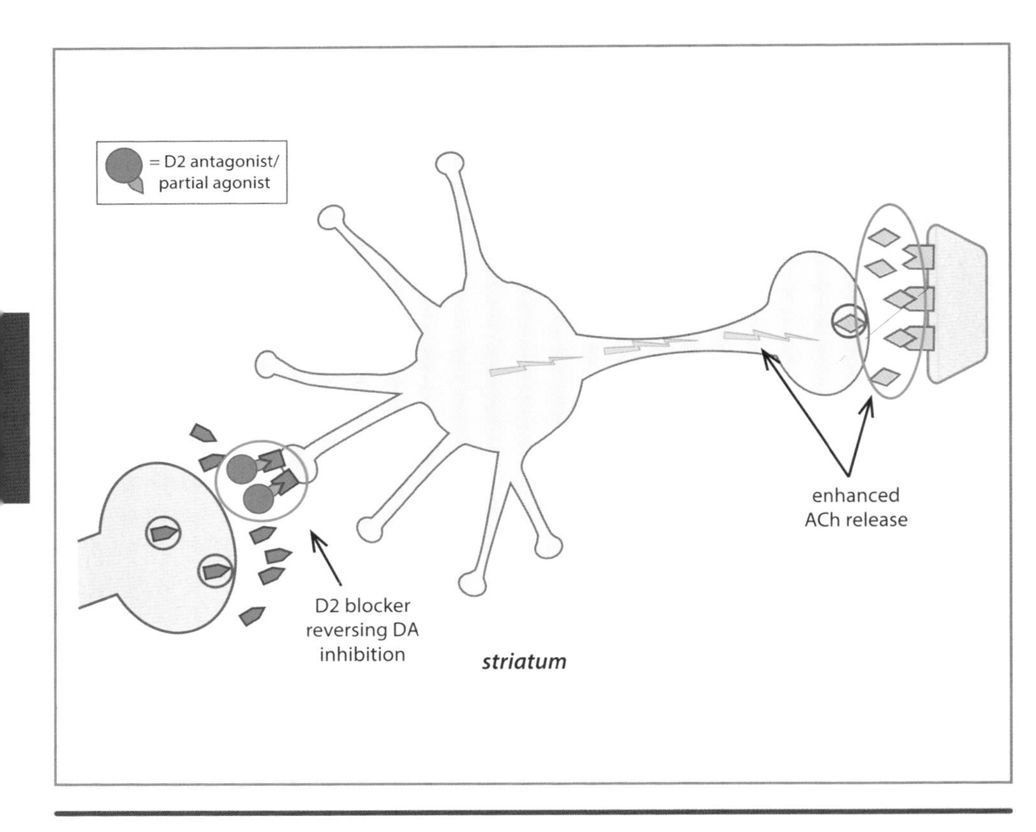


**FIGURE 3.9.** Since DA normally suppresses ACh activity, removal of DA inhibition causes an increase in ACh activity. As shown here, if D2 receptors are blocked on the cholinergic dendrite on the left, then ACh release from the cholinergic axon on the right is enhanced. This is associated with the production of drug-induced parkinsonism (Stahl, 2021).

# D2 Antagonism and Anticholinergic Agents

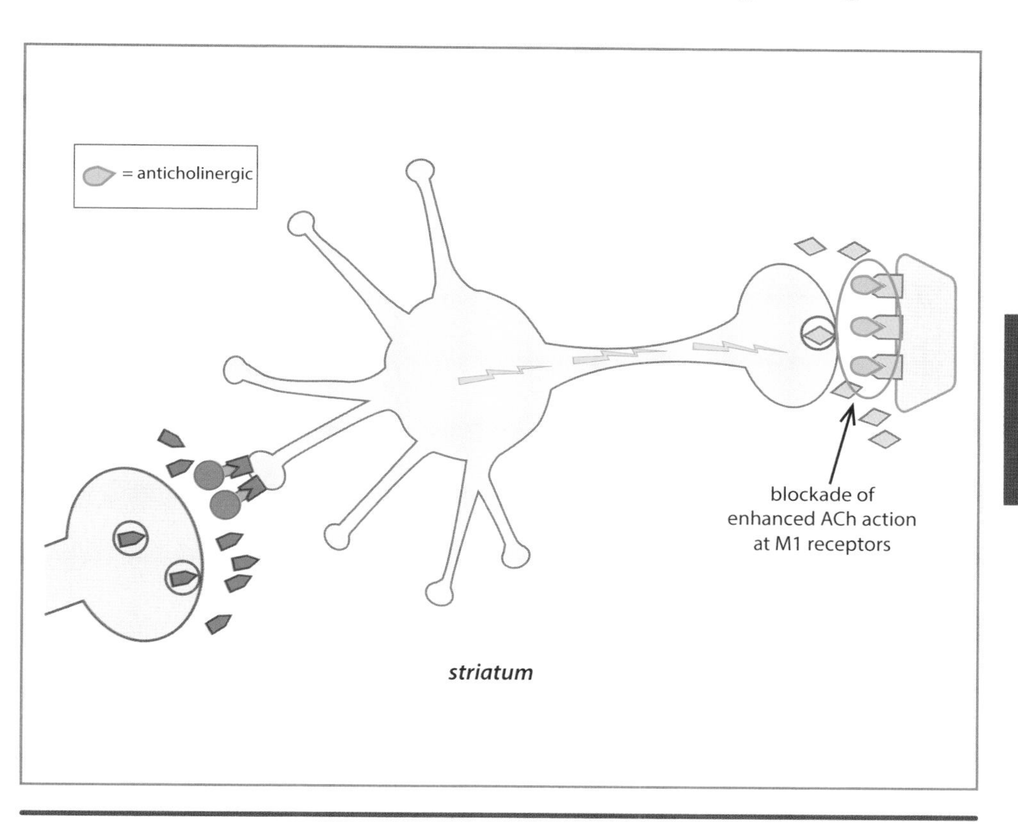


**FIGURE 3.10.** One compensation for the overactivity that occurs when D2 receptors are blocked is to block the muscarinic cholinergic receptors with an anticholinergic agent (M1 receptors being blocked by an anticholinergic on the far right). This hypothetically restores in part the normal balance between DA and ACh and can reduce symptoms of drug-induced parkinsonism (Stahl, 2021).

# Side Effects of Muscarinic (M1) Cholinergic Receptor Blockade

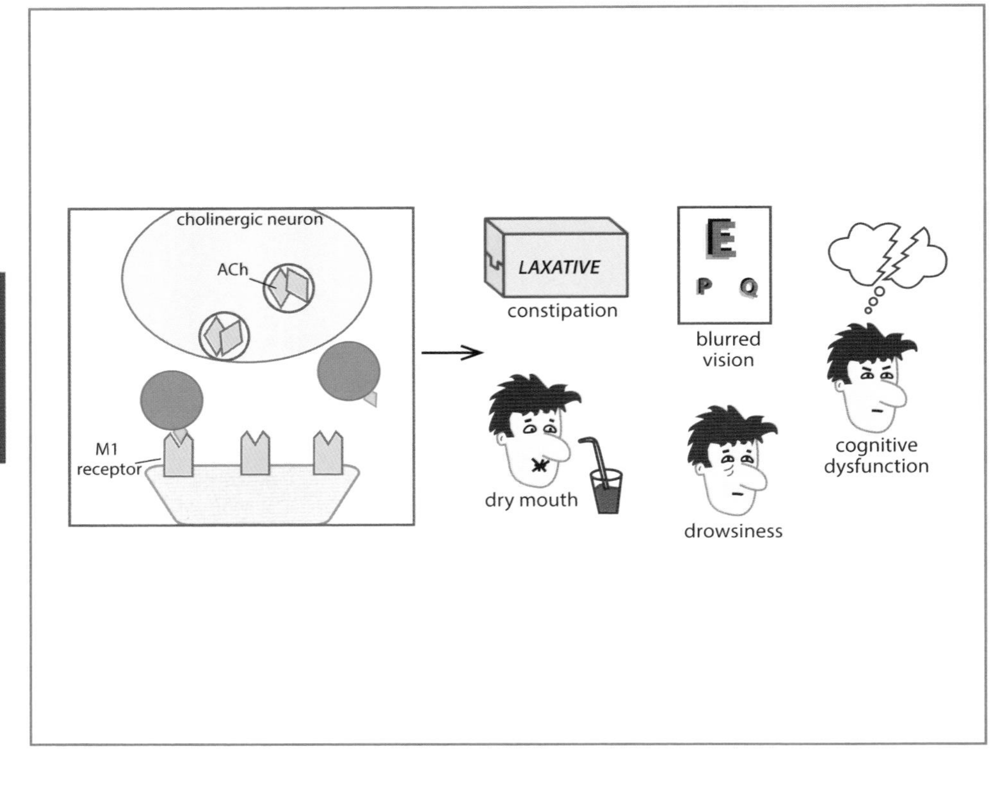

# Side Effects of Muscarinic (M1) Cholinergic Receptor Blockade

**FIGURE 3.11.** Blockade of muscarinic cholinergic receptors can reduce drug-induced parkinsonism, but can also induce side effects such as constipation, blurred vision, dry mouth, drowsiness, and cognitive dysfunction (problems with memory and concentration, slowed cognitive processing) (Stahl, 2021).

# D2 Receptor Inhibition of the CSTC Stop Pathway

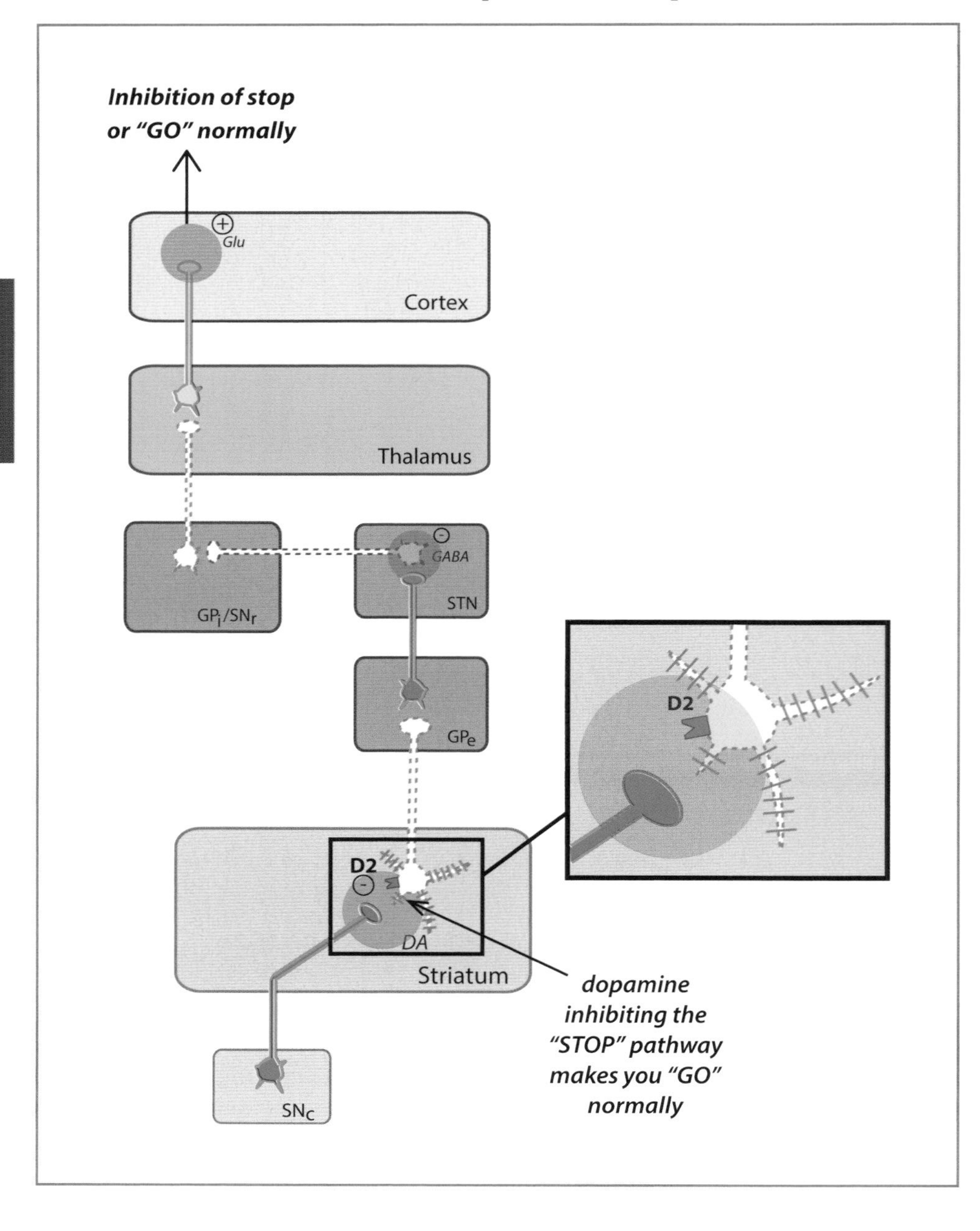

# D2 Receptor Inhibition of the CSTC Stop Pathway

**FIGURE 3.12.** DA released from the nigrostriatal pathway binds to postsynaptic D2 receptors on a γ-aminobutyric acid (GABA) neuron projecting to the globus pallidus externa. This causes inhibition of the indirect (stop) pathway, thus instead telling it to "go" (Stahl, 2017; Stahl, 2021). GPe: globus pallidus externa; GPi: globus pallidus interna; SNc: substantia nigra compacta; SNr: substantia nigra reticulata; STN: subthalamic nucleus.

# D2 Receptor Blockade Activates the CSTC Stop Pathway

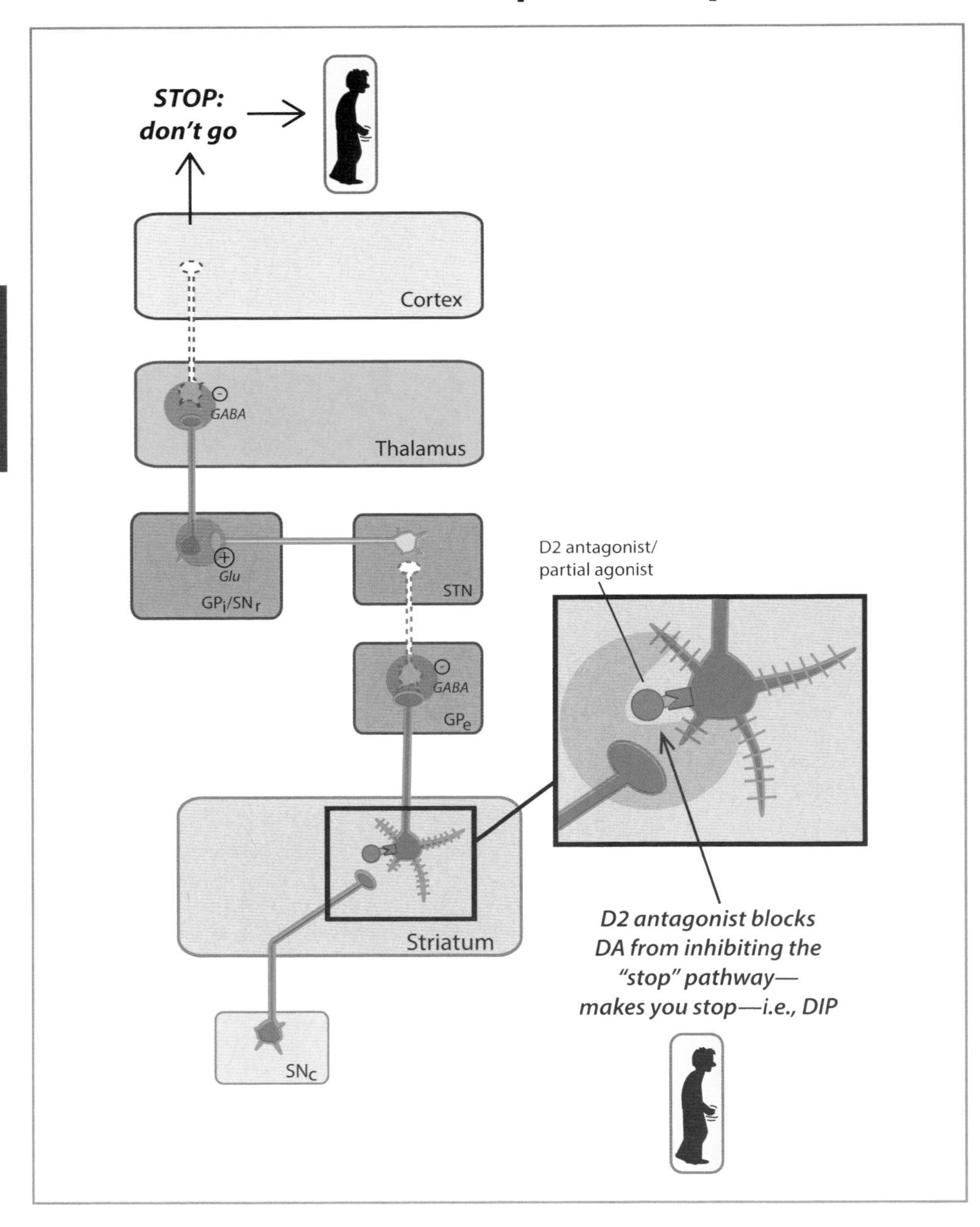

# D2 Receptor Blockade Activates the CSTC Stop Pathway

**FIGURE 3.13.** DA released from the nigrostriatal pathway is blocked from binding to postsynaptic D2 receptors on a γ-aminobutyric acid (GABA) neuron projecting to the globus pallidus externa. This prevents inhibition of the indirect (stop) pathway; in other words, D2 antagonists activate the indirect (stop) pathway. Too much stop can result in drug-induced parkinsonism (DIP) (Stahl, 2017; Stahl, 2021).

# Chronic D2 Receptor Blockade of the CSTC Stop Pathway

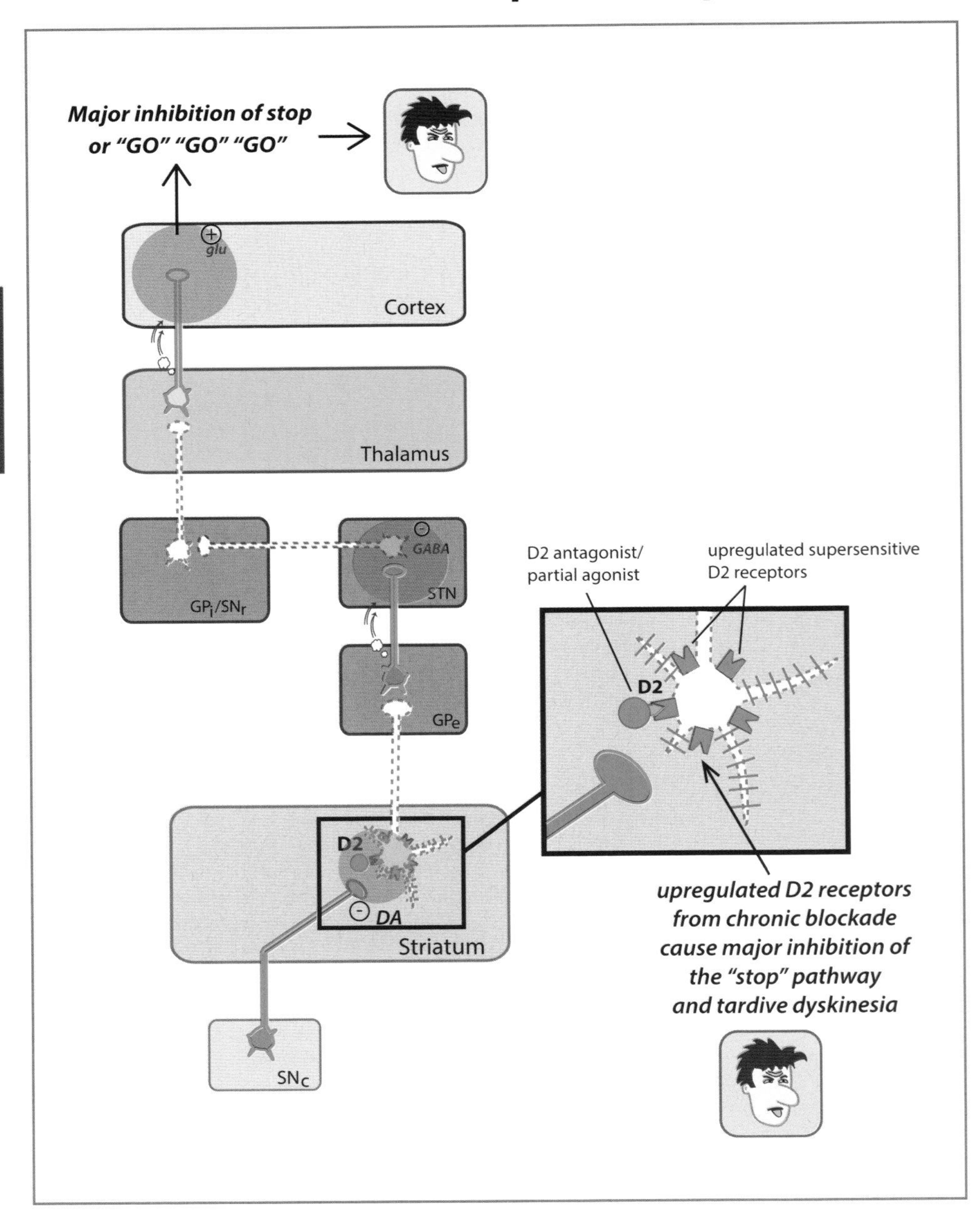

# Chronic D2 Receptor Blockade of the CSTC Stop Pathway

**FIGURE 3.14.** DA released from the nigrostriatal pathway is blocked from binding to postsynaptic D2 receptors on a $\gamma$-aminobutyric acid (GABA) neuron projecting to the globus pallidus externa. Chronic blockade of these receptors can lead to their upregulation; the upregulated receptors may also be "supersensitive" to DA. DA can now exert its inhibitory effects in the indirect (stop) pathway, and in fact cause so much inhibition of the "stop" signal that the "go" signal is overactive, leading to the hyperkinetic involuntary movements of tardive dyskinesia (Stahl, 2017; Stahl, 2021).

# Storage of DA by Vesicular Monoamine Transporter 2 (VMAT2)

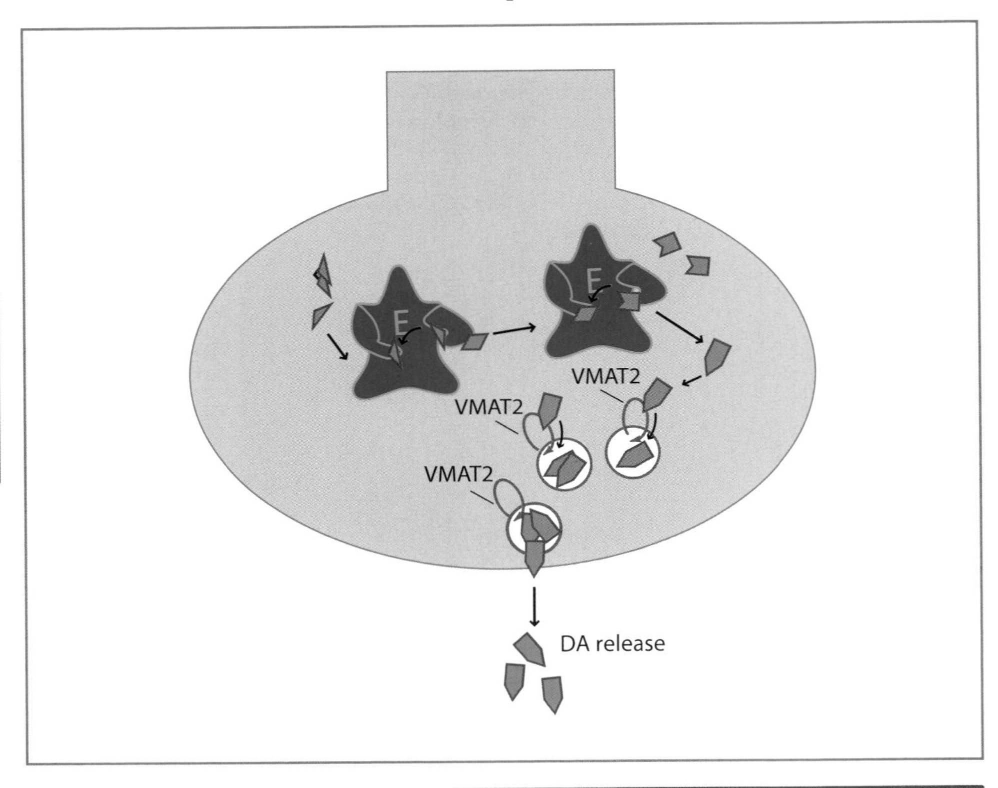


**FIGURE 3.15.** The VMAT2 is an intraneuronal transporter located on synaptic vesicles. VMAT2 takes intraneuronal monoamines, including DA, up into the synaptic vesicles so that they can be stored until they are needed for release during neurotransmission (Stahl, 2021).

# DA Depletion by VMAT2 Inhibition

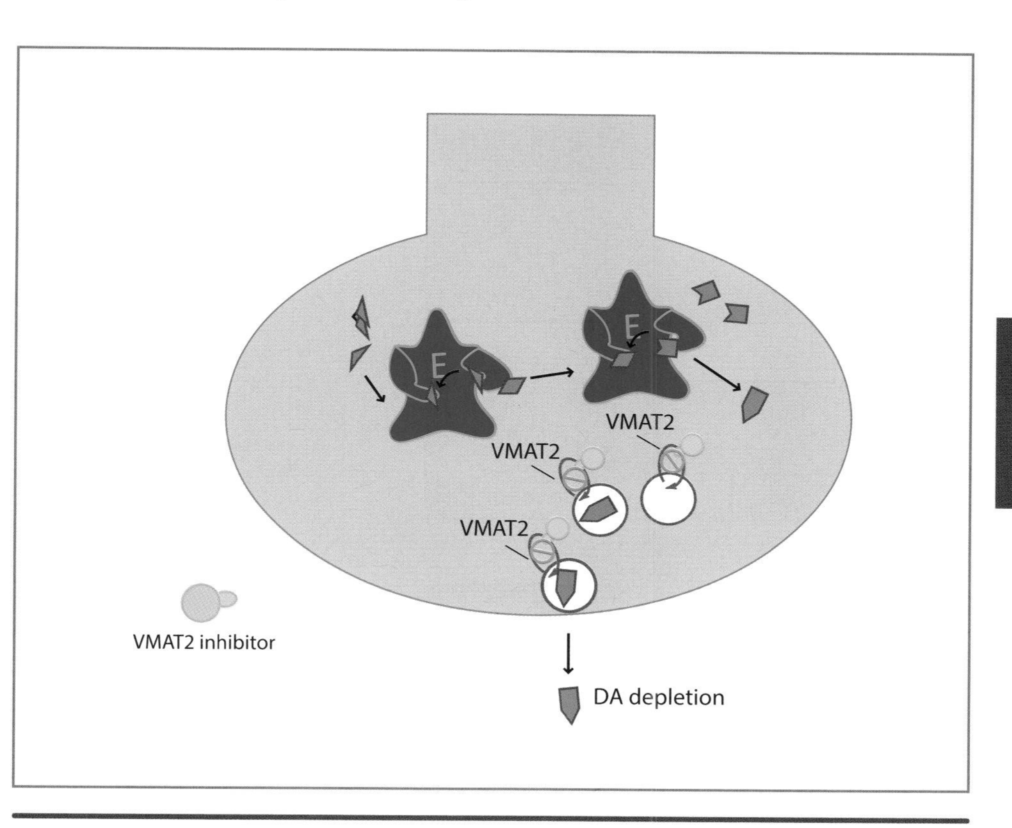


**FIGURE 3.16.** Inhibition of VMAT2 prevents DA from being taken up into synaptic vesicles. The intraneuronal DA is therefore metabolized, leading to depletion of DA stores. Tetrabenazine-related drugs reversely inhibit VMAT2 and preferentially affect dopamine transport at clinical doses. Deutetrabenazine and valbenazine are VMAT2 inhibitors that are FDA approved for treating tardive dyskinesia (Niemann & Jankovic, 2018; Stahl, 2018; Stahl, 2021).

# TD: Upregulation of D2 Receptors in the CSTC Indirect Pathway

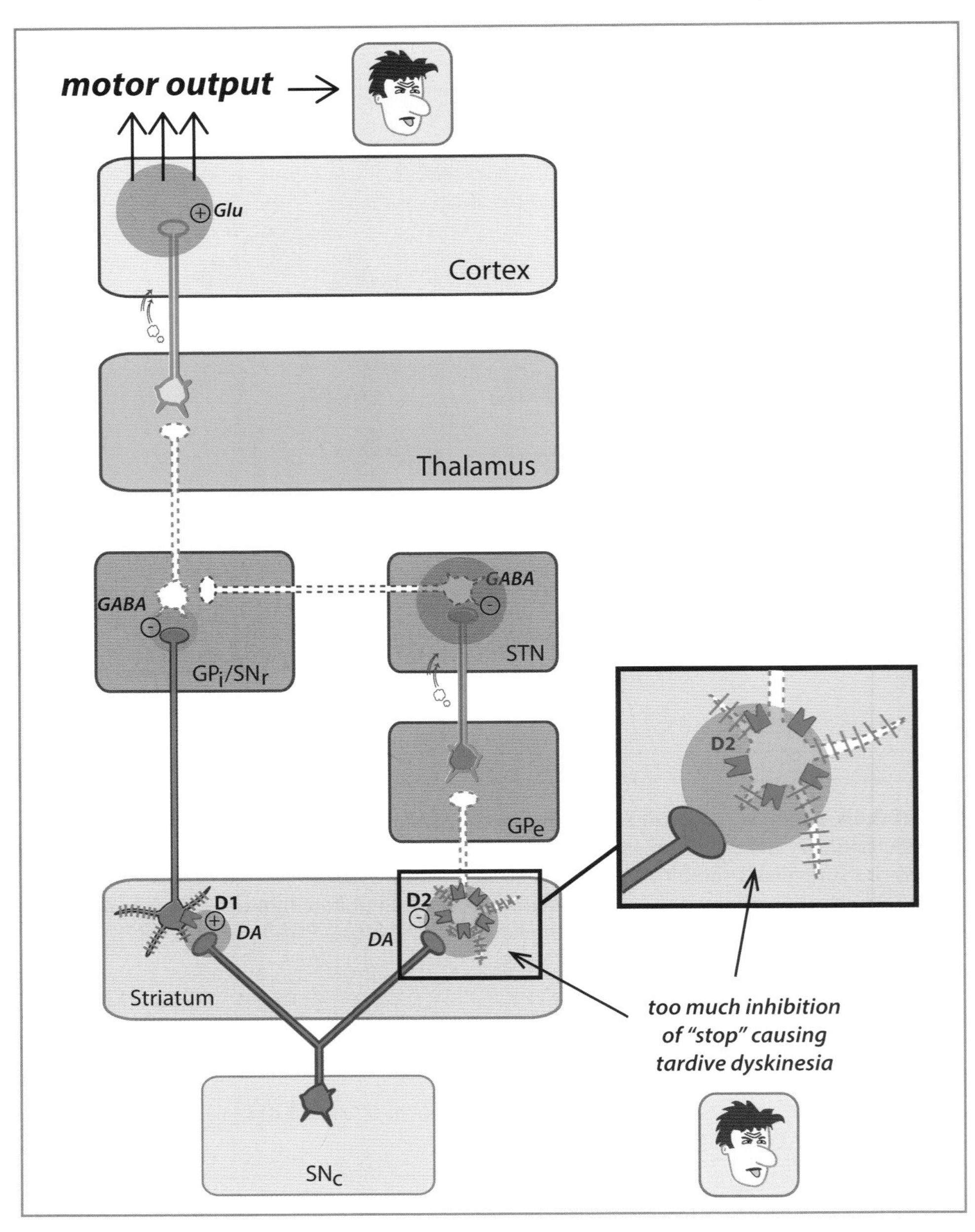

# TD: Upregulation of D2 Receptors in the CSTC Indirect Pathway

**FIGURE 3.17.** Chronic blockade of D2 receptors can lead to their upregulation; the upregulated receptors may also be supersensitive to DA. In the indirect (stop) pathway, this can lead to so much inhibition of the "stop" signal that the "go" signal is overactive, leading to the hyperkinetic involuntary movements of tardive dyskinesia (Stahl, 2017; Stahl, 2021).

# VMAT2 Inhibition in the CSTC Indirect Pathway

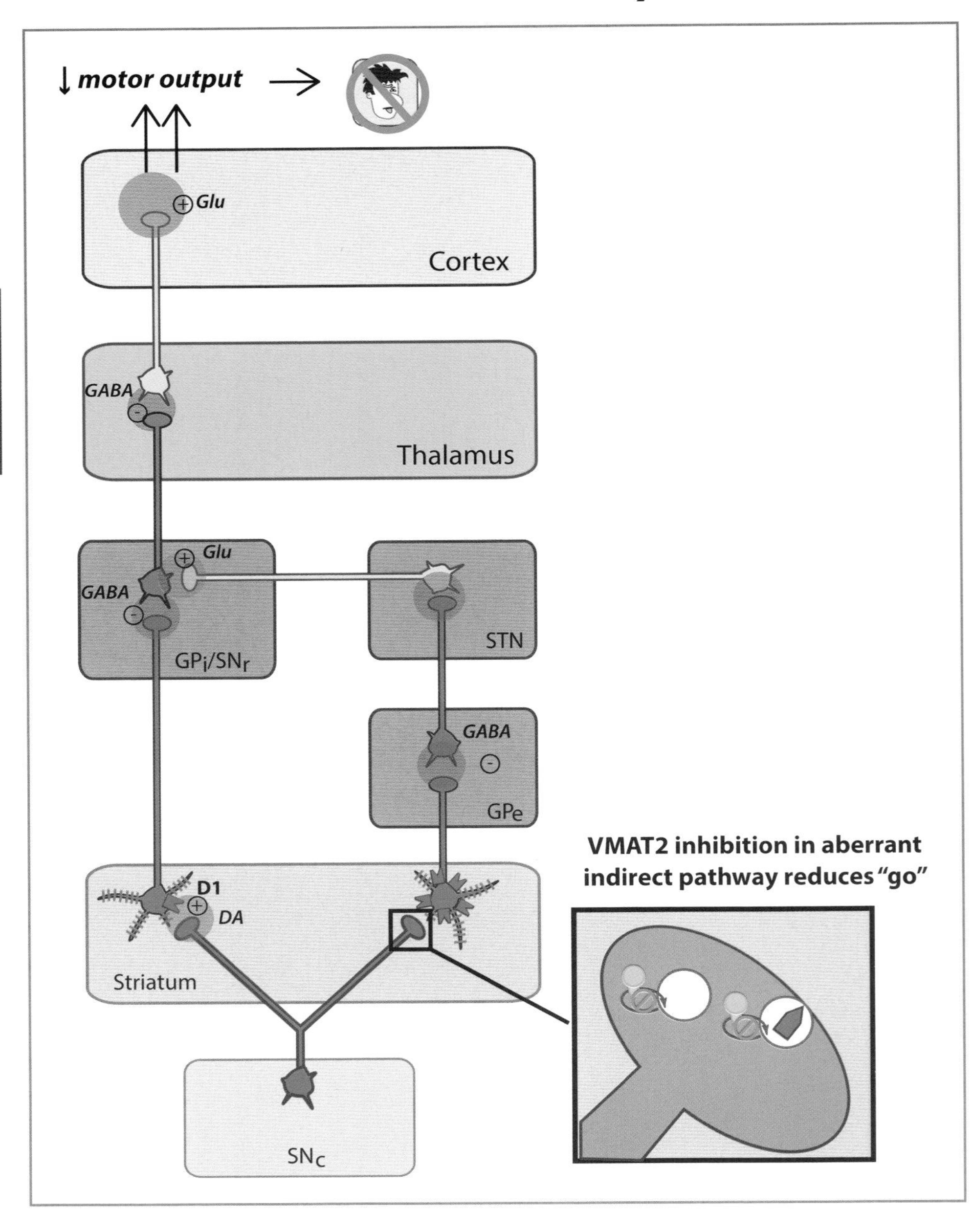

# VMAT2 Inhibition in the CSTC Indirect Pathway

**FIGURE 3.18.** VMAT2 inhibition reduces dopaminergic output; thus, it can reduce the overstimulation of inhibitory D2 receptors in the indirect (stop) pathway. This disinhibits the indirect (stop) pathway and therefore can reduce the hyperkinetic movements of tardive dyskinesia (Niemann & Jankovic, 2018; Stahl, 2018; Stahl, 2021).

# VMAT2 Inhibition in the CSTC Direct Pathway

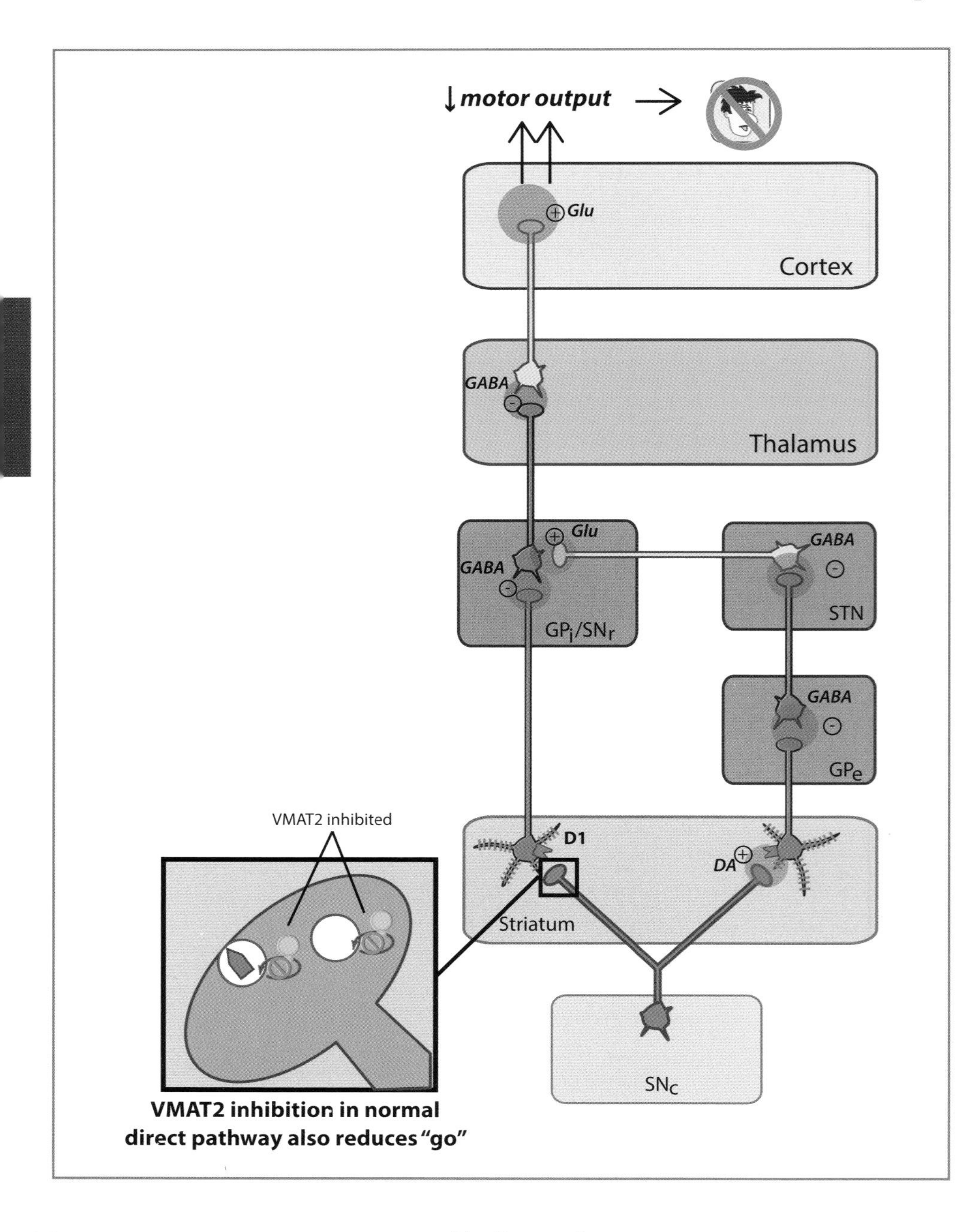

# VMAT2 Inhibition in the CSTC Direct Pathway

**FIGURE 3.19.** VMAT2 inhibition reduces dopaminergic output; thus, it can reduce activation of excitatory D1 receptors in the direct (go) pathway. This inhibits the direct (go) pathway and therefore can reduce the hyperkinetic movements of tardive dyskinesia (Niemann & Jankovic, 2018; Stahl, 2018; Stahl, 2021).

# Blockade of Histamine 1 (H1) and α1-Adrenergic Receptors

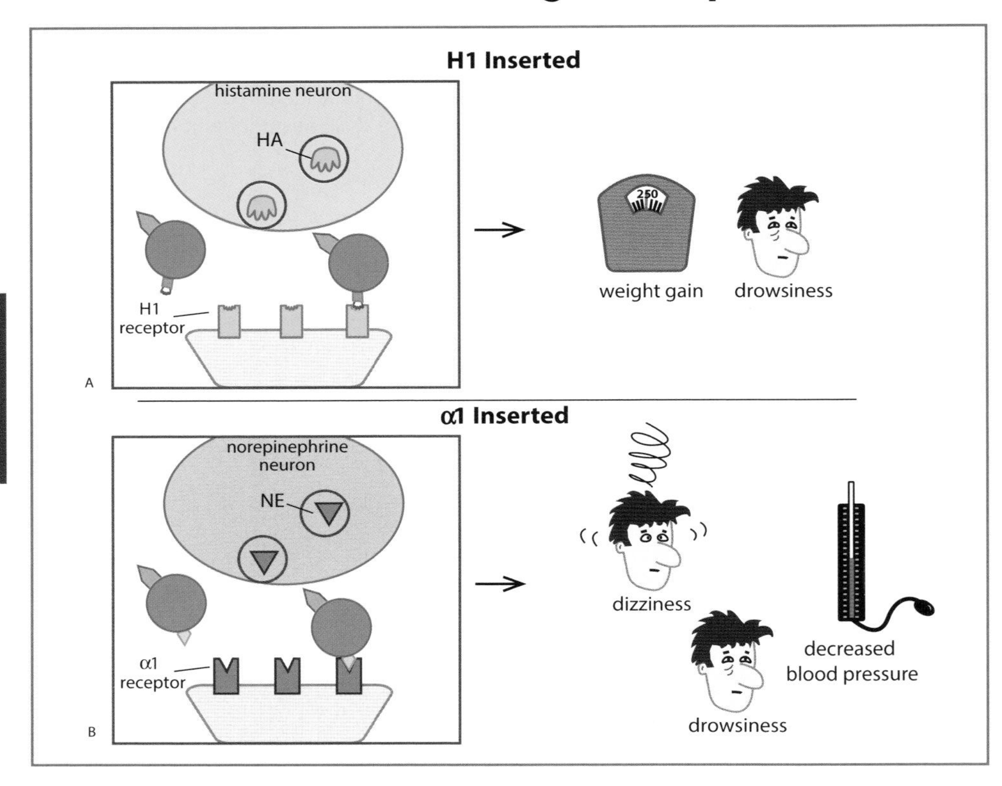


**FIGURE 3.20.** The majority of D2 antagonists have additional pharmacological properties; the specific receptor profiles differ for each agent and contribute to divergent side effect profiles. Many of the early D2 antagonists also block H1 receptors (A), which can contribute to weight gain and drowsiness, and/or α1-adrenergic receptors (B), which can contribute to dizziness, drowsiness, and decreased blood pressure (Stahl, 2021).

# Neurotransmitters of Cortical Arousal

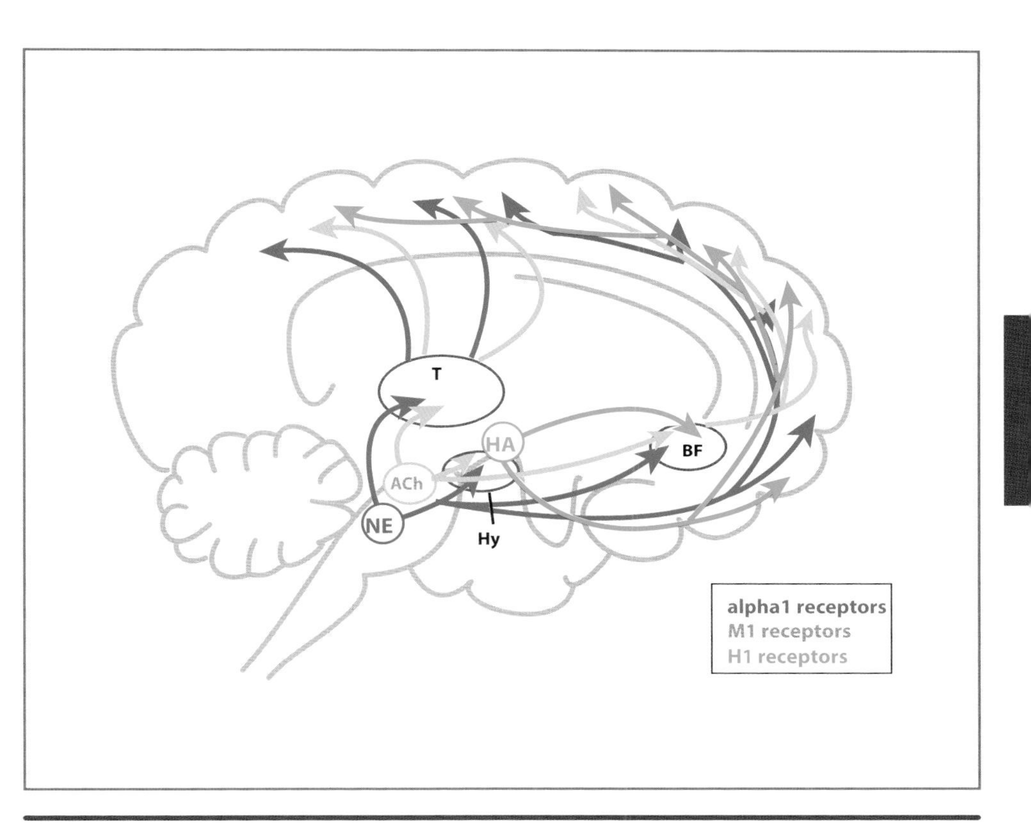


**FIGURE 3.21.** The neurotransmitters acetylcholine (ACh), histamine (HA), and norepinephrine (NE) are all involved in arousal pathways connecting neurotransmitter centers with the thalamus (T), hypothalamus (Hy), basal forebrain (BF), and cortex. Thus, pharmacological actions at their receptors could influence arousal. In particular, antagonism of muscarinic M1, histamine H1, and $\alpha$1-adrenergic receptors are all associated with sedating effects (Stahl, 2021).

# Earliest Agents Used to Treat Psychosis

| Generic name | Trade name | Comment |
|---|---|---|
| Chlorpromazine | Thorazine | Low potency |
| Cyamemazine | Tercian | Popular in France; not available in the US |
| Flupenthixol | Depixol | Depot; not available in the US |
| Haloperidol | Haldol | High potency; depot |
| Loxapine | Loxitane | |
| Mesoridazine | Serentil | Low potency; QTc issues; discontinued |
| Perphenazine | Trilafon | High potency |
| Pimozide | Orap | High potency; Tourette syndrome; QTc issues; second line |
| Pipotiazine | Piportil | Depot; not available in the US |
| Sulpiride | Dolmatil | Not available in the US |
| Thioridazine | Mellaril | Low potency; QTc issues; second line |
| Thiothixene | Navane | High potency |
| Trifluoperazine | Stelazine | High potency |
| Zuclopenthixol | Clopixol | Depot; not available in the US |

**TABLE 3.1.**

# Agonist Spectrum for Drugs to Treat Psychosis

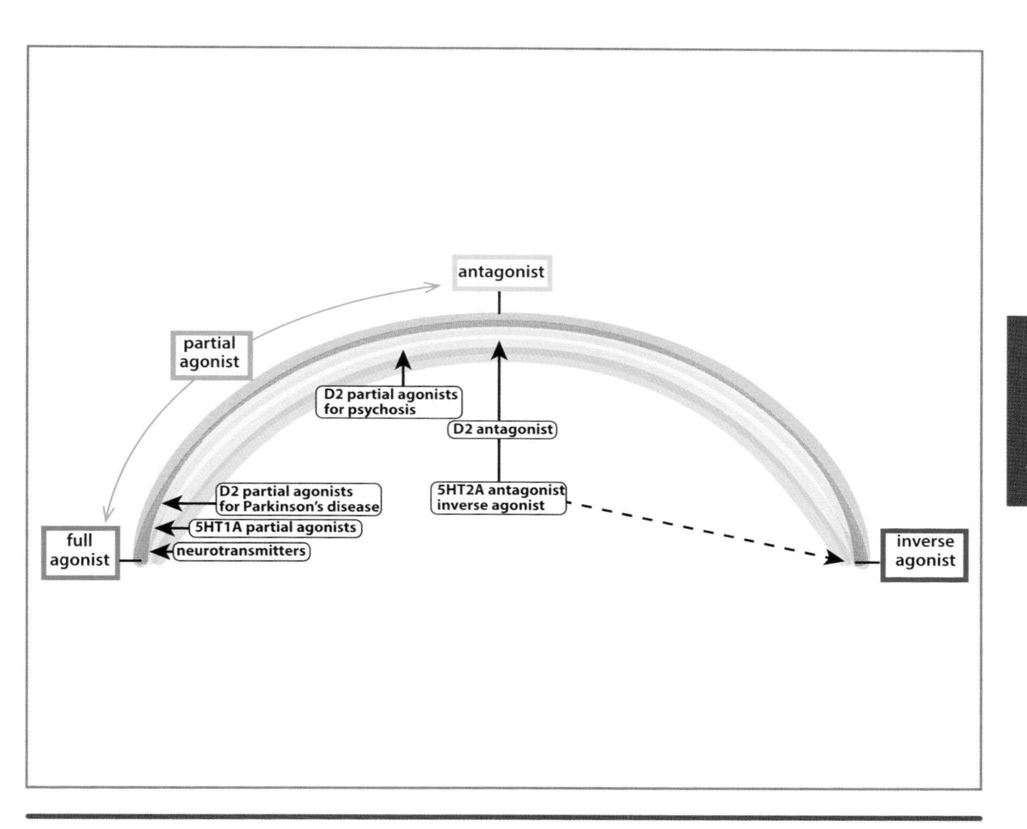


**FIGURE 3.22.** Drugs used to treat psychosis may fall along a spectrum, with some having actions closer to a silent antagonist and others having actions closer to a full agonist. For dopamine 2 (D2) binding, agents with too much agonism may be psychotomimetic and thus not ideal for treating psychosis but may be useful within Parkinson's disease. D2 partial agonists that are closer to the antagonist end of the spectrum may be preferred for treating psychosis, as are D2 antagonists. Many drugs used to treat psychosis are serotonin 5HT2A antagonists, either in conjunction with D2 binding or without D2 binding. Some preclinical data suggest that they may actually be inverse agonists, but the clinical significance of this distinction is unclear. 5HT1A partial agonism is also a common property of many drugs used to treat psychosis, in particular many D2 partial agonists (Stahl, 2021).

# 5HT2A Receptor Regulation of Downstream DA Release

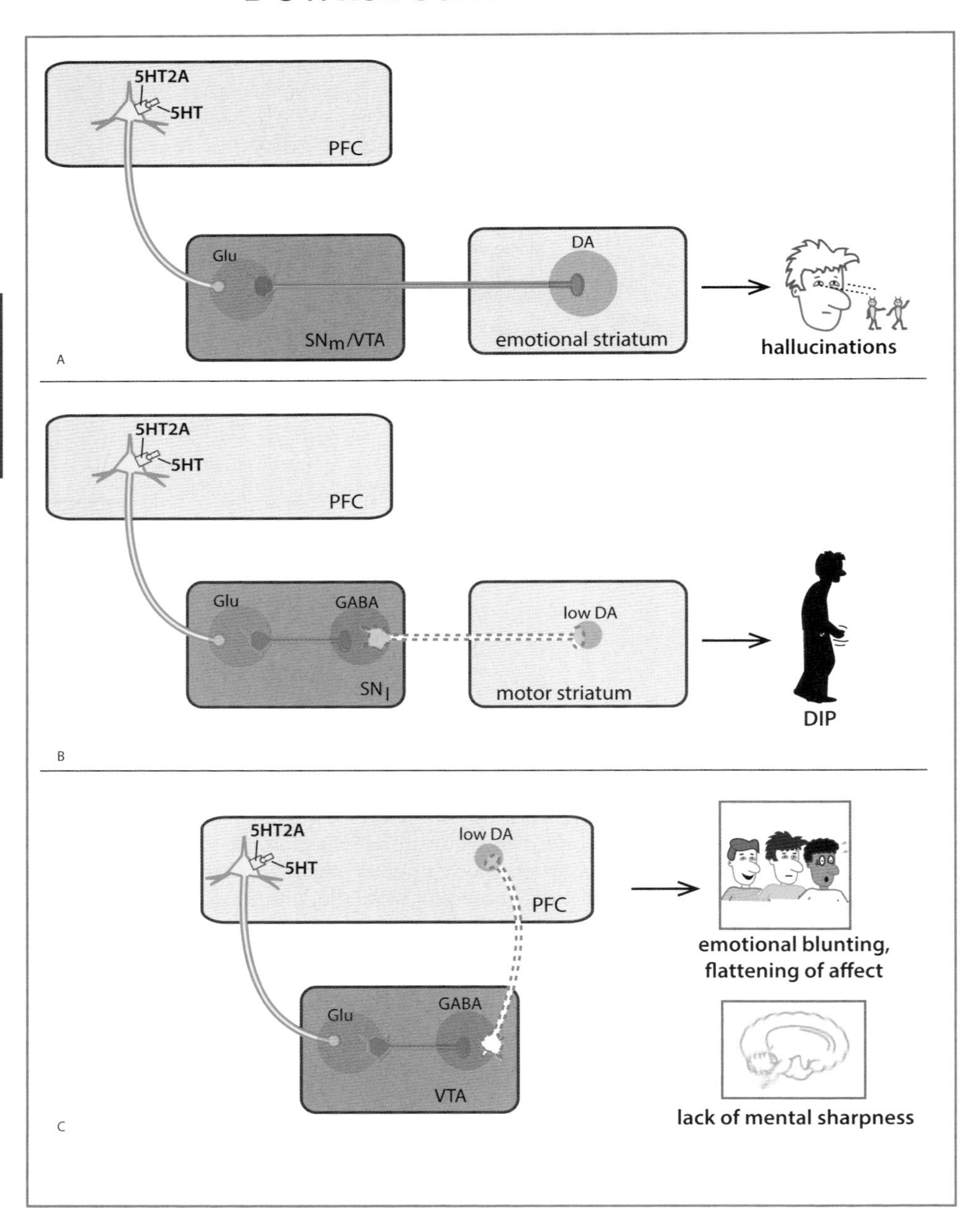

# 5HT2A Receptor Regulation of Downstream DA Release

**FIGURE 3.23.** 5HT2A receptors, which are postsynaptic and excitatory, are relevant to the treatment of psychosis because of their presence on three separate populations of descending Glu neurons. (A) 5HT2A receptors are located on descending glutamatergic pyramidal neurons that directly innervate mesolimbic/mesostriatal DA neurons projecting to the emotional striatum. Excessive activity in this pathway can lead to the positive symptoms of psychosis. (B) 5HT2A receptors are located on descending glutamatergic pyramidal neurons that indirectly innervate nigrostriatal DA neurons via a GABAergic interneuron in the substantia nigra. Excessive stimulation of these 5HT2A receptors leads to a reduction in DA release in the motor striatum and can cause side effects such as drug-induced parkinsonism (DIP). (C) 5HT2A receptors are located on descending glutamatergic pyramidal neurons that indirectly innervate mesocortical DA neurons via a GABAergic interneuron in the ventral tegmental area. Excessive stimulation of these 5HT2A receptors leads to a reduction in DA release in the prefrontal cortex (PFC), which could lead to cognitive dysfunction as well as negative symptoms such as emotional blunting and flattened affect (Stahl, 2018; Stahl, 2021). SNl: lateral substantia nigra; SNm: medial substantia nigra; VTA: ventral tegmental area.

# 5HT2A Receptor Antagonism and Downstream DA Release

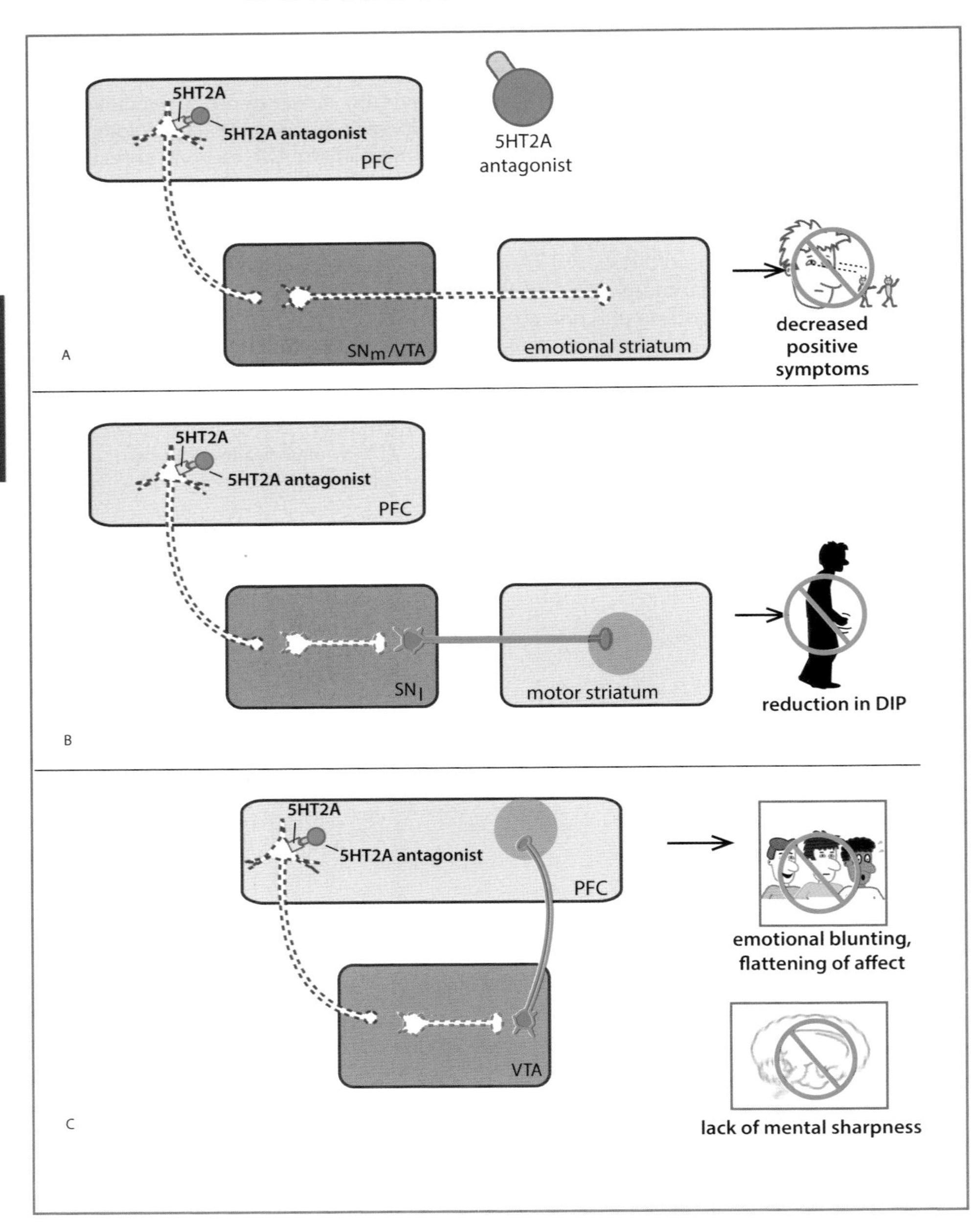

# 5HT2A Receptor Antagonism and Downstream DA Release

**FIGURE 3.24.** 5HT2A antagonism can modulate downstream DA release via three key pathways. (A) 5HT2A antagonism reduces glutamatergic output from a descending neuron that directly innervates mesolimbic/mesostriatal DA neurons. This in turn reduces DA output in the emotional striatum and can therefore decrease the positive symptoms of psychosis. (B) 5HT2A antagonism reduces glutamatergic output in the substantia nigra, leading to reduced activity of the GABA interneuron and therefore disinhibition of the nigrostriatal DA pathway. The increased DA release in the motor striatum can reduce motor side effects caused by D2 antagonism, because there is more DA to compete with the D2 antagonist. (C) 5HT2A antagonism reduces glutamatergic output in the ventral tegmental area, leading to reduced activity of the GABA interneuron and therefore disinhibition of the mesocortical DA pathway. Increased dopamine release in the prefrontal cortex (PFC) can potentially reduce cognitive and negative symptoms of psychosis (Stahl, 2018; Stahl, 2021). DIP: drug-induced parkinsonism; SNl: lateral substantia nigra; SNm: medial substantia nigra; VTA: ventral tegmental area.

# DA and 5HT Have Reciprocal Regulatory Action on Prolactin

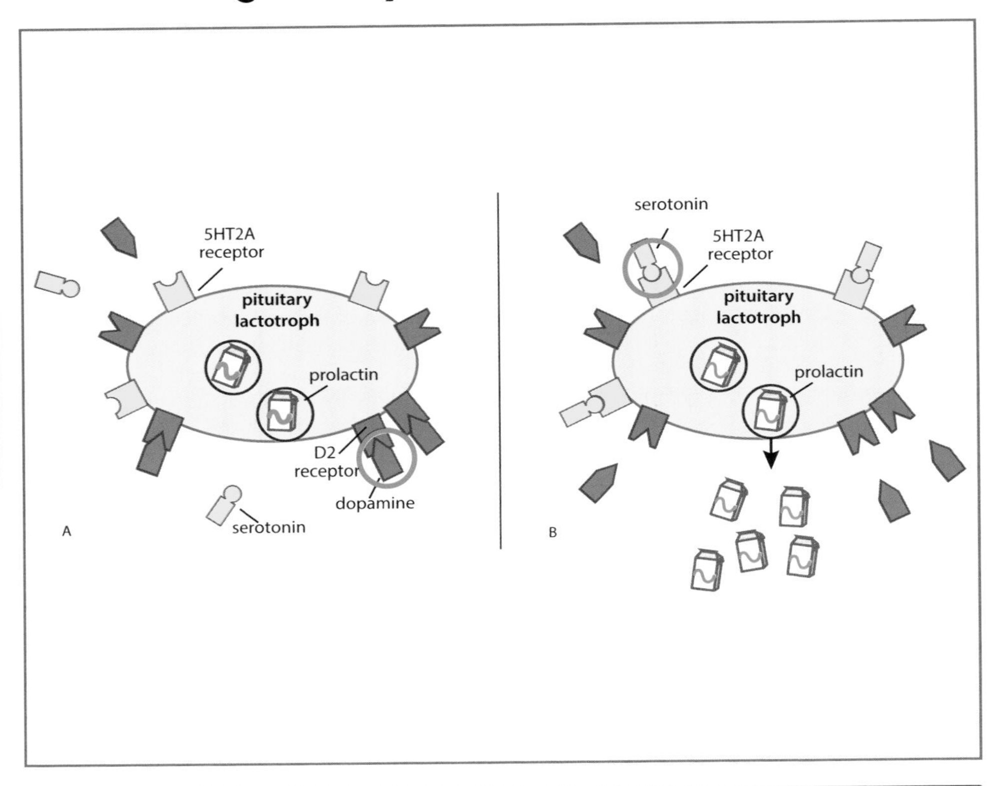


**FIGURE 3.25.** (A) DA binding at inhibitory D2 receptors (red circle) prevents prolactin release from pituitary lactotroph cells in the pituitary gland. (B) 5HT binding at excitatory 5HT2A receptors (red circle) stimulates prolactin release from pituitary lactotroph cells in the pituitary gland. Thus, DA and 5HT have a reciprocal regulatory action on prolactin release (Stahl, 2021).

# 5HT2A Antagonism Reverses Effect of D2 Antagonism to Raise Prolactin

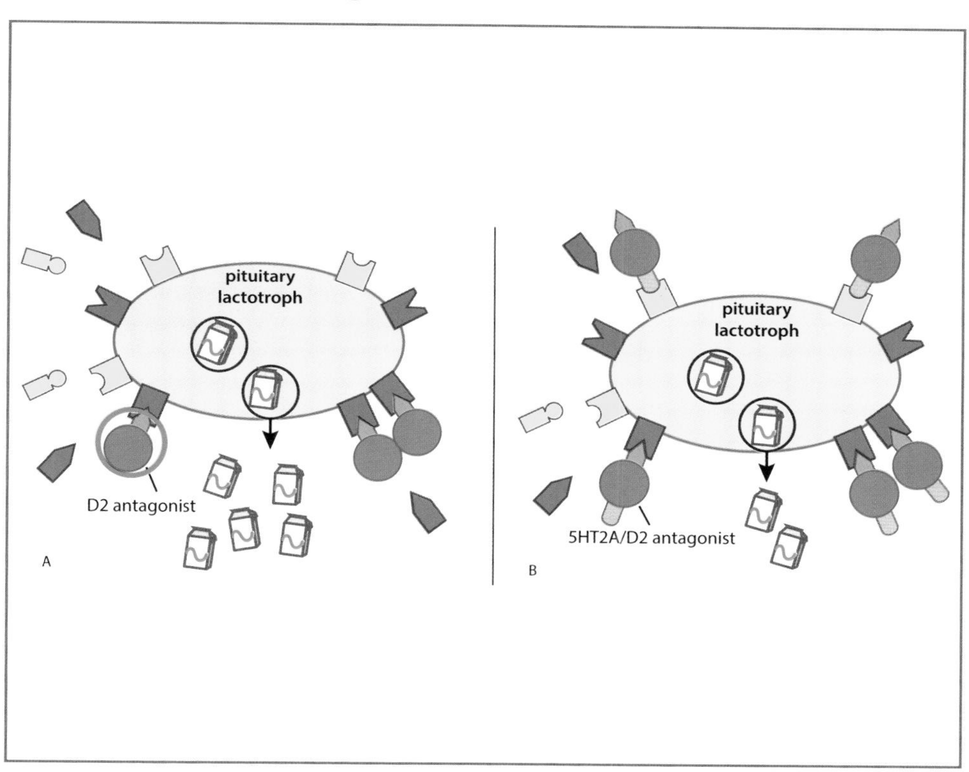


**FIGURE 3.26.** (A) D2 antagonism (red circle) blocks DA's inhibitory effect on prolactin secretion from pituitary lactotrophs. Thus, these drugs increase prolactin levels. (B) As DA and 5HT have reciprocal regulatory roles in the control of prolactin secretion, one cancels the other. Thus, 5HT2A antagonism reverses the ability of D2 antagonism to increase prolactin secretion (Stahl, 2021).

# Spectrum of DA Neurotransmission

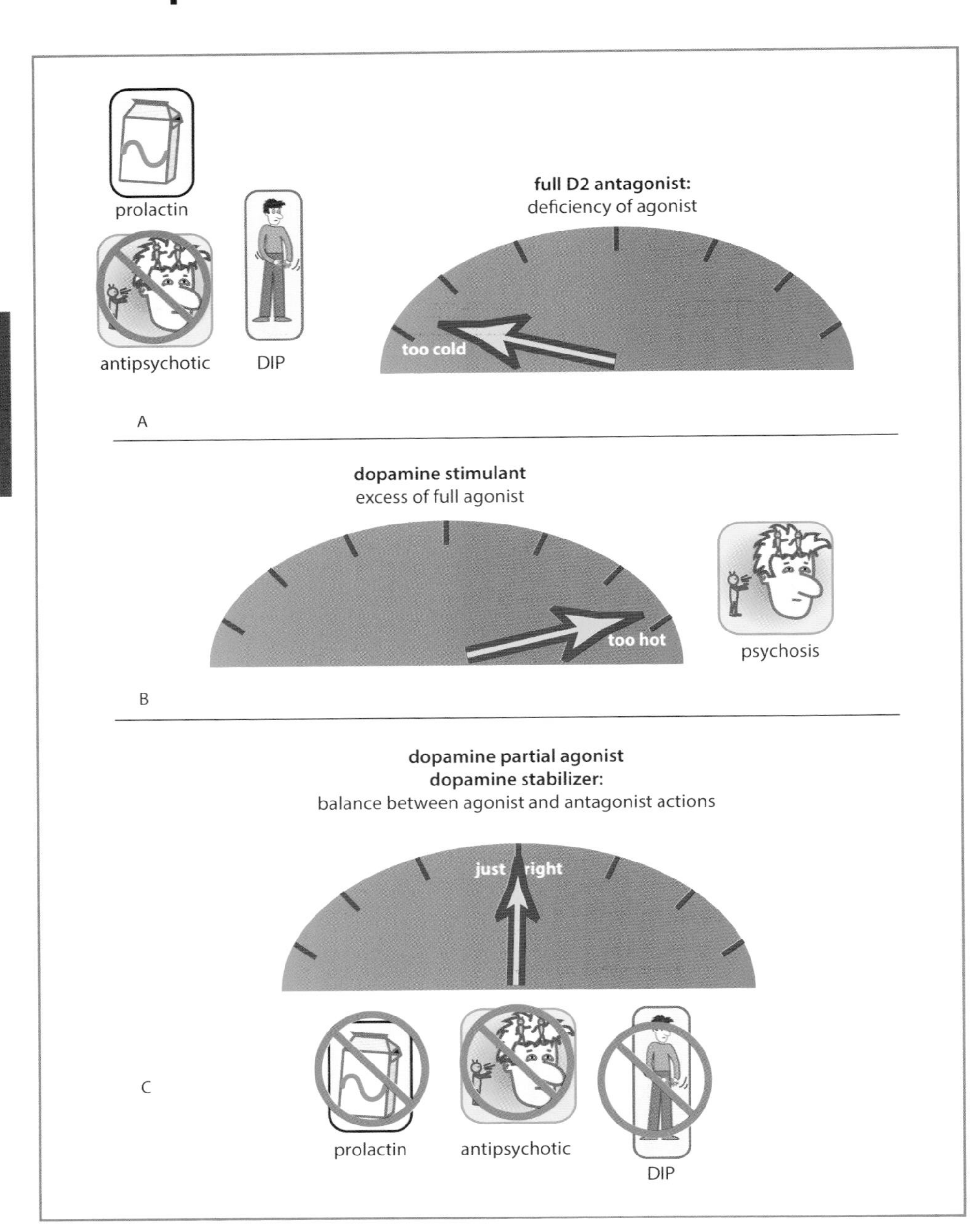

# Spectrum of DA Neurotransmission

**FIGURE 3.27.** Simplified explanation of actions on DA. (A) Full D2 antagonists bind to the D2 receptor in a manner that is "too cold"; that is, they have powerful antagonist actions while preventing agonist actions and thus can reduce positive symptoms of psychosis but also cause drug-induced parkinsonism (DIP) and prolactin elevation. (B) D2 receptor agonists, such as dopamine itself, are "too hot" and can therefore lead to positive symptoms. (C) D2 partial agonists bind in an intermediary manner to the D2 receptor and are therefore "just right," with antipsychotic actions but without DIP or prolactin elevation (Stahl, 2021).

# 5HT1A Receptor Partial Agonism and Downstream DA Release

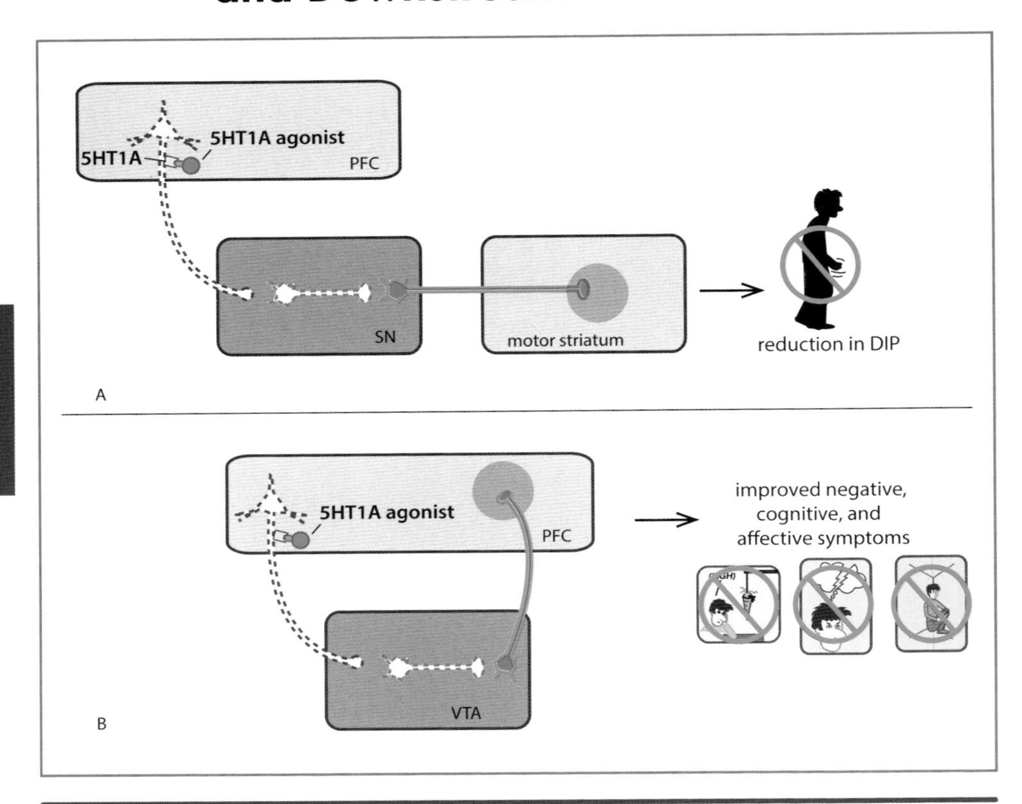


**FIGURE 3.28.** 5HT1A receptors are inhibitory and can be located both presynaptically on 5HT neurons and postsynaptically on other neurons. (A) 5HT1A receptors are located on descending glutamatergic pyramidal neurons that indirectly innervate nigrostriatal DA neurons via a GABAergic interneuron in the substantia nigra (SN). Partial agonism of these 5HT1A receptors reduces glutamatergic output in the substantia nigra, leading to reduced activity of the GABA interneuron and therefore disinhibition of the nigrostriatal DA pathway. The increased DA release in the motor striatum can reduce motor side effects caused by D2 antagonism/partial agonism because there is more DA to compete with the D2 binding agents. (B) 5HT1A receptors are located on descending glutamatergic pyramidal neurons that indirectly innervate mesocortical DA neurons via a GABAergic interneuron in the ventral tegmental area (VTA). 5HT1A partial agonism reduces glutamatergic output in the VTA, leading to reduced activity of the GABA interneuron and therefore disinhibition of the mesocortical DA pathway. Increased DA release in the prefrontal cortex (PFC) can potentially reduce cognitive, negative, and affective symptoms of psychosis (Stahl, 2021).

# Other Therapeutic and Side Effects of Drugs for Psychosis

| Therapeutic Effect | Binding Property |
|---|---|
| Antimanic | D2 antagonism |
| | D2 partial agonism |
| Antidepressant | Monoamine reuptake blocking |
| | α2 antagonism |
| | D3 partial agonism |
| | 5HT2C antagonism |
| | 5HT3 antagonism |
| | 5HT7 antagonism |
| Anxiolytic | H1 antagonism |
| | ACh antagonism |
| Anti-agitation in dementia | α1B antagonism |

| Side Effect | Binding Property |
|---|---|
| Sedation | H1 antagonism |
| | ACh antagonism |
| | α1 antagonism |
| Weight gain | H1 antagonism |
| | 5HT2C antagonism |

**TABLE 3.2.**

# Insulin Resistance Caused by Tissue Actions at an Unknown Receptor?

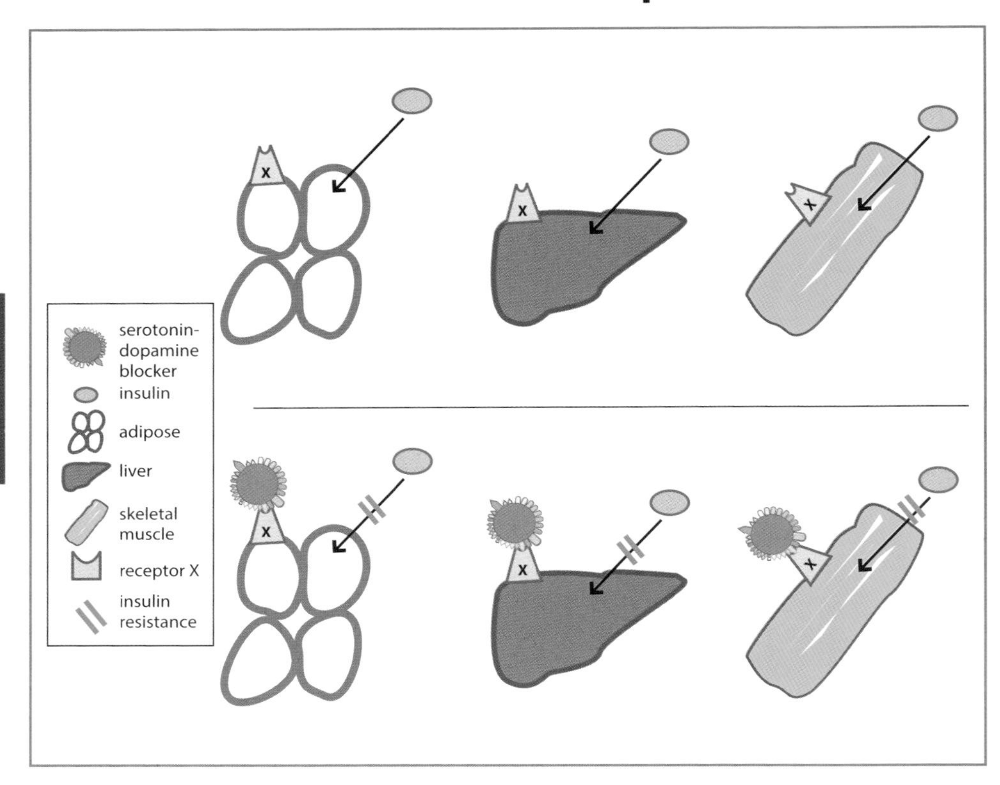


**FIGURE 3.29.** All D2/5HT2A/5HT1A drugs for treating psychosis share a class warning for causing weight gain and risks for obesity, dyslipidemia, and hyperglycemia/diabetes mellitus. It appears that cardiometabolic risk cannot simply be explained by increased appetite and weight gain, nor by antagonist actions at the 5HT2C and histamine 1 receptors. Immediate increase in insulin resistance may be a second mechanism acting to cause weight gain, dyslipidemia, and diabetes. Some drugs used to treat psychosis may lead to insulin resistance and elevated triglycerides, independently of weight gain, although the mechanism is not yet established. This figure depicts a hypothesized mechanism in which an agent binds to receptor X at adipose tissue, liver, and skeletal muscle to cause insulin resistance. Several factors influence whether an individual develops insulin resistance, including genetic makeup, age, lifestyle, diet, and selection of medications that either do or do not cause insulin resistance (Grajales et al., 2019; Kowalchuk et al., 2017; Stahl, 2021).

Stahl's Illustrated | Chapter 4

# Pharmacological Properties of Selected Dopamine Receptor Blocking Agents

This chapter will describe currently available selected drugs for psychosis in terms of binding properties, side effect profile, dosing tips, and drug interactions. As with all drugs for psychosis discussed in this chapter, binding properties vary greatly with technique and from one laboratory to another; they are constantly being revised and updated. Thus, it is important to remain up to date on the specifics of each drug. Binding profiles are also presented by receptor, including the second-generation drugs for psychosis that bind to the specific receptor (**FIGURE 4.6** to **FIGURE 4.16**).

| ***Symbols Used in This Chapter*** | | | |
|---|---|---|---|
| | Life-threatening or dangerous side effects | | Drug interactions |
| | Tips and pearls | | Cardiac impairment |
| | Children and adolescents | | Renal impairment |
| | Pregnancy and lactation | | Hepatic impairment |

# First-Generation D2 Antagonists: Chlorpromazine

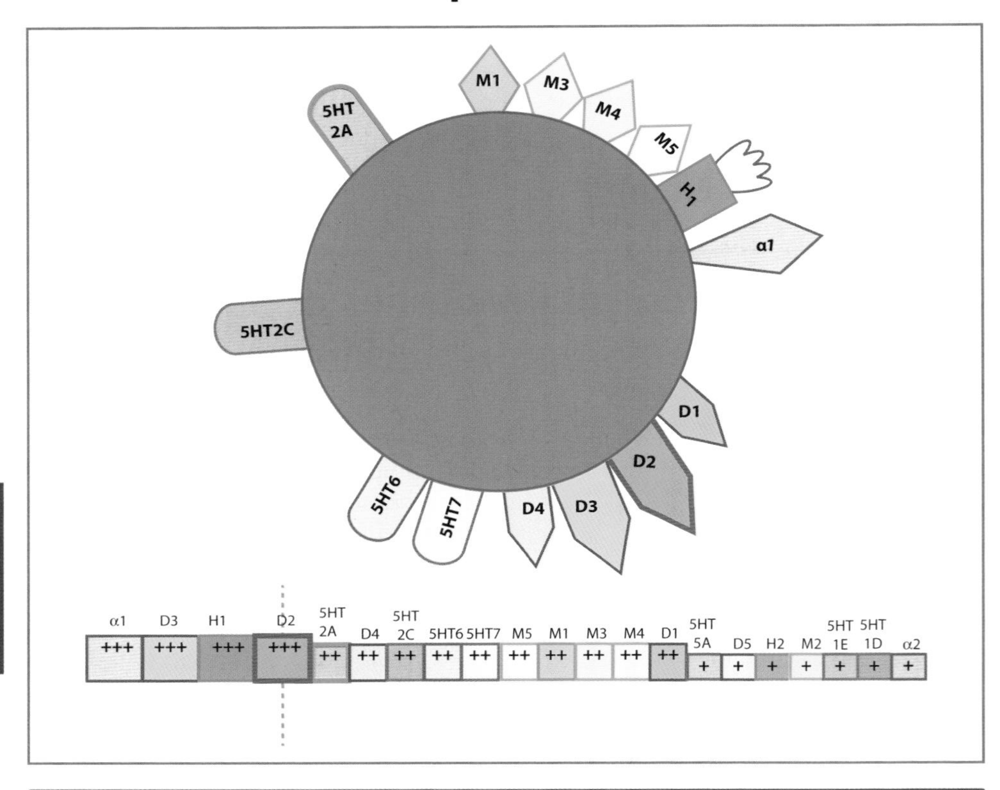


**FIGURE 4.1.** Chlorpromazine, in the chemical class of phenothiazine, was the first truly effective drug for psychosis, discovered by accident in the 1950s. In addition to binding at the D2 receptor as an antagonist, chlorpromazine has strong binding at the histamine H1, dopamine D3, and α1-adrenergic receptors (Stahl, 2020; Stahl, 2021).

# Chlorpromazine: Tips and Pearls

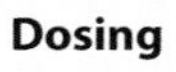

## Dosing

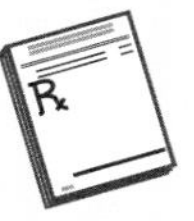

***Formulation:***
10, 25, 50, 100, and 200 mg tablets
25 mg/mL; 1 and 2 mL ampoule

***Dosage Range:***
200–800 mg/day

***Approved For:***
Schizophrenia (PO), acute psychosis (IM), severe behavioral problems associated with oppositional defiant disorder or other disruptive behavioral disorders, or for attention-deficit hyperactivity disorder in pediatric patients who show excessive motor activity with accompanying conduct disorders (PO, IM for acute, severe agitation in hospitalized patients)

## Side effects I

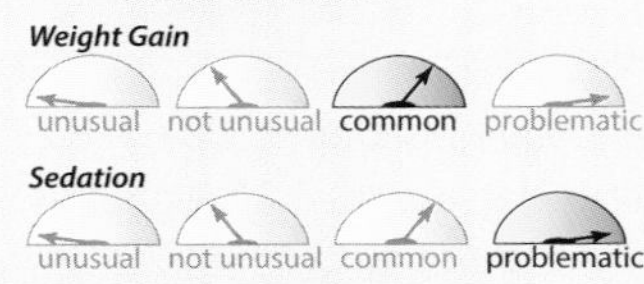


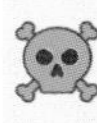

Rare neuroleptic malignant syndrome, jaundice, agranulocytosis, seizures, elderly patients with dementia-related psychosis are at increased risk of death, drug-induced movement disorders

## Pearls

Adding chlorpromazine as the choice for patients who require sedation or behavioral control, either as a daily or as-needed treatment, should be avoided in order to reduce the chances of potentially fatal paralytic ileus in patients on concomitant anticholinergics, including antipsychotic drugs with anticholinergic properties such as clozapine

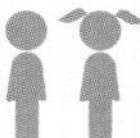

Can be used cautiously in children or adolescents over age 1 with severe behavioral problems

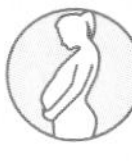

Some animal studies show adverse effects; no controlled studies in pregnant women; recommended either to discontinue drug or bottle feed

## Side effects II

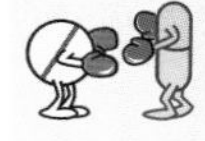

May decrease the effects of levodopa and other dopamine agonists; may increase the effects of antihypertensive drugs except for guanethidine, whose antihypertensive actions chlorpromazine may antagonize; plasma levels of chlorpromazine and propranolol may increase if used concomitantly

Cardiovascular toxicity can occur, especially orthostatic hypotension, in patients with cardiac impairments

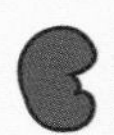

Use with caution in patients with renal impairments

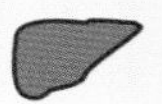

Use with caution in patients with hepatic impairments

# First-Generation D2 Antagonists: Fluphenazine

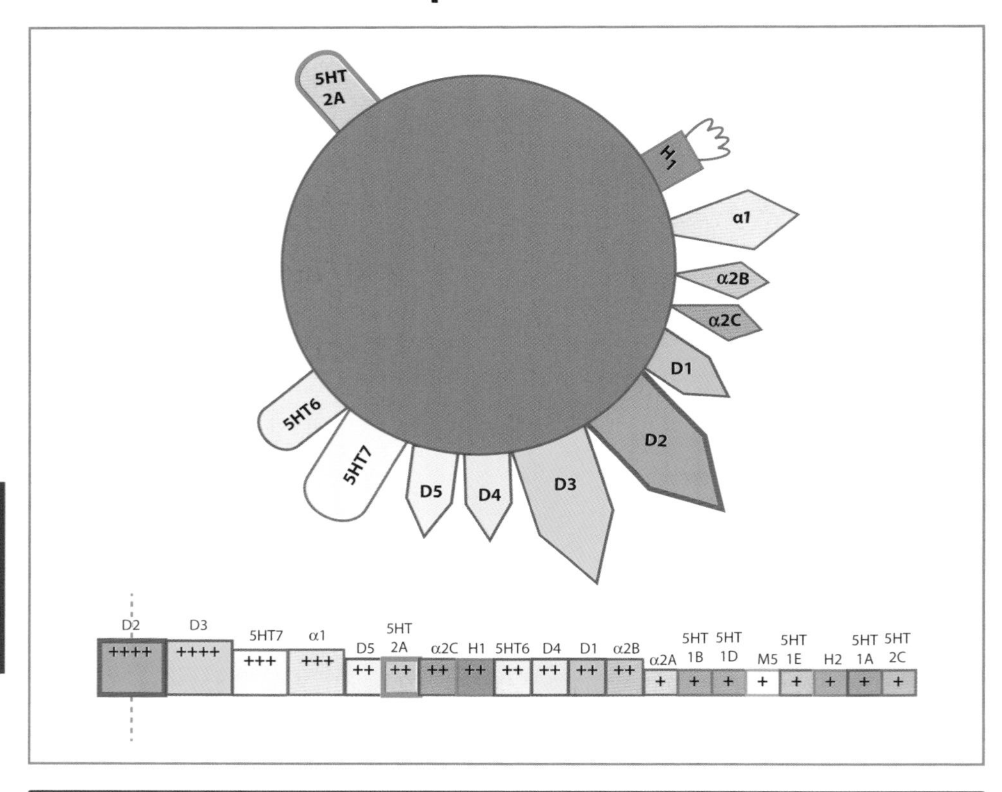


**FIGURE 4.2.** Along with D2 antagonism, fluphenazine has potent actions at D3, 5HT7, and α1-adrenergic receptors, and binds at numerous other receptors as well. Fluphenazine is in the chemical class of phenothiazine. It is more potent and less sedating than chlorpromazine (Stahl, 2020; Stahl, 2021).

# Fluphenazine: Tips and Pearls

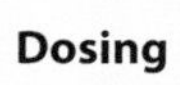

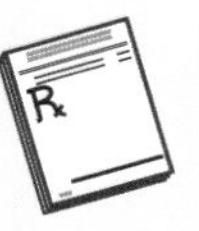

## Dosing

*Formulation:*
1, 2.5, 5, and 10 mg tablets
2.5 mg/mL injection for acute IM administration
2.5 mg/5 mL elixir
5 mg/mL concentrate
Also available in an LAI formulation (fluphenazine decanoate)

*Dosage Range:*
PO: 1–20 mg/day
IM: 1/3 to 1/2 the oral dose

*Approved For:*
Psychotic disorders

## Side effects I

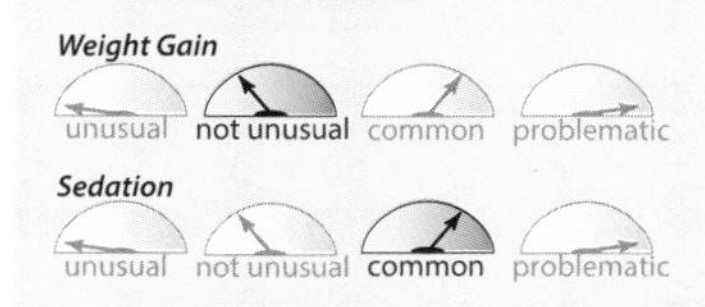


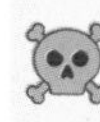

Rare neuroleptic malignant syndrome, jaundice, agranulocytosis, and seizures; elderly patients with dementia-related psychosis are at increased risk of death; drug-induced movement disorders; hyperprolactinemia

## Pearls

Fluphenazine is a high-potency phenothiazine; less risk of sedation and orthostatic hypotension but greater risk of drug-induced parkinsonism than with low-potency phenothiazines like chlorpromazine; not shown to be effective for behavioral problems in those with intellectual disability

Safety and efficacy not established; generally considered second line after second-generation drugs for psychosis

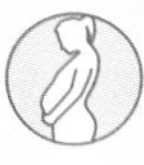

Some animal studies show adverse effects; no controlled studies in pregnant women; recommended either to discontinue drug or bottle feed

## Side effects II

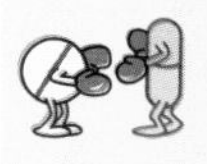

May decrease the effects of levodopa and other dopamine agonists; may increase the effects of antihypertensive drugs except for guanethidine, whose antihypertensive actions fluphenazine may antagonize; additive anticholinergic effects may occur if used with atropine or related compounds

Cardiovascular toxicity can occur, especially orthostatic hypotension

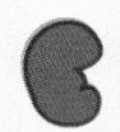

Use with caution; titration should be slower

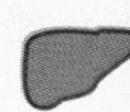

Use with caution; titration should be slower

# First-Generation D2 Antagonists: Haloperidol

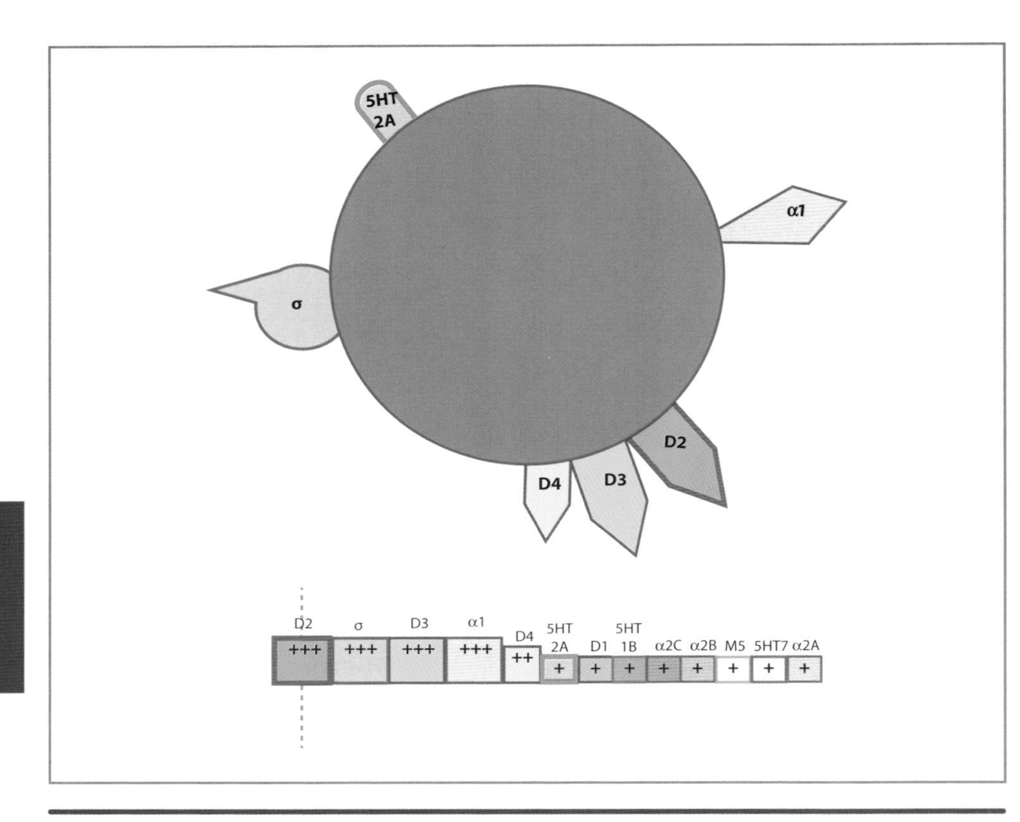


**FIGURE 4.3.** Haloperidol binds potently to D2 receptors as well as to omega, D3, and α1-adrenergic receptors. Haloperidol is one of the most potent D2 antagonists and less sedating than others (Stahl, 2020; Stahl, 2021).

# Haloperidol: Tips and Pearls

## Dosing

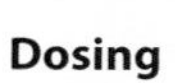
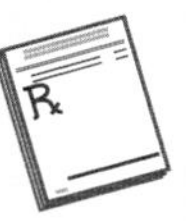

***Formulation:***
0.5, 1, 2, 5, 10, and 20 mg tablets
2 mg/mL concentrate
5 mg/mL immediate-release injection
Also available in an LAI formulation (haloperidol decanoate)

***Dosage Range:***
PO: 1–40 mg/day
Immediate-release injection: 2–5 mg

***Approved For:***
Psychotic disorders (PO, immediate-release injection, LAI), Tourette's syndrome (PO, immediate-release injection), second-line treatment of severe hyperactive behavior or behavior problems in children (PO)

## Side effects I

***Weight Gain***

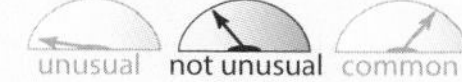
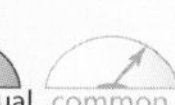
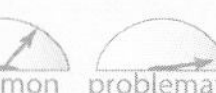


***Sedation***

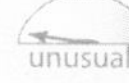
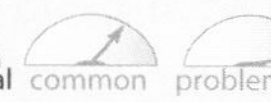


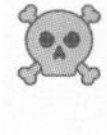

Rare neuroleptic malignant syndrome, jaundice, agranulocytosis, leukopenia, seizures; elderly patients with dementia-related psychosis are at increased risk of death; drug-induced movement disorders; hyperprolactinemia

## Pearls

Low doses may not induce negative symptoms, but high doses may; not clearly effective for improving cognitive or affective symptoms of schizophrenia; less sedating than many other first-generation drugs for psychosis, especially low-potency phenothiazines

Safety and efficacy have not been established; not intended for use under age 3

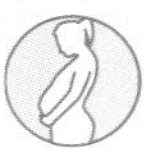

Some animal studies show adverse effects; no controlled studies in pregnant women; recommended either to discontinue drug or bottle feed

## Side effects II

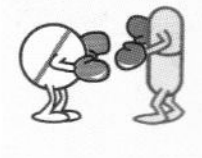

May decrease the effects of levodopa and other dopamine agonists; may increase the effects of antihypertensive drugs except for guanethidine, whose antihypertensive actions haloperidol may antagonize; use with anticholinergic agents may increase intraocular pressure

Use with caution because of risk of orthostatic hypertension; possible increased risk of QT prolongation or torsades de pointes at higher doses or with IV administration

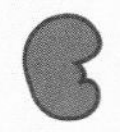

Use with caution in patients with renal impairments

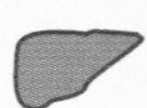

Use with caution in patients with hepatic impairments

# First-Generation D2 Antagonists: Sulpiride

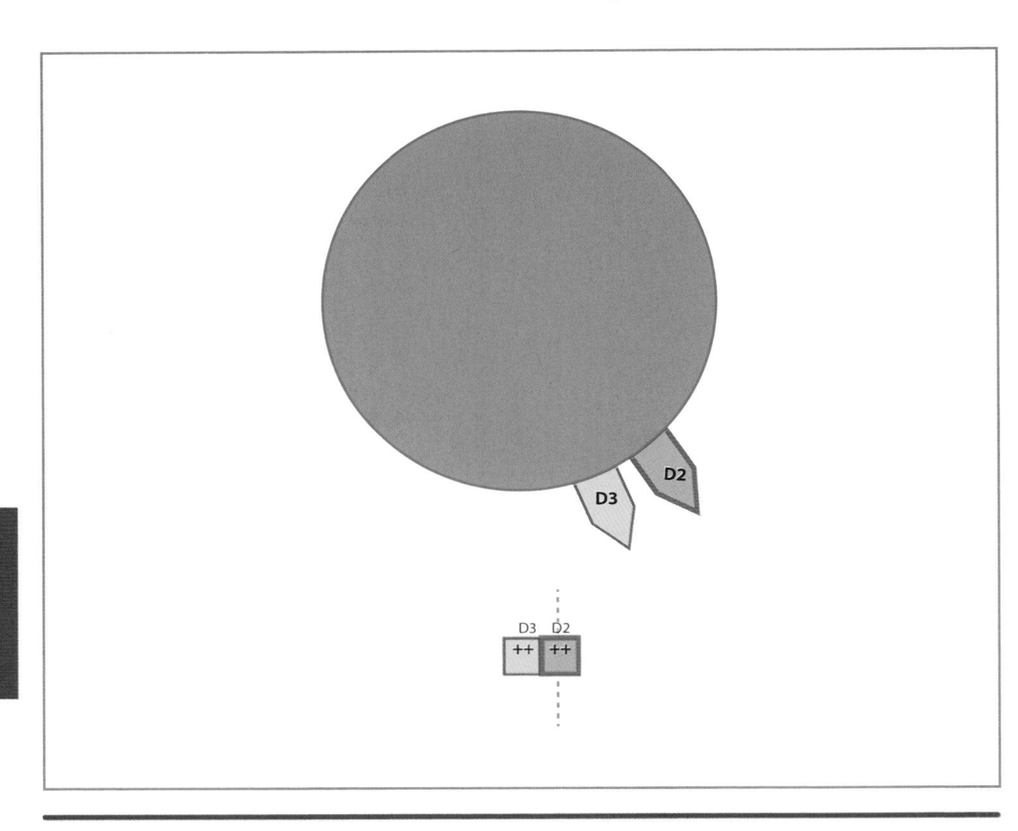


**FIGURE 4.4.** At usual antipsychotic doses, sulpiride is a D2 antagonist and has D3 antagonist/ partial agonist actions. At lower doses, sulpiride may be a bit activating and have efficacy for negative symptoms of schizophrenia and for depression. Sulpiride remains a popular option for treating psychosis in countries outside the US, such as the UK, as it may be better tolerated than some of the other original D2 agents (Stahl, 2020; Stahl, 2021).

# Sulpiride: Tips and Pearls

## Dosing

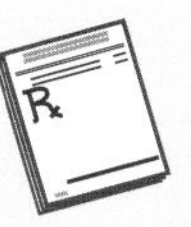

***Formulation:***
200, 400, and 500 mg tablets
50, 100 mg/mL IM injection

***Dosage Range:***
400–800 mg/day in 2 doses (PO) for schizophrenia
50–300 mg/day (PO) for predominantly negative symptoms
150–300 mg/day (PO) for depression
600–800 mg/day (IM injection)

***Approved For:***
Not available in the US

## Side effects I

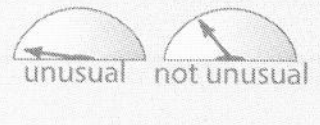
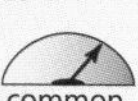
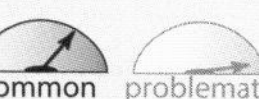


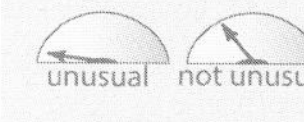
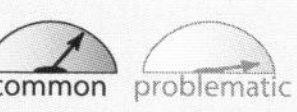

Rare neuroleptic malignant syndrome, seizures; elderly patients with dementia-related psychosis are at increased risk of death; drug-induced movement disorders

## Pearls

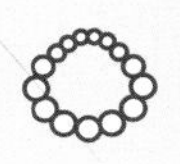
Sulpiride is poorly absorbed from the gastrointestinal tract and penetrates the blood–brain barrier poorly, which can lead to highly variable clinical responses, especially at lower doses; some patients with inadequate response to clozapine may benefit from augmentation with sulpiride

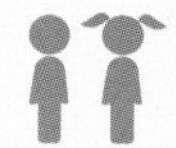
Not recommended for use in children under age 15

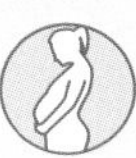
Potential risks should be weighed against the potential benefits, and sulpiride should be used only if deemed necessary; recommended either to discontinue drug or bottle feed

## Side effects II

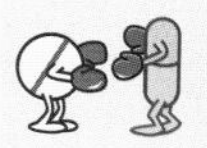
May decrease the effects of levodopa and other dopamine agonists; may increase the effects of antihypertensive drugs; antacids or sucralfate may reduce the absorption of sulpiride

Use with caution due to risk of orthostatic hypotension

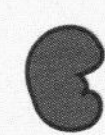
Use with caution; drug may accumulate; in cases of severe renal insufficiency, the dose should be decreased and intermittent treatment or switching to another drug for psychosis should be considered

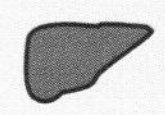
Use with caution in patients with hepatic impairments

# First-Generation D2 Antagonists: Amisulpride

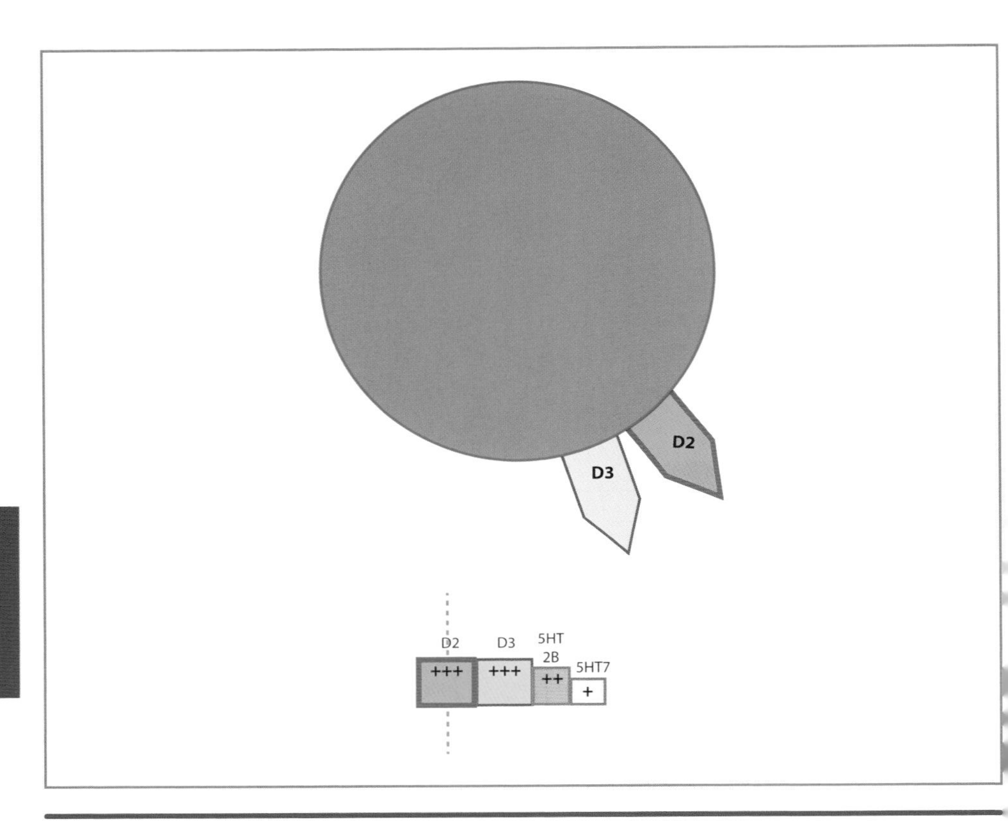


**FIGURE 4.5.** Amisulpride is structurally related to sulpiride and was developed and marketed outside the US. In addition to its actions at D2 receptors, amisulpride has some D3 antagonist actions and some weak 5HT7 antagonist actions (Stahl, 2020; Stahl, 2021).

# Amisulpride: Tips and Pearls

## Dosing

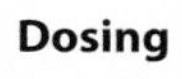

*Formulation:*
50, 100, 200, and 400 mg tablets
100 mg/mL oral solution

*Dosage Range:*
400–800 mg/day in 2 doses (schizophrenia)
50–300 mg/day (negative symptoms only)
50 mg/day (dysthymia)

*Approved For:*
Not available for psychosis in the US

## Pearls

Efficacy has been particularly well demonstrated in patients with predominantly negative symptoms; the increase in prolactin caused by amisulpride may cause menstruation to stop; for treatment-resistant patients with inadequate responses to clozapine, amisulpride may be a preferred augmentation option; very low doses may be useful in dysthymia

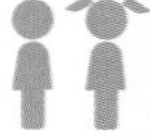

Efficacy and safety not established under the age of 18

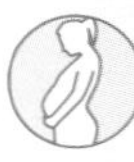

Not recommended during pregnancy or breastfeeding

## Side effects I

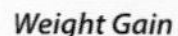

*Weight Gain*

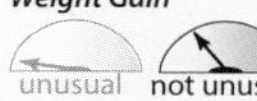

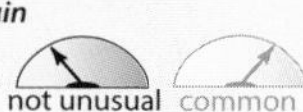

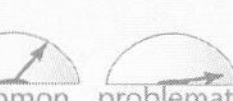


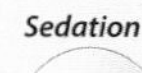

*Sedation*

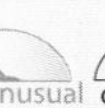

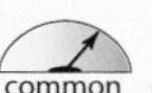

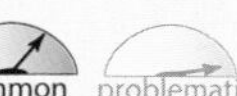


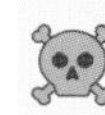

Rare neuroleptic malignant syndrome, seizures; dose-dependent QTc prolongation; elderly patients with dementia-related psychosis are at increased risk of death; drug-induced movement disorders

## Side effects II

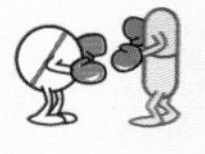

Increases effect of antihypertensive drugs and decreases effects of dopamine agonists; as it is weakly metabolized, few drug interactions exist

Dose-dependent prolongation of QTc interval

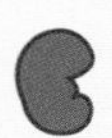

Use with caution if renal insufficiency is present; drug can accumulate, as it is eliminated by the kidneys

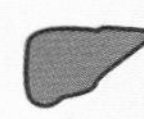

Use with caution in patients with hepatic impairments

# 5HT2A Binding by Drugs Used to Treat Psychosis

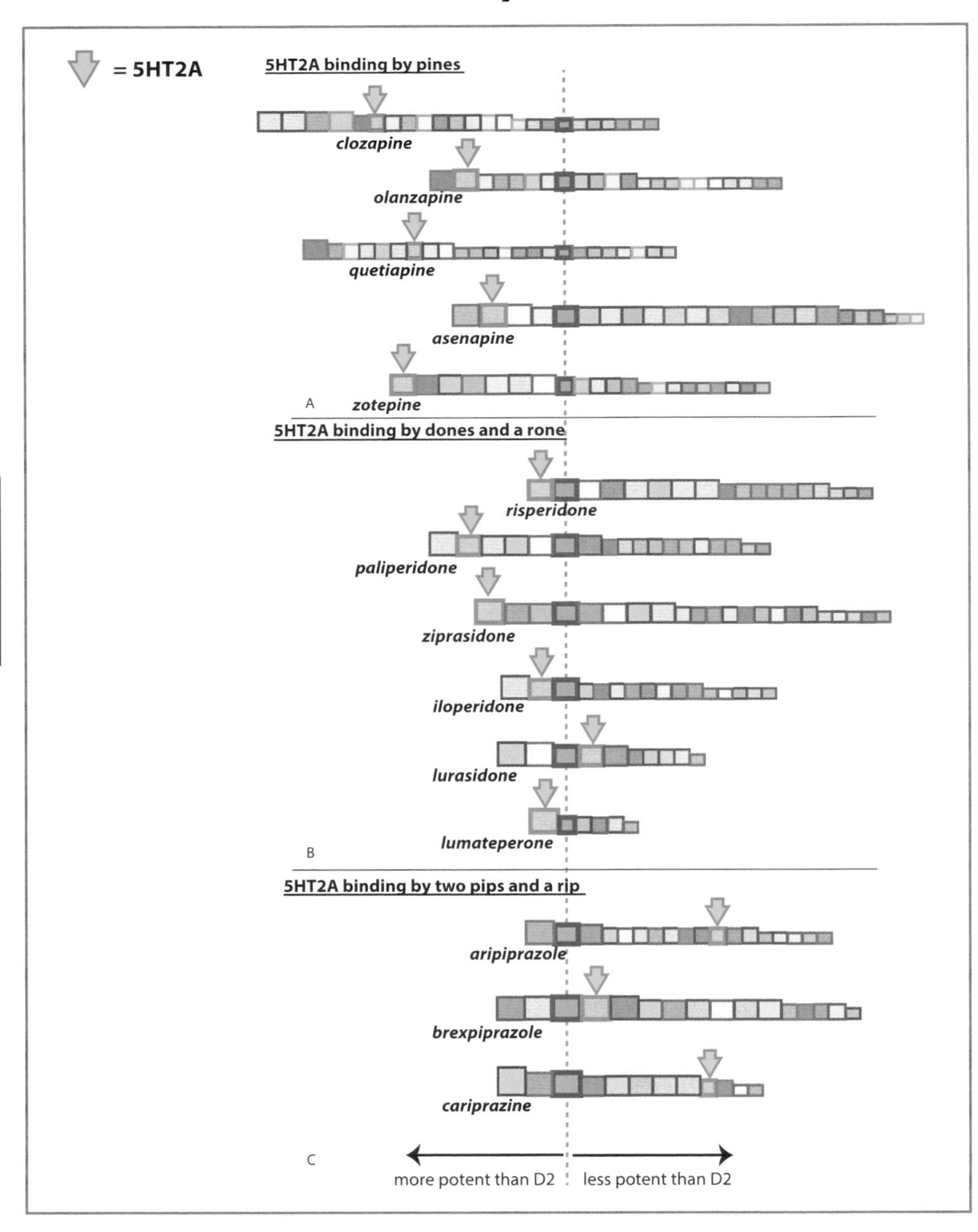

# 5HT2A Binding by Drugs Used to Treat Psychosis

**FIGURE 4.6.** Shown here is a visual depiction of the binding profiles of drugs used to treat psychosis. Description of graphic: Each colored box represents a different binding property, with the size and positioning of the box reflecting the binding potency of the property (i.e., size indicates potency relative to a standard Ki scale, while position reflects potency relative to the other binding properties of that drug). The vertical dotted line cuts through the D2 receptor binding box, with binding properties that are more potent than D2 on the left and those that are less potent than D2 on the right. Interestingly, D2 binding is not the most potent property for any of the agents shown here. (A) The "pines" (i.e., clozapine, olanzapine, quetiapine, asenapine, and zotepine) all bind much more potently to the 5HT2A receptor than they do to the D2 receptor. (B) The "dones" and "rone" (i.e., risperidone, paliperidone, ziprasidone, iloperidone, lurasidone, and lumateperone) also bind more or as potently to the 5HT2A receptor as they do to the D2 receptor. (C) Aripiprazole and cariprazine both bind more potently to the D2 receptor than to the 5HT2A receptor, while brexpiprazole has similar potency at both receptors (Stahl, 2021).

# 5HT1A Binding by Drugs Used to Treat Psychosis

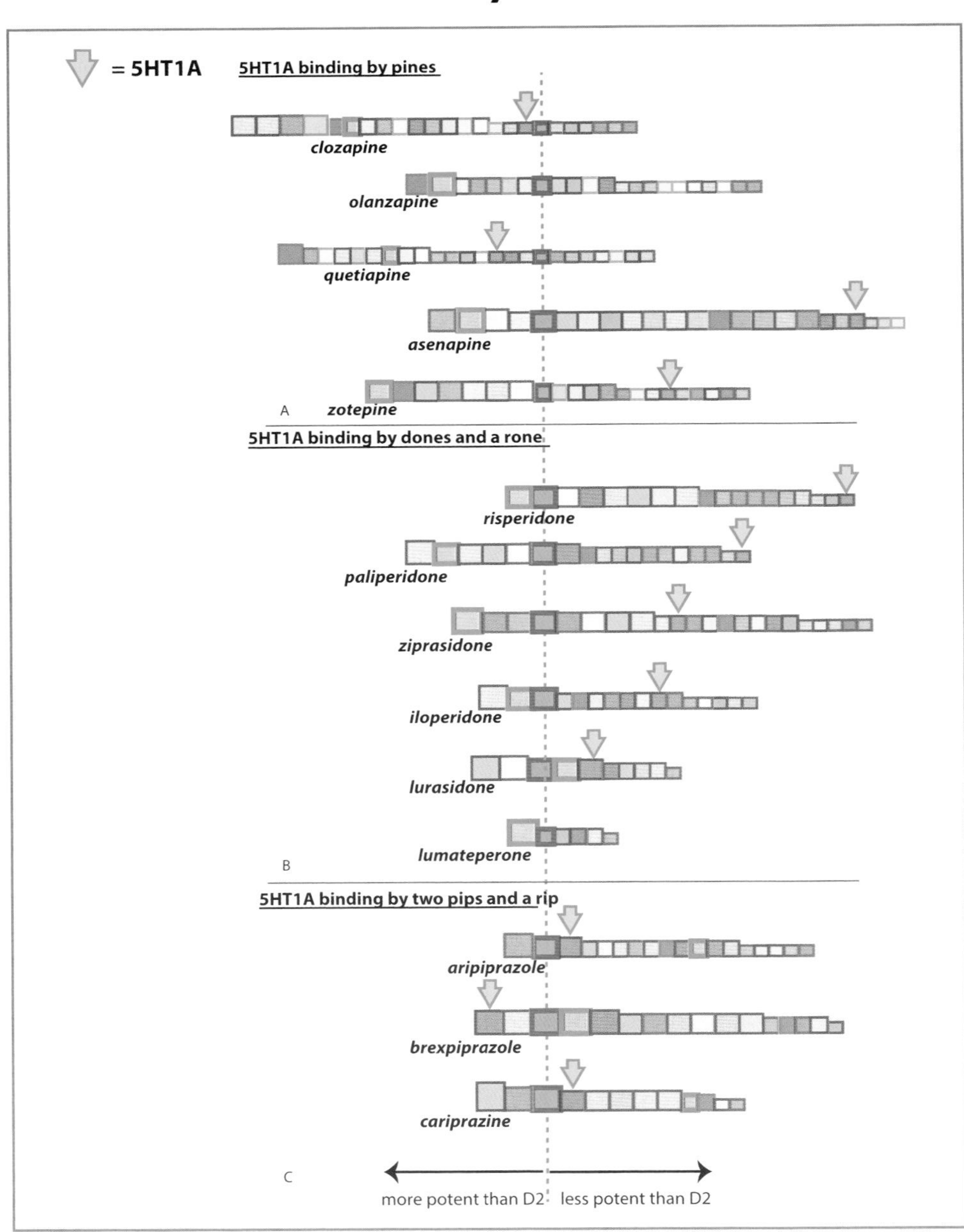

# 5HT1A Binding by Drugs Used to Treat Psychosis

**FIGURE 4.7.** Shown here is a visual depiction of the binding profiles of drugs used to treat psychosis. (A) Clozapine and quetiapine both bind more potently to the 5HT1A receptor than they do to the D2 receptor, while asenapine and zotepine bind less potently to the 5HT1A receptor and olanzapine does not bind to it at all. (B) All of the "dones" (i.e., risperidone, paliperidone, ziprasidone, iloperidone, and lurasidone) bind to the 5HT1A receptor with less potency than they do to the D2 receptor; lumateperone does not bind the 5HT1A receptor. (C) Aripiprazole, brexpiprazole, and cariprazine each have similar relative potency for the D2 and 5HT1A receptors. 5HT1A binding is actually the most potent property of brexpiprazole. Description of graphic: Each colored box represents a different binding property, with the size and positioning of the box reflecting the binding potency of the property (i.e., size indicates potency relative to a standard Ki scale, while position reflects potency relative to the other binding properties of that drug). The vertical dotted line cuts through the D2 receptor binding box, with binding properties that are more potent than D2 on the left and those that are less potent than D2 on the right. Binding at 5HT2A (see **FIGURE 4.6**) is indicated by an orange outline around the box (Stahl, 2021).

# Monoamine Transporter Binding by Drugs Used to Treat Psychosis

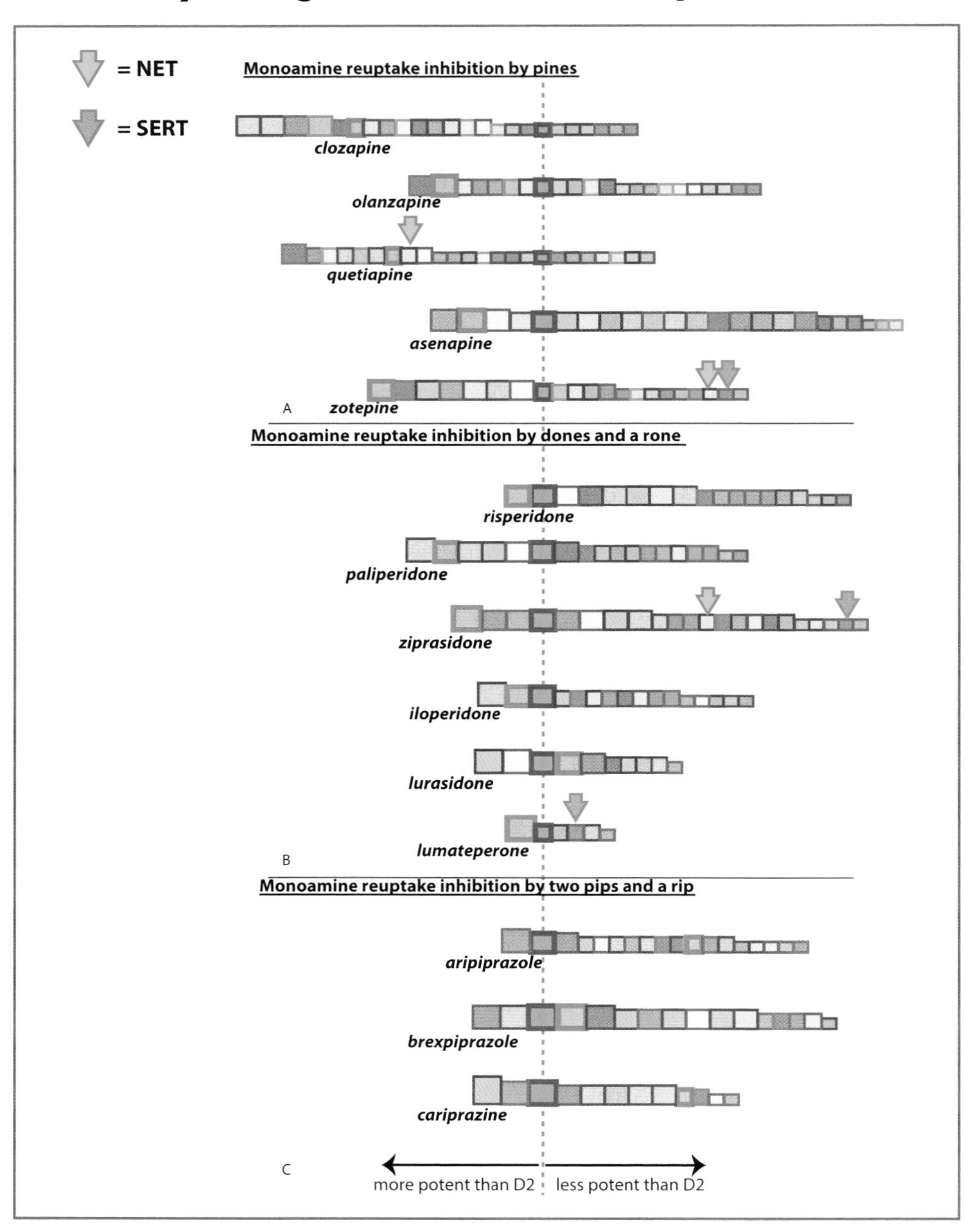

# Monoamine Transporter Binding by Drugs Used to Treat Psychosis

**FIGURE 4.8.** Shown here is a visual depiction of the binding profiles of drugs used to treat psychosis. (A) Of the "pines," quetiapine is the only one with any relevant monoamine reuptake inhibition. Specifically, it binds to the norepinephrine transporter (NET) with similar potency as it does to the 5HT2A receptor, and greater potency than to the D2 receptor. (B) Ziprasidone binds to NET and the serotonin transporter (SERT), though with less potency than to the D2 receptor. Lumateperone binds to SERT with similar potency as to the D2 receptor. (C) Aripiprazole, brexpiprazole, and cariprazine do not bind to any of the monoamine transporters. Description of graphic: Each colored box represents a different binding property, with the size and positioning of the box reflecting the binding potency of the property (i.e., size indicates potency relative to a standard Ki scale, while position reflects potency relative to the other binding properties of that drug). The vertical dotted line cuts through the dopamine 2 (D2) receptor binding box, with binding properties that are more potent than D2 on the left and those that are less potent than D2 on the right. Binding at 5HT2A (see **FIGURE 4.6**) is indicated by an orange outline around the box (Stahl, 2021).

# Alpha-2 Binding by Drugs Used to Treat Psychosis

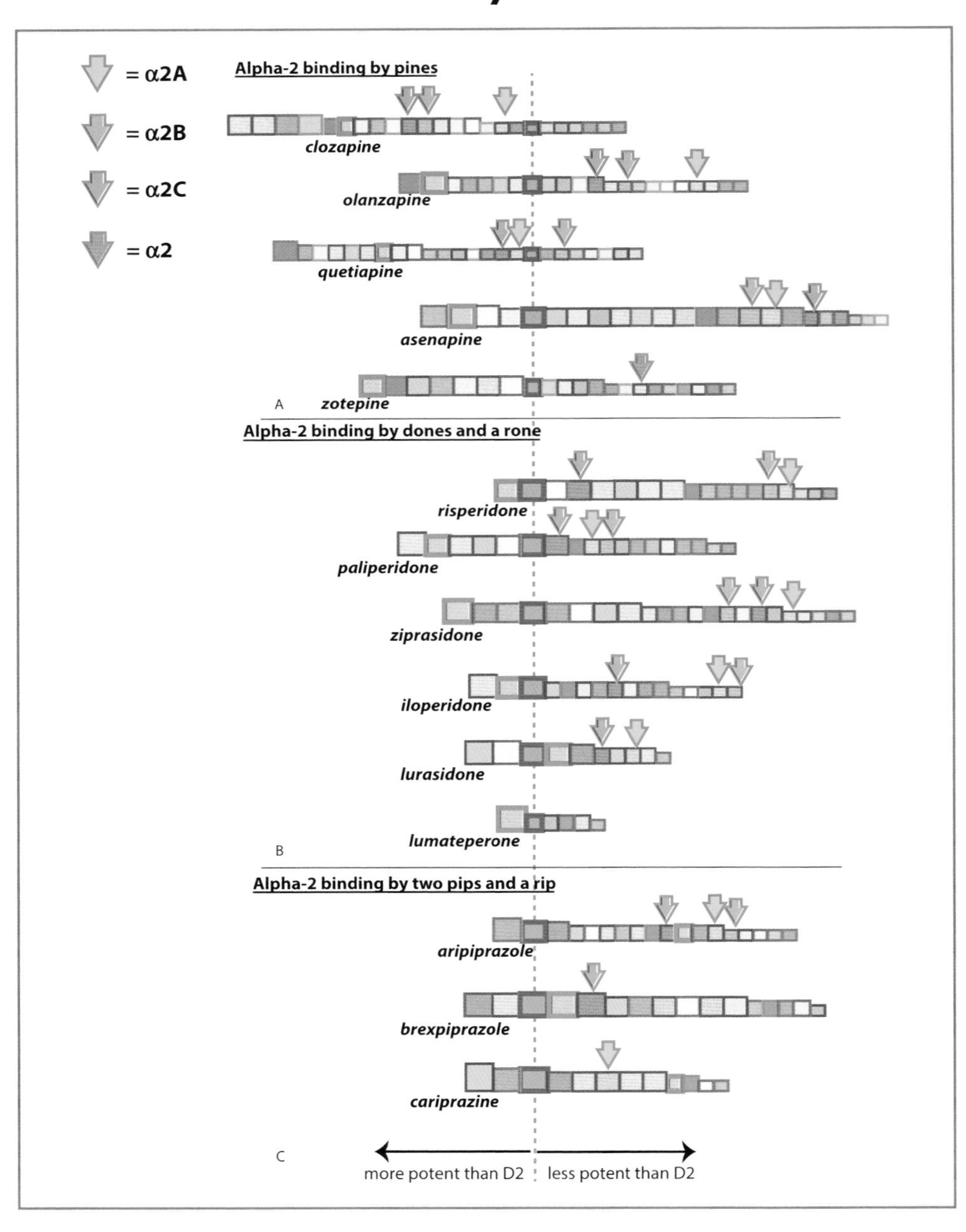

# Alpha-2 Binding by Drugs Used to Treat Psychosis

**FIGURE 4.9.** Shown here is a visual depiction of the binding profiles of drugs used to treat psychosis. (A) All of the "pines" (i.e., clozapine, olanzapine, quetiapine, asenapine, zotepine) bind to α2 receptors to varying degrees. Clozapine and quetiapine in particular bind to some α2 receptor subtypes with greater potency than they do to the D2 receptor. (B) All of the "dones" (i.e., risperidone, paliperidone, ziprasidone, iloperidone, lurasidone) bind to α2 receptors to varying degrees. Risperidone and paliperidone bind to the α2C receptor with similar potency as to the D2 receptor. Lumateperone does not bind to any α2 receptors. (C) Aripiprazole binds to α2 receptors with less potency than it does to the D2 receptor. Brexpiprazole binds to α2C receptors, and cariprazine has some affinity for α2A receptors. Description of graphic: Each colored box represents a different binding property, with the size and positioning of the box reflecting the binding potency of the property (i.e., size indicates potency relative to a standard Ki scale, while position reflects potency relative to the other binding properties of that drug). The vertical dotted line cuts through the dopamine 2 (D2) receptor binding box, with binding properties that are more potent than D2 on the left and those that are less potent than D2 on the right. Binding at 5HT2A (see **FIGURE 4.6**) is indicated by an orange outline around the box (Stahl, 2021).

# D3 Binding by Drugs Used to Treat Psychosis

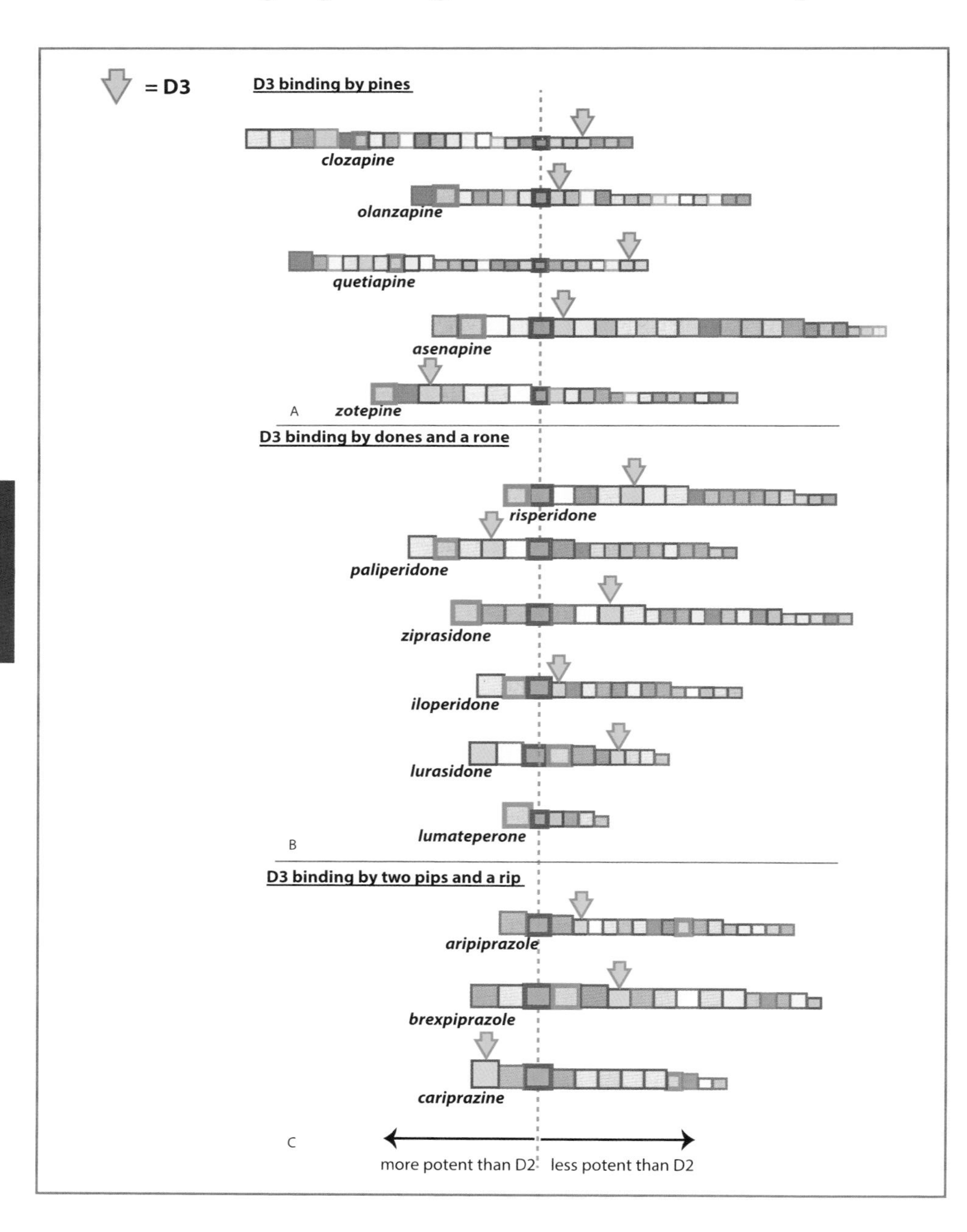

# D3 Binding by Drugs Used to Treat Psychosis

**FIGURE 4.10.** Shown here is a visual depiction of the binding profiles of drugs used to treat psychosis. (A) All of the "pines" bind to D3 receptors, but with varying degrees of potency. (B) Likewise, all of the "dones" bind to D3 receptors, again with varying degrees of potency. Lumateperone, however, does not bind to D3 receptors at all. (C) D3 receptor partial agonism is actually the most potent binding property of cariprazine. Aripiprazole and brexpiprazole also bind to D3 receptors less potently than they do to D2 receptors. Description of graphic: Each colored box represents a different binding property, with the size and positioning of the box reflecting the binding potency of the property (i.e., size indicates potency relative to a standard Ki scale, while position reflects potency relative to the other binding properties of that drug). The vertical dotted line cuts through the dopamine 2 (D2) receptor binding box, with binding properties that are more potent than D2 on the left and those that are less potent than D2 on the right. Binding at 5HT2A (see **FIGURE 4.6**) is indicated by an orange outline around the box (Stahl, 2021).

# 5HT2C Binding by Drugs Used to Treat Psychosis

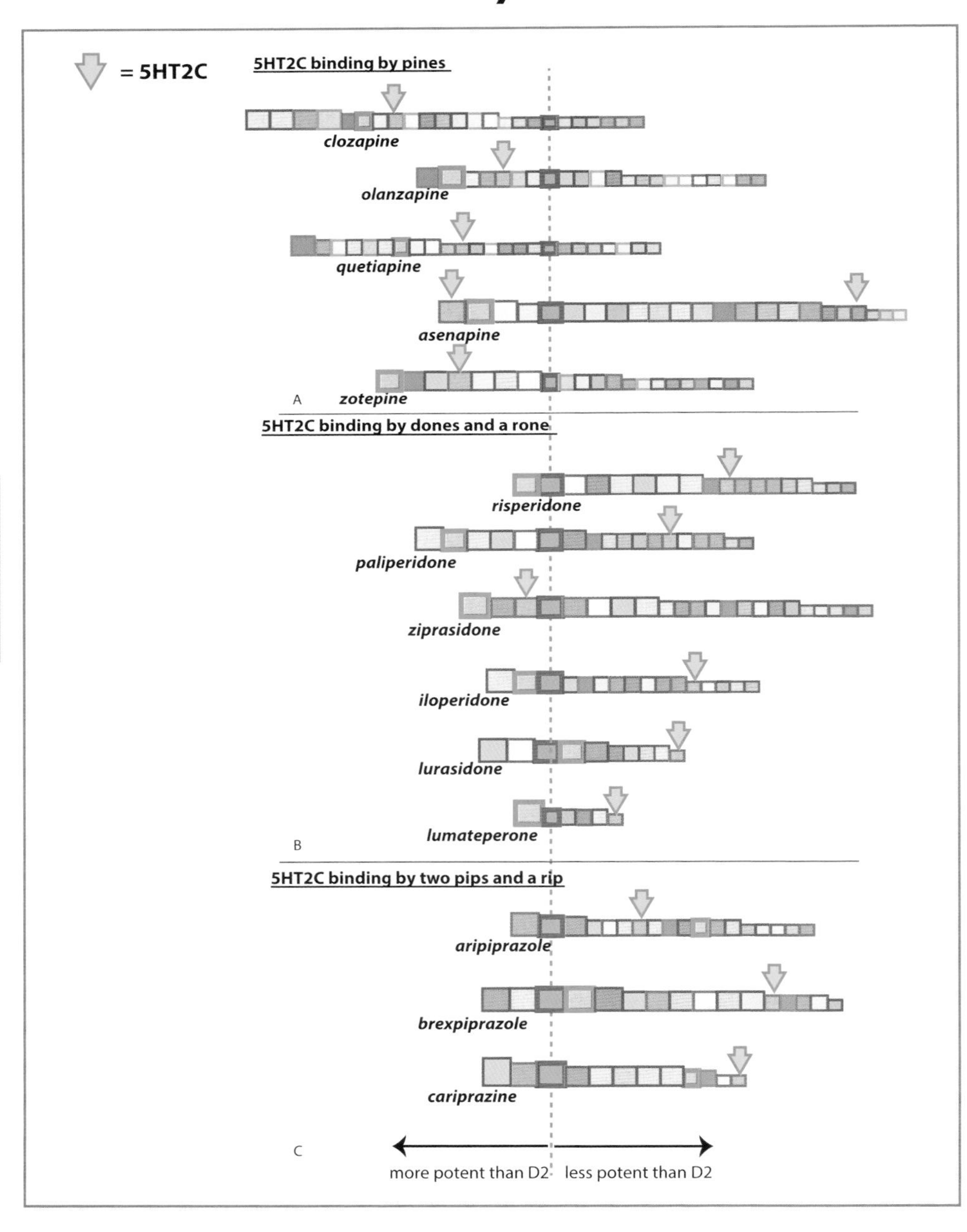

# 5HT2C Binding by Drugs Used to Treat Psychosis

**FIGURE 4.11.** Shown here is a visual depiction of the binding profiles of drugs used to treat psychosis. (A) All of the "pines" (i.e., clozapine, olanzapine, quetiapine, asenapine, zotepine) bind more potently to the 5HT2C receptor than they do to the D2 receptor. (B) All of the "dones" (i.e., risperidone, paliperidone, ziprasidone, iloperidone, lurasidone) as well as lumateperone have some affinity for the 5HT2C receptor, although only ziprasidone binds with comparable potency as at the D2 receptor. (C) Aripiprazole, brexpiprazole, and cariprazine all have relatively weak affinity for the 5HT2C receptor. Description of graphic: Each colored box represents a different binding property, with the size and positioning of the box reflecting the binding potency of the property (i.e., size indicates potency relative to a standard Ki scale, while position reflects potency relative to the other binding properties of that drug). The vertical dotted line cuts through the dopamine 2 (D2) receptor binding box, with binding properties that are more potent than D2 on the left and those that are less potent than D2 on the right. Binding at 5HT2A (see **FIGURE 4.6**) is indicated by an orange outline around the box (Stahl, 2021).

# 5HT3 Binding by Drugs Used to Treat Psychosis

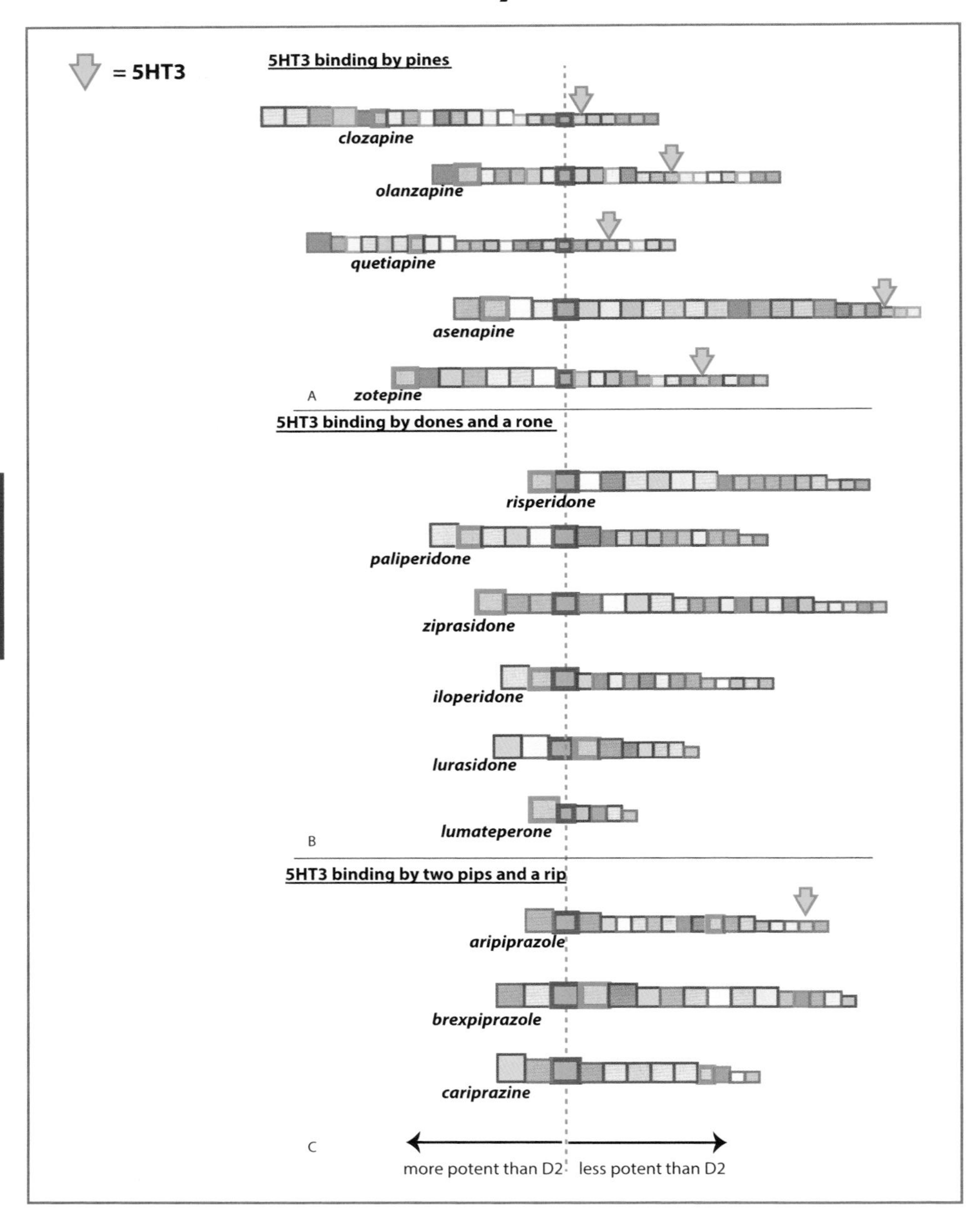

# 5HT3 Binding by Drugs Used to Treat Psychosis

**FIGURE 4.12.** Shown here is a visual depiction of the binding profiles of drugs used to treat psychosis. (A) All of the "pines" bind to 5HT3 with less affinity than they have for the D2 receptor. (B) None of the "dones" or "rone" have any binding activity at 5HT3 receptors. (C) Aripiprazole binds weakly to 5HT3 receptors. Description of graphic: Each colored box represents a different binding property, with the size and positioning of the box reflecting the binding potency of the property (i.e., size indicates potency relative to a standard Ki scale, while position reflects potency relative to the other binding properties of that drug). The vertical dotted line cuts through the dopamine 2 (D2) receptor binding box, with binding properties that are more potent than D2 on the left and those that are less potent than D2 on the right. Binding at 5HT2A (see **FIGURE 4.6**) is indicated by an orange outline around the box (Stahl, 2021).

# 5HT6 and 5HT7 Binding by Drugs Used to Treat Psychosis

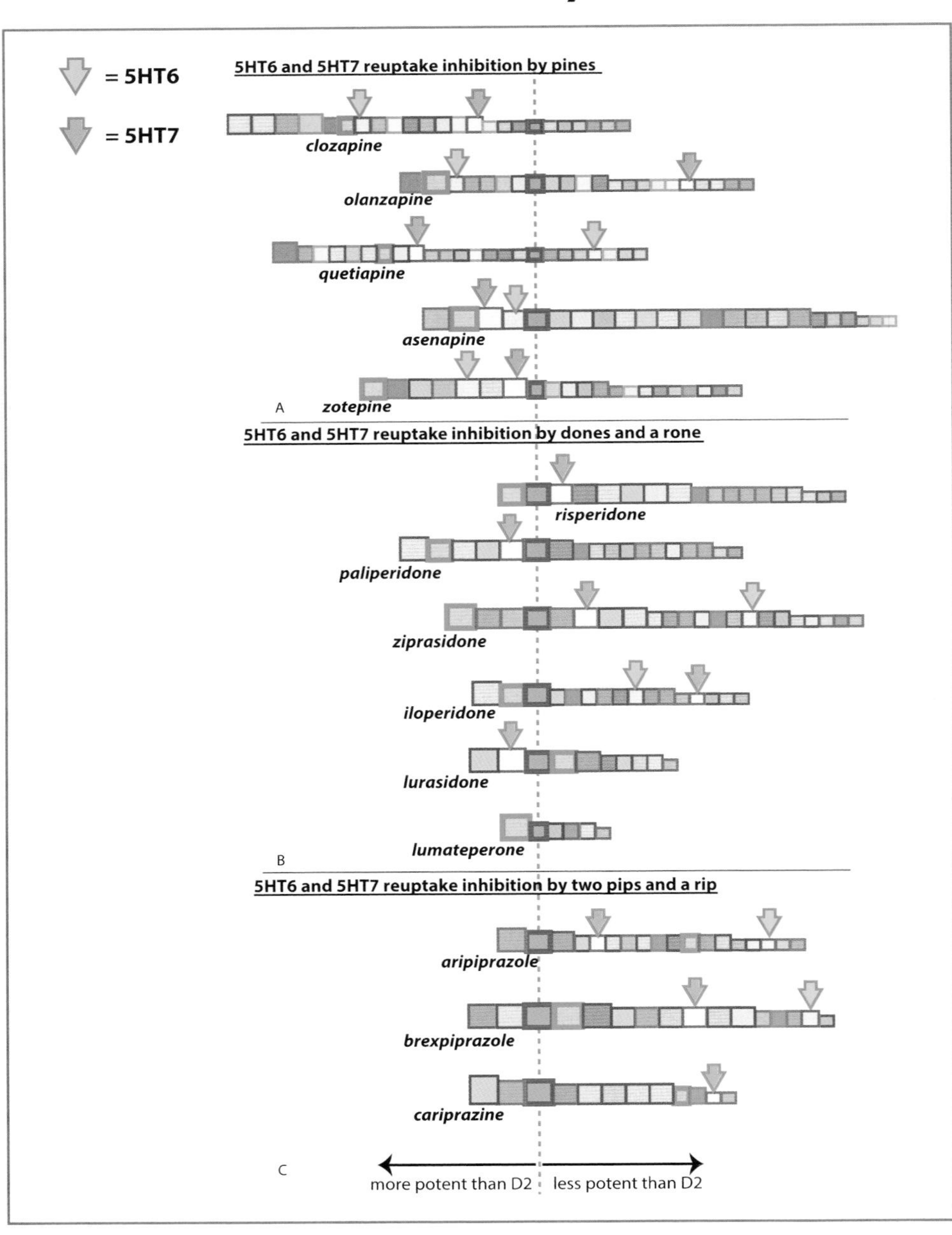

# 5HT6 and 5HT7 Binding by Drugs Used to Treat Psychosis

**FIGURE 4.13.** Shown here is a visual depiction of the binding profiles of drugs used to treat psychosis. (A) Clozapine, quetiapine, asenapine, and zotepine each have greater or similar potency for the 5HT7 receptor compared to the D2 receptor, while clozapine, olanzapine, asenapine, and zotepine each have greater or similar potency for the 5HT6 receptor compared to the D2 receptor. (B) Risperidone, paliperidone, ziprasidone, and lurasidone all bind potently to the 5HT7 receptor. In fact, lurasidone has greater affinity for the 5HT7 receptor than for the D2 receptor. Ziprasidone and iloperidone also bind to the 5HT6 receptor. (C) Aripiprazole, brexpiprazole, and cariprazine all bind to the 5HT7 receptor, though none with more potency than for the D2 receptor. Description of graphic: Each colored box represents a different binding property, with the size and positioning of the box reflecting the binding potency of the property (i.e., size indicates potency relative to a standard Ki scale, while position reflects potency relative to the other binding properties of that drug). The vertical dotted line cuts through the dopamine 2 (D2) receptor binding box, with binding properties that are more potent than D2 on the left and those that are less potent than D2 on the right. Binding at 5HT2A (see **FIGURE 4.6**) is indicated by an orange outline around the box (Stahl, 2021).

# 5HT1B/D Binding by Drugs Used to Treat Psychosis

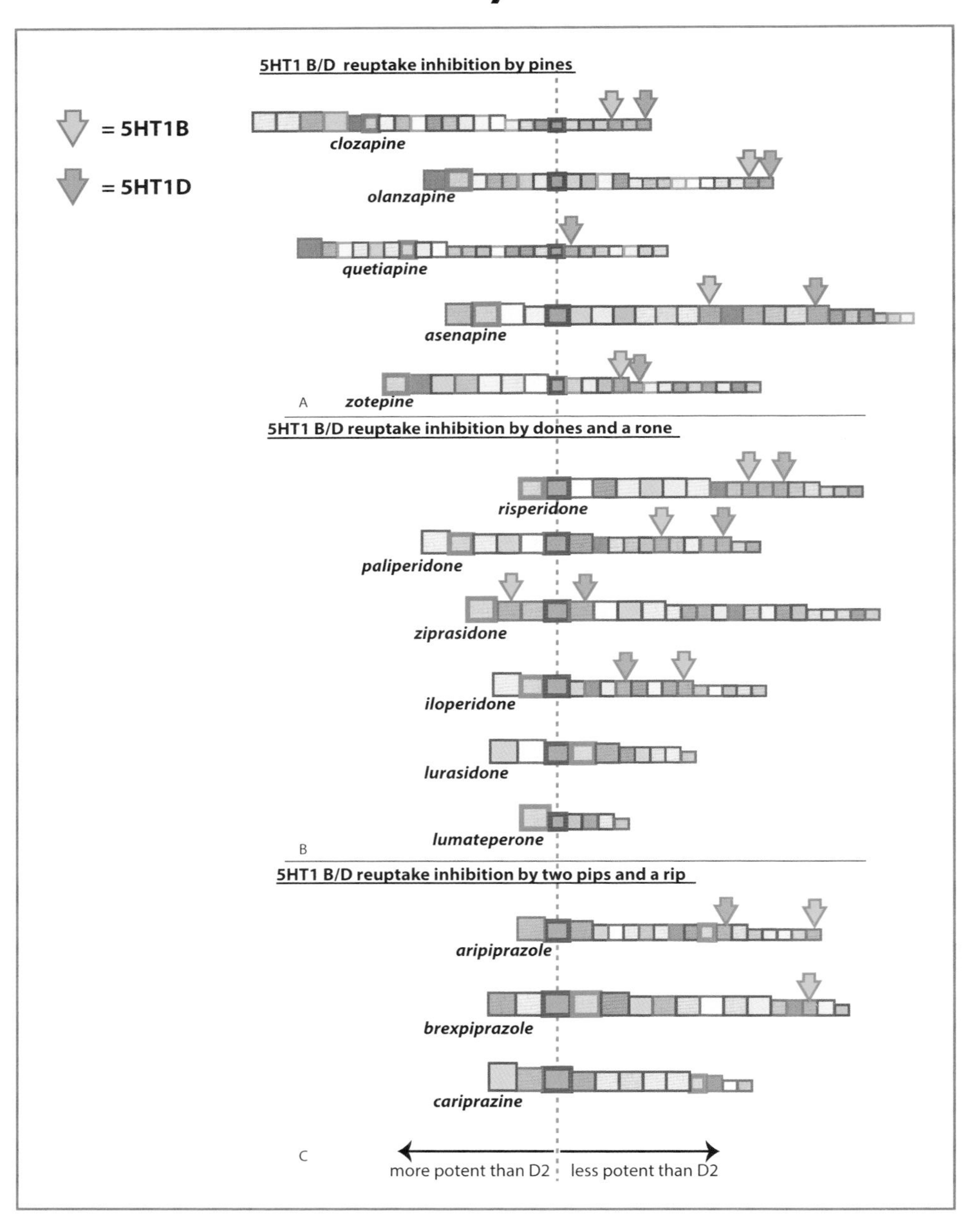

# 5HT1B/D Binding by Drugs Used to Treat Psychosis

**FIGURE 4.14.** Shown here is a visual depiction of the binding profiles of drugs used to treat psychosis. (A) Clozapine, olanzapine, asenapine, and zotepine all bind relatively weakly to the 5HT1B and 5HT1D receptors, while quetiapine binds relatively weakly only to the 5HT1D receptor. (B) Risperidone, paliperidone, ziprasidone, and iloperidone all have some affinity for the 5HT1B and 5HT1D receptors. In particular, ziprasidone binds with similar potency to these two receptors as it does to the D2 receptor. Lurasidone and lumateperone do not bind to 5HT1B/D receptors. (C) Aripiprazole and brexpiprazole each bind weakly to the 5HT1B receptor; aripiprazole also binds to the 5HT1D receptor. Cariprazine does not bind to 5HT1B/D receptors. Description of graphic: Each colored box represents a different binding property, with the size and positioning of the box reflecting the binding potency of the property (i.e., size indicates potency relative to a standard Ki scale, while position reflects potency relative to the other binding properties of that drug). The vertical dotted line cuts through the dopamine 2 (D2) receptor binding box, with binding properties that are more potent than D2 on the left and those that are less potent than D2 on the right. Binding at 5HT2A (see **FIGURE 4.6**) is indicated by an orange outline around the box (Stahl, 2021).

# Antihistamine/Anticholinergic Binding by Drugs Used to Treat Psychosis

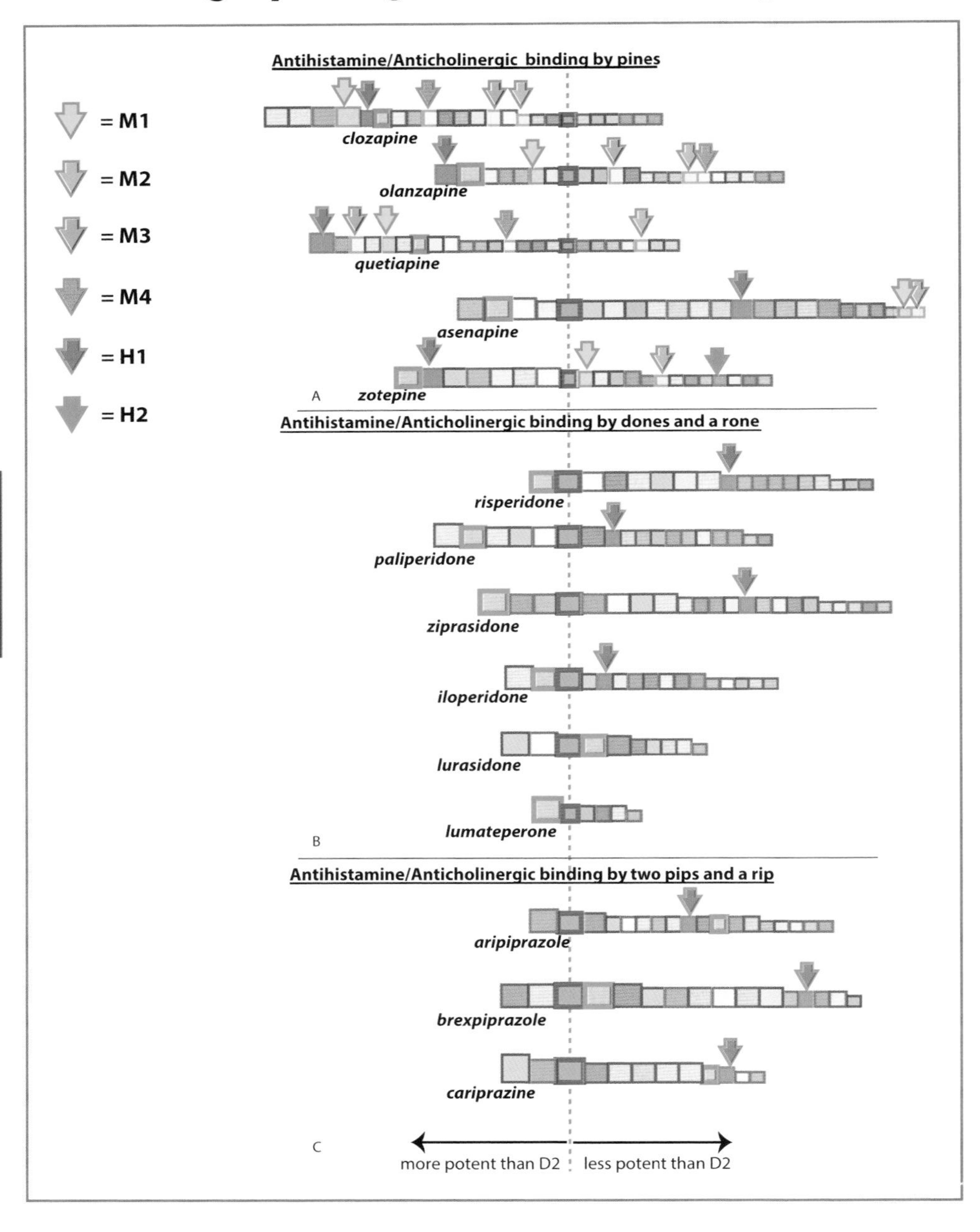

# Antihistamine/Anticholinergic Binding by Drugs Used to Treat Psychosis

**FIGURE 4.15.** Shown here is a visual depiction of the binding profiles of drugs used to treat psychosis. (A) Clozapine, olanzapine, quetiapine, and zotepine all have strong potency for histamine 1 receptors; clozapine, olanzapine, and quetiapine also have strong potency for muscarinic receptors. Asenapine has some affinity for histamine H1 receptors and weak affinity for muscarinic receptors. (B) None of the "dones" or "rones" have anticholinergic properties. Risperidone, paliperidone, ziprasidone, and iloperidone all have some potency for H1 receptors. (C) Aripiprazole, brexpiprazole, and cariprazine all bind at the H1 receptor with less potency than they do to the D2 receptor, and do not bind to muscarinic receptors. Description of graphic: Each colored box represents a different binding property, with the size and positioning of the box reflecting the binding potency of the property (i.e., size indicates potency relative to a standard Ki scale, while position reflects potency relative to the other binding properties of that drug). The vertical dotted line cuts through the dopamine 2 (D2) receptor binding box, with binding properties that are more potent than D2 on the left and those that are less potent than D2 on the right. Binding at 5HT2A (see **FIGURE 4.6**) is indicated by an orange outline around the box (Stahl, 2021).

# Alpha-1 Binding by Drugs Used to Treat Psychosis

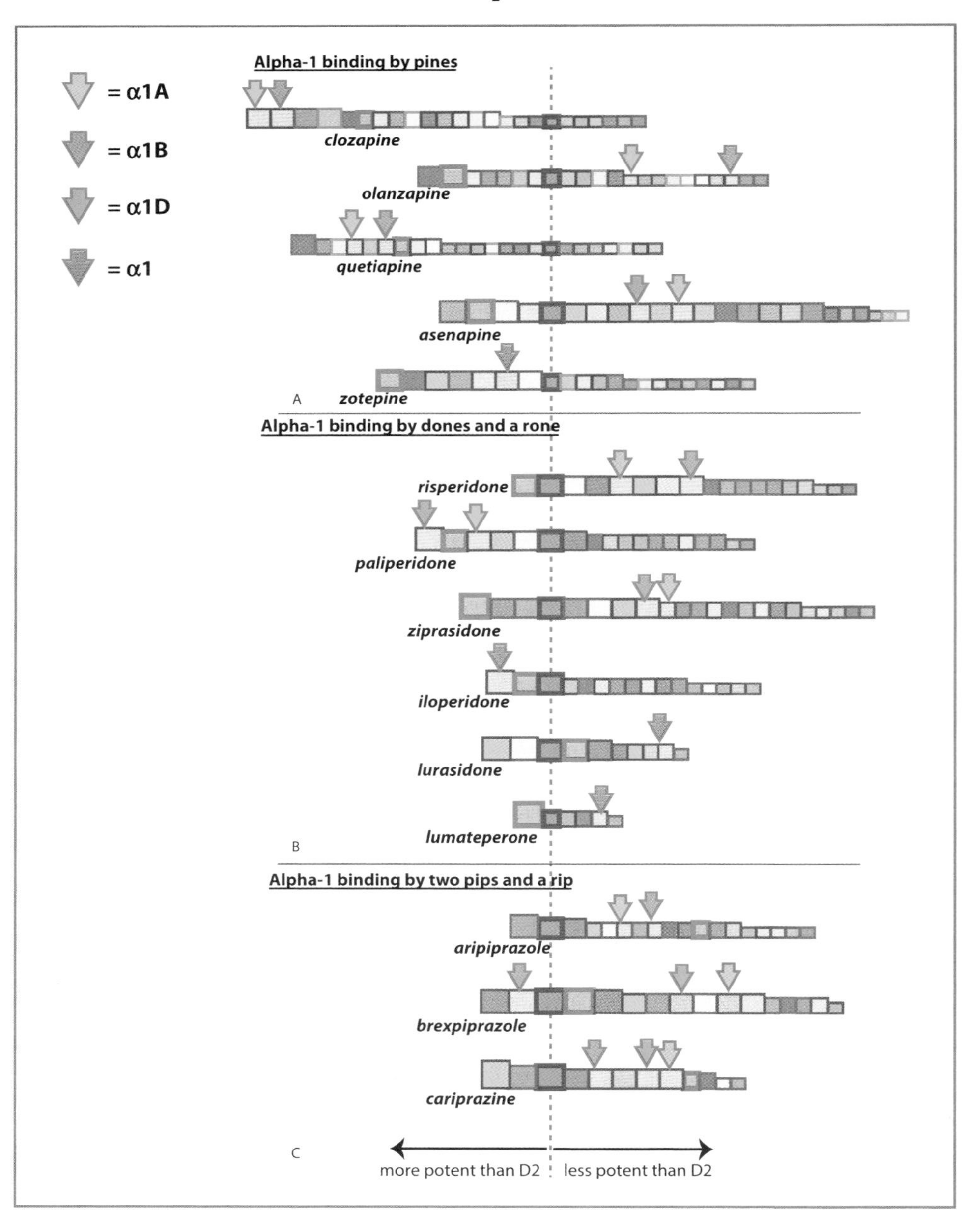

# Alpha-1 Binding by Drugs Used to Treat Psychosis

**FIGURE 4.16.** Shown here is a visual depiction of the binding profiles of drugs used to treat psychosis. (A) Clozapine, quetiapine, and zotepine each have greater potency for α1 receptors than for the D2 receptor, while asenapine binds with similar potency to the α1 and the D2 receptors. (B) All of the "dones" (i.e., risperidone, paliperidone, ziprasidone, iloperidone, lurasidone) as well as lumateperone bind to the α1 receptor. In particular, paliperidone and iloperidone bind with greater potency than they do to the D2 receptor. (C) Aripiprazole, brexpiprazole, and cariprazine each have some binding potency at α1 receptors. Description of graphic: Each colored box represents a different binding property, with the size and positioning of the box reflecting the binding potency of the property (i.e., size indicates potency relative to a standard Ki scale, while position reflects potency relative to the other binding properties of that drug). The vertical dotted line cuts through the dopamine 2 (D2) receptor binding box, with binding properties that are more potent than D2 on the left and those that are less potent than D2 on the right. Binding at 5HT2A (see **FIGURE 4.6**) is indicated by an orange outline around the box (Stahl, 2021).

# The Pines (Peens): Clozapine

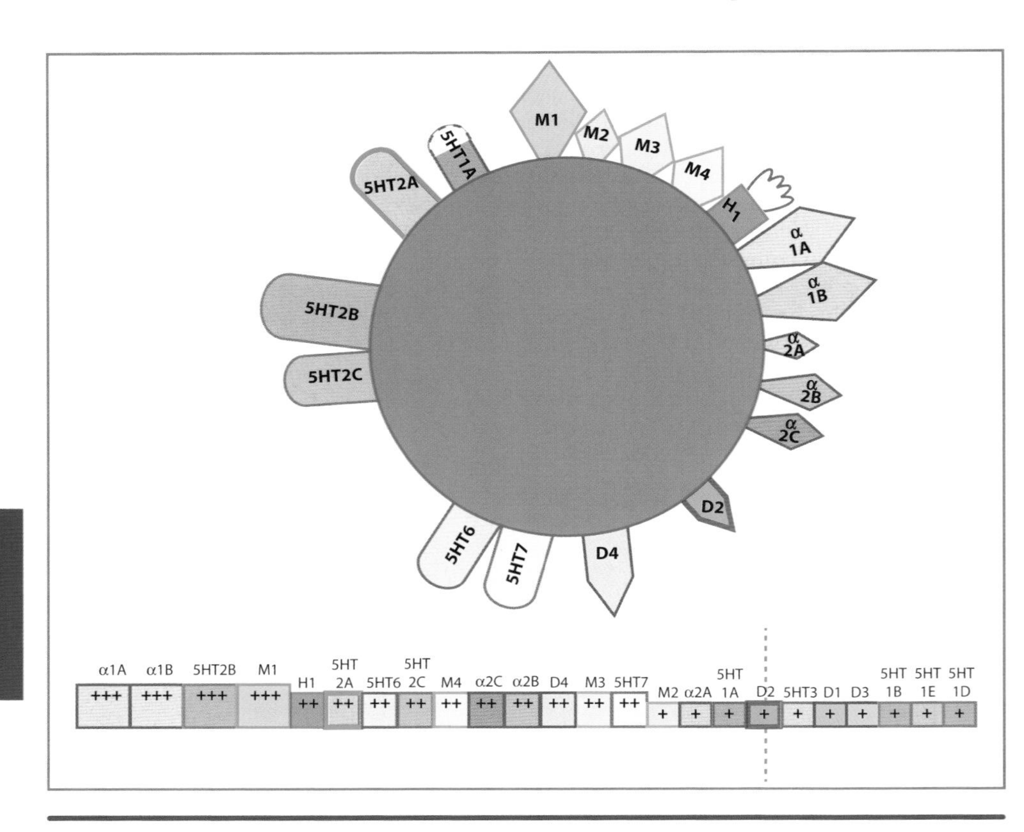


**FIGURE 4.17.** Clozapine is widely recognized as being particularly effective when other drugs for psychosis fail and is thus the "gold standard" for efficacy in schizophrenia. Clozapine is also the only drug for psychosis that has been documented to reduce the risk of suicide in schizophrenia and may have a particular niche in treating aggression and violence in psychotic patients. Even though it is very effective for psychosis, clozapine is not considered first-line due to its side effects that require expert management. These include neutropenia, constipation/paralytic ileus, sedation, orthostasis, tachycardia, excessive salivation (sialorrhea), seizures, weight gain, dyslipidemia, hyperglycemia, myocarditis, cardiomyopathy, interstitial nephritis, DRESS (drug reaction with eosinophilia and systemic symptoms), and serositis. In addition to 5HT2A/D2 antagonism, numerous other binding properties have been identified for clozapine, most of which are more potent than its binding at the D2 receptor. It is unknown which of these contribute to clozapine's special efficacy or to its unique side effects (Meyer & Stahl, 2019; Stahl, 2020; Stahl, 2021).

# Clozapine: Tips and Pearls

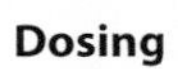

## Dosing

***Formulation:***
12.5, 25, 50, and 100 mg tablets
12.5, 25, 50, and 100 mg orally disintegrating tablets
50 mg/mL oral suspension

***Dosage Range:***
300–450 mg/day; depends on plasma levels, but threshold for response is trough plasma level of 350 ng/mL

***Approved For:***
Treatment-resistant schizophrenia; reduction in risk of recurrent suicidal behavior in patients with schizophrenia or schizoaffective disorder

## Side effects I

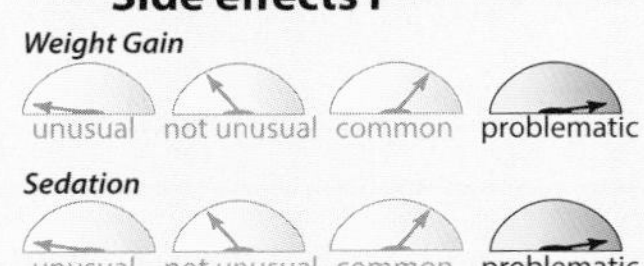


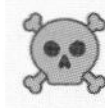

Severe neutropenia, myocarditis (only in first 6 weeks of treatment), paralytic ileus, seizures (risk increases with dose), hyperglycemia, ketoacidosis, pulmonary embolism, dilated cardiomyopathy, rare neuroleptic malignant syndrome, increased risk of death in elderly

## Pearls

The gold standard treatment for refractory schizophrenia; not used first line due to side effects and monitoring burden; rapid discontinuation can lead to rebound psychosis; most efficacious but most dangerous; reduced suicide in schizophrenia; may reduce violence and aggression in difficult cases, including forensic cases

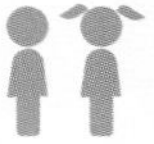

Potentially efficacious in early-onset treatment-resistant schizophrenia; children and adolescents should be monitored more often than adults

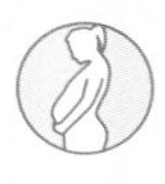

Animal studies have not shown adverse effects; no controlled studies in pregnant women; recommended either to discontinue drug or bottle feed

## Side effects II

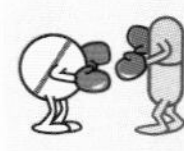

CYP450 1A2, 3A4, and 2D6 inhibitors increase its plasma levels; CYP450 1A2 inducers decrease plasma levels; clozapine enhances effects of antihypertensives

Use with caution, especially if patient takes concomitant medication

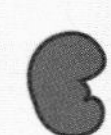

Use with caution in patients with renal impairments

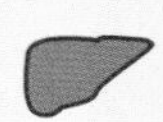

Use with caution in patients with hepatic impairments

# The Pines (Peens): Olanzapine

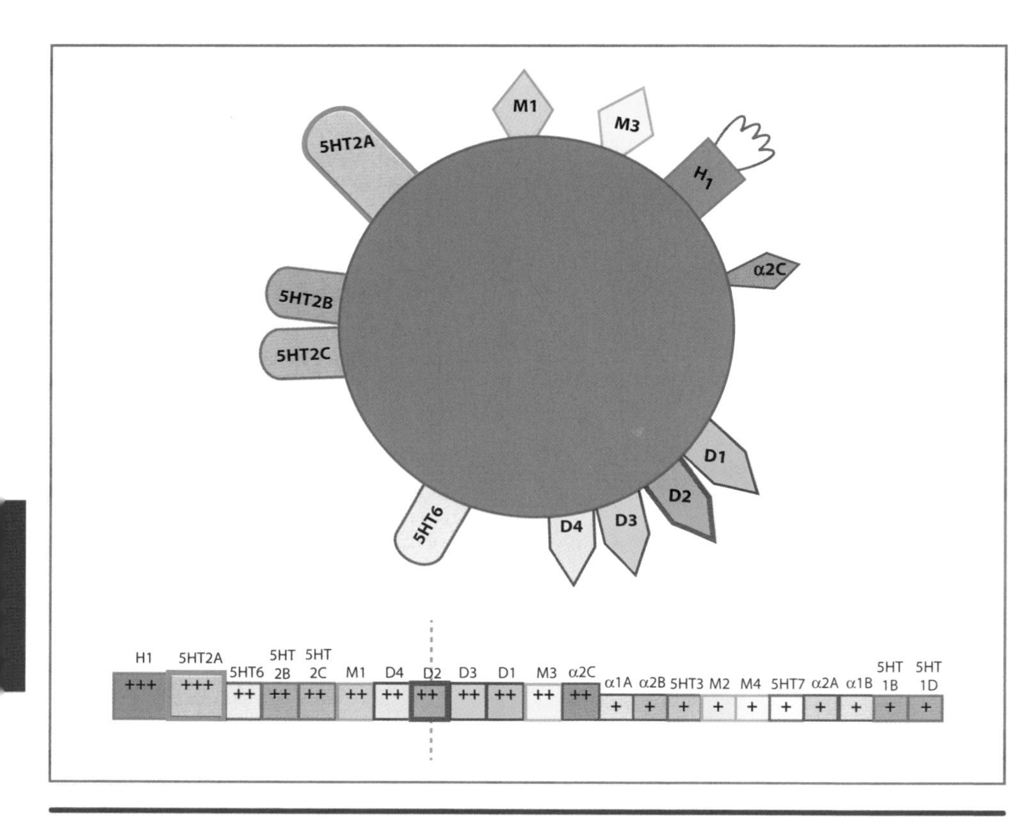


**FIGURE 4.18.** Olanzapine binds at several receptors more potently than it does at the D2 receptor; in fact, it has strongest potency for the H1 and 5HT2A receptors. Olanzapine's 5HT2C antagonist properties may contribute to its efficacy for mood and cognitive symptoms, although together with its H1 antihistamine properties they could also contribute to its propensity to cause weight gain. Clinical experience indicates that except for clozapine, olanzapine is the most effective agent in this class for treating symptoms of psychosis. However, it also has a higher risk for metabolic side effects (Stahl, 2020; Stahl, 2021).

# Olanzapine: Tips and Pearls

## Dosing

***Formulation:***
2.5, 5, 7.5, 10, 15, and 20 mg tablets
5, 10, 15, and 20 mg orally disintegrating tablets
5 mg/mL vials (IM)
Also available in an LAI formulation (olanzapine pamoate)

***Dosage Range:***
10–20 mg/day (PO or IM)

***Approved For:***
Schizophrenia, schizophrenia and bipolar maintenance, acute agitation associated with schizophrenia and bipolar I mania (IM), acute mania/mixed mania

## Side effects I

***Weight Gain***

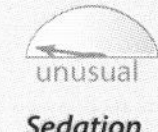

unusual not unusual common **problematic**

***Sedation***

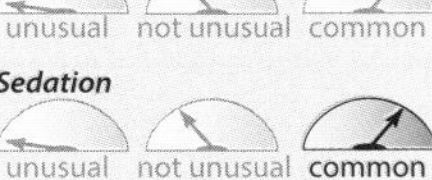

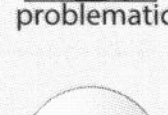

unusual not unusual **common** problematic

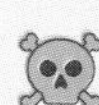

Rare Drug Reaction with Eosinophilia and Systemic Symptoms (DRESS), neuroleptic malignant syndrome, seizures, tardive dyskinesia; hyperglycemia, ketoacidosis; elderly patients with dementia-related psychosis are at increased risk of death

## Pearls

Greater efficacy but greater metabolic side effects compared to other drugs for psychosis; utility in treatment-refractory cases, especially at higher doses

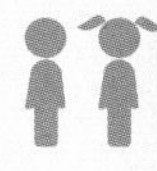

Approved for use in schizophrenia and manic/mixed episodes (ages 13 and older); IM formulation not recommended; may need to be monitored more often than adults

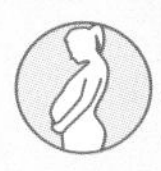

Some animal studies show adverse effects; no controlled studies in pregnant women; recommend either to discontinue drug or bottle feed

## Side effects II

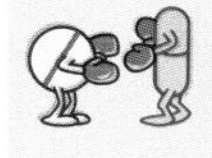

May increase effect of antihypertensive agents; may antagonize levodopa and other dopamine agonists; dose may need to be lowered if given with CYP450 1A2 inhibitors and raised if given with CYP450 1A2 inducers

Should be used with caution because of risk of orthostatic hypotension

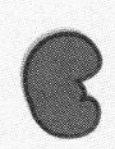

No dose adjustment required for oral formulation; not removed by hemodialysis; consider lower starting dose for IM formulation

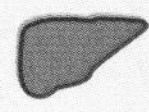

Patients with liver disease should have liver function tests a few times a year; lower starting dose (5 mg) for moderate-to-severe hepatic impairment and increase dose with caution; consider lower starting dose (5 mg) for IM formulation

# The Pines (Peens): Olanzapine-Samidorphan

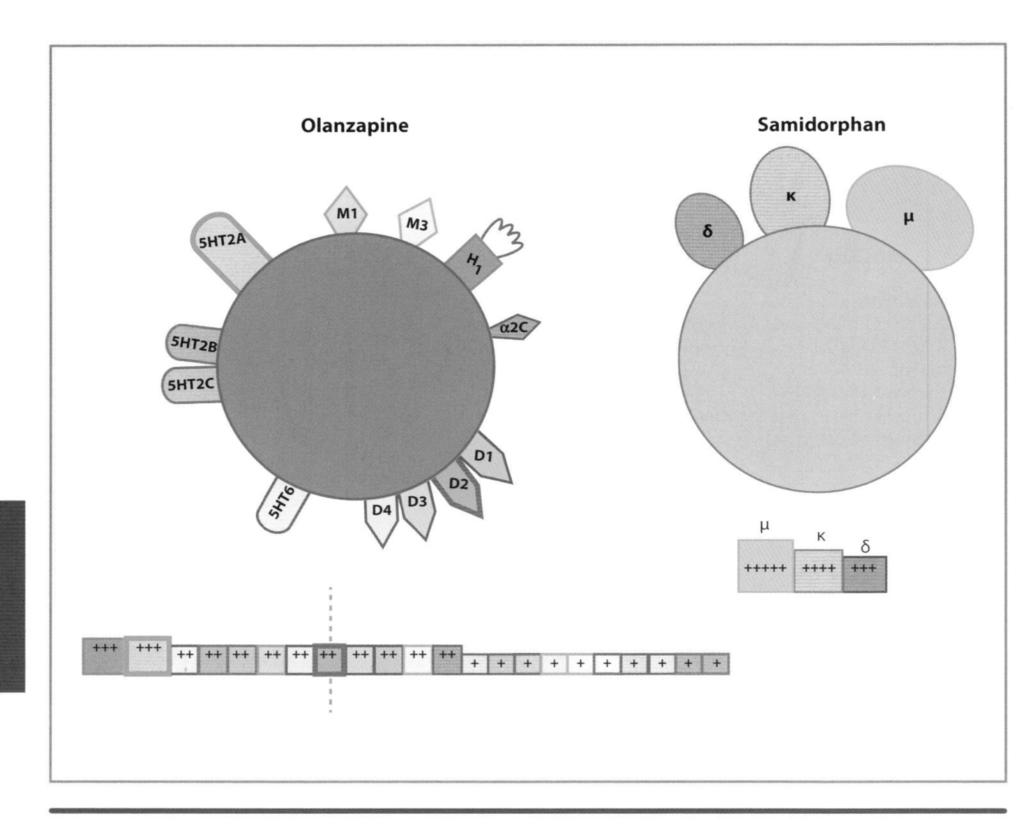


**FIGURE 4.19.** The combination of olanzapine and samidorphan was developed to capitalize on the efficacy of olanzapine while minimizing its metabolic side effects. Samidorphan is a mu-opioid receptor antagonist (Wentland et al., 2005) that mitigates olanzapine-induced weight gain and possibly metabolic abnormalities, including among patients early in their illness. It was approved by the Food and Drug Administration for the treatment of schizophrenia and bipolar I disorder in 2021 (Jawad et al., 2022; Kahn et al., 2023).

# Olanzapine-Samidorphan: Tips and Pearls

## Dosing

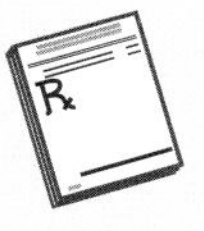

***Formulation:***
5 mg/10 mg, 10 mg/10 mg, 15 mg/10 mg, and 20 mg/10 mg olanzapine/samidorphan capsules

***Dosage Range:***
5 mg/10 mg–20 mg/10 mg olanzapine/samidorphan

***Approved For:***
Schizophrenia, bipolar I disorder acute mania/mixed mania monotherapy and adjunct to lithium or valproate, bipolar I disorder maintenance monotherapy

## Side effects I

*Weight Gain*

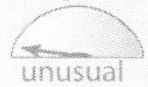
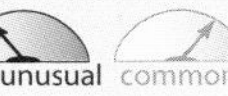
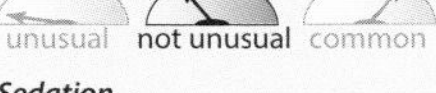


*Sedation*

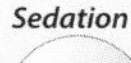
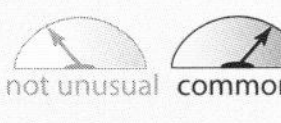


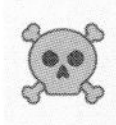

Rare Drug Reaction with Eosinophilia and Systemic Symptoms (DRESS), neuroleptic malignant syndrome, seizures, tardive dyskinesia; hyperglycemia, ketoacidosis; elderly patients with dementia-related psychosis are at increased risk of death; vulnerability to life-threatening opioid overdose; precipitation of opioid withdrawal in patients who are dependent on opioids

## Pearls

Head-to-head study shows smaller increases in weight and waist circumference and similar efficacy compared to olanzapine monotherapy; consider opioid urine screen prior to initiating drug to avoid causing withdrawal in opioid users

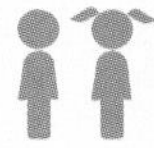

Safety and efficacy have not been established in pediatric patients

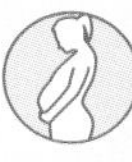

Some animal studies show adverse effects; no controlled studies in pregnant women; recommend either to discontinue drug or bottle feed

## Side effects II

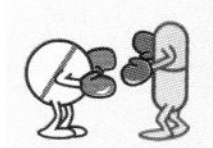

May increase effect of antihypertensive agents; not recommended when using levodopa, dopamine agonists; dose may need to be lowered if given with CYP450 1A2 inhibitors and raised if given with CYP450 1A2 inducers; not recommended when using strong CYP450 3A4 inducers

Use with caution in patients with cardiac impairments

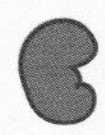

No dosage adjustment is needed in patient with mild, moderate, or severe renal impairment; not recommended in patients with end-stage renal disease

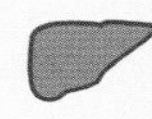

No dose adjustment is needed in patients with hepatic impairment

# The Pines (Peens): Quetiapine

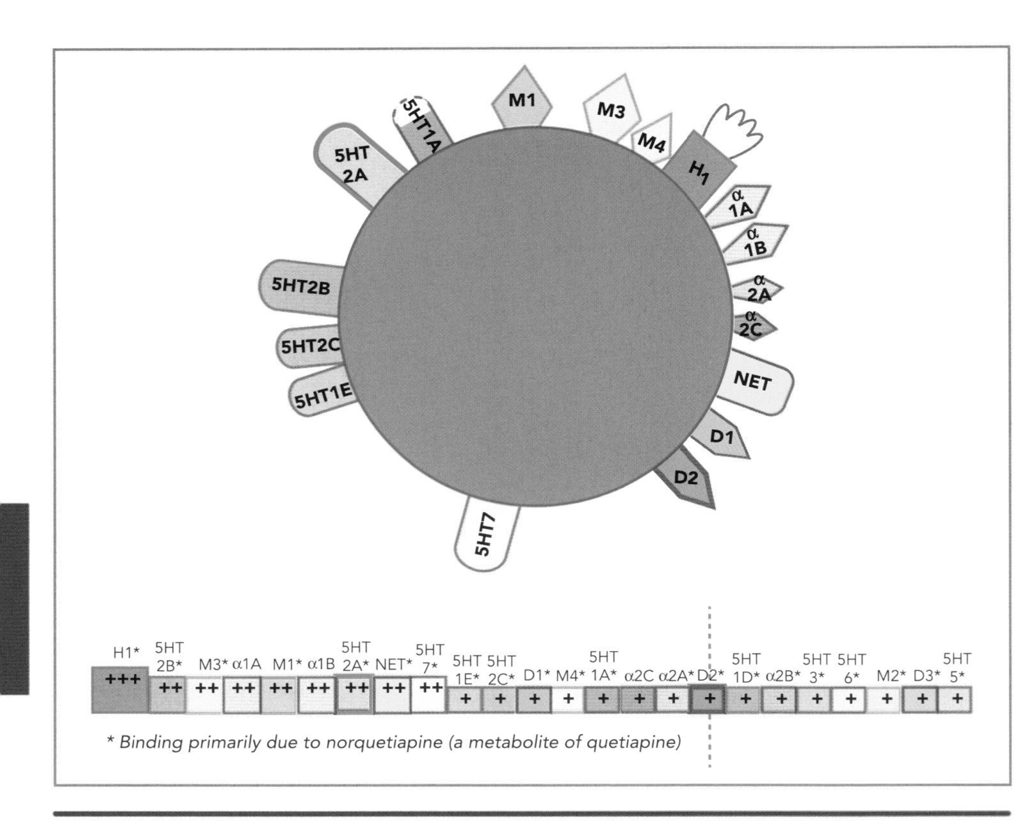


**FIGURE 4.20.** Quetiapine does not have particularly potent binding at D2 receptors. Its prominent H1 antagonist properties probably contribute to its ability to enhance sleep. However, this property can also contribute to daytime sedation, especially combined with M1 antimuscarinic and α1-adrenergic antagonist properties. 5HT1A partial agonist actions, norepinephrine transporter (NET) inhibition, and 5HT2C, α2, and 5HT7 antagonist actions may all contribute to mood-improving properties of quetiapine. However, 5HT2C antagonist actions combined with H1 antagonist actions may contribute to weight gain. The binding properties of quetiapine vary depending on the dose used. At antipsychotic doses (i.e., up to 800 mg/day), quetiapine has a relatively wide binding profile, with actions at multiple serotonergic, muscarinic, and α-adrenergic receptors. H1 receptor blockade is also present. At antidepressant doses (i.e., approximately 300 mg/day), the binding profile of quetiapine is more selective and includes norepinephrine reuptake inhibition, 5HT1A partial agonism, and 5HT2A, α2, 5HT2C, and 5HT7 antagonism. At sedative hypnotic doses (i.e., 50 mg/day), the most prominent pharmacological property of quetiapine is H1 antagonism (Stahl, 2020; Stahl, 2021).

# Quetiapine: Tips and Pearls

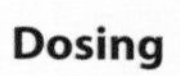

## Dosing

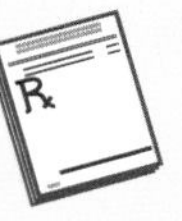

***Formulation:***
25, 50, 100, 150, 200, 300, and 400 mg tablets
50, 150, 200, 300, and 400 mg XR tablets

***Dosage Range:***
400–800 mg/day in 1 (quetiapine XR) or 2 (quetiapine) doses for schizophrenia

***Approved For:***
Acute schizophrenia in adults and ages 13–17, schizophrenia maintenance, acute mania in adults and ages 10–17, bipolar maintenance, bipolar depression, depression

## Side effects I

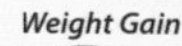

***Weight Gain***

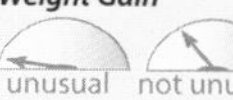
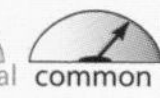
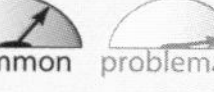


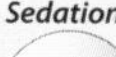

***Sedation***

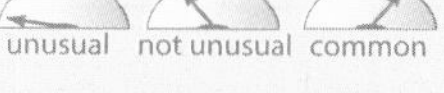
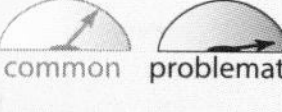

Rare neuroleptic malignant syndrome, seizures; hyperglycemia, ketoacidosis; increased risk of death and cerebrovascular events in elderly patients with dementia

## Pearls

Efficacy may be underestimated for psychosis and mania since quetiapine is often underdosed in clinical practice; essentially no motor side effects or prolactin elevation; may be the preferred antipsychotic for psychosis in Parkinson's disease and Lewy body dementia

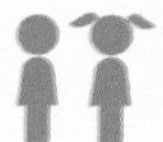

Children and adolescents may need to be monitored more often than adults and may tolerate lower doses better

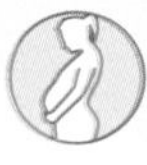

Some animal studies show adverse effects; no controlled studies in pregnant women; recommend either to discontinue drug or bottle feed

## Side effects II

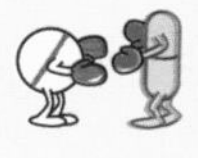

CYP450 3A4 inhibitors and CYP450 2D6 inhibitors may reduce clearance of quetiapine and thus raise quetiapine plasma levels, but dosage reduction of quetiapine usually not necessary; may enhance the effects of antihypertensive drugs; may antagonize levodopa, dopamine agonists

Use with caution in patients with cardiac impairments

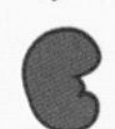

No dose adjustment required

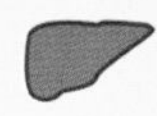

Downward dose adjustment may be necessary

# The Pines (Peens): Asenapine

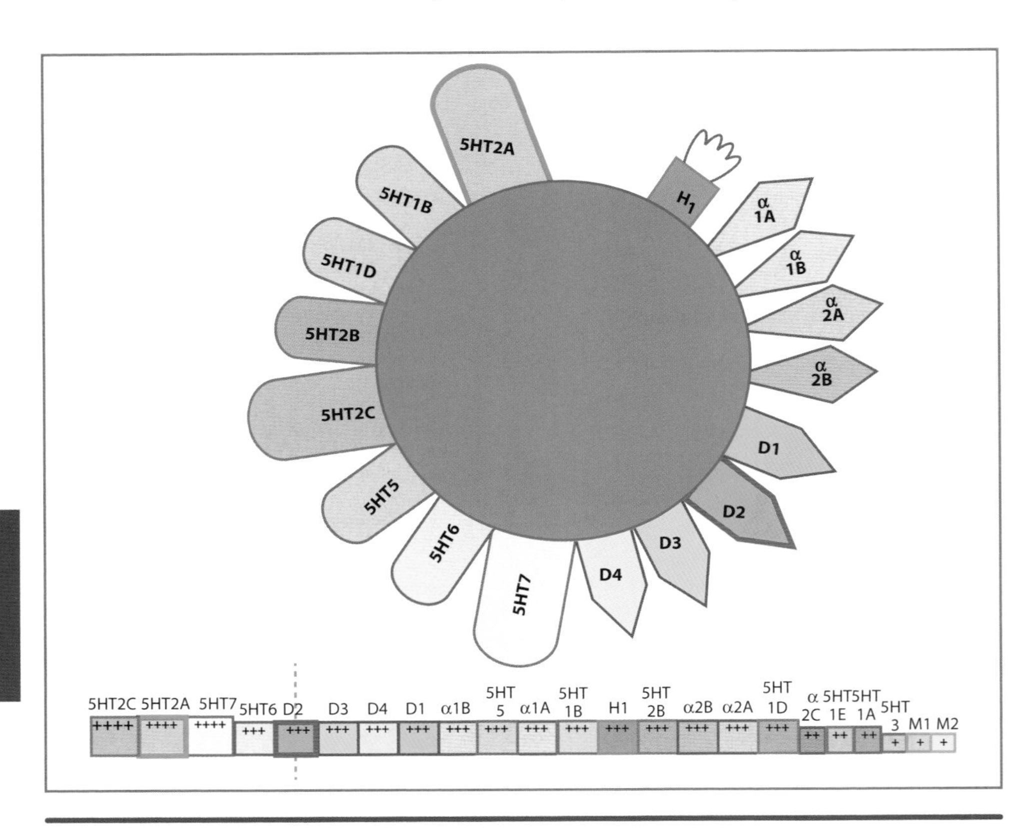


**FIGURE 4.21.** Asenapine has a complex binding profile, with potent binding at multiple serotonergic and dopaminergic receptors, α1 and α2 receptors, and H1 histamine receptors. 5HT2C antagonist properties may contribute to its efficacy for mood and cognitive symptoms, while 5HT7 antagonist properties may contribute to its efficacy for mood, cognitive, and sleep symptoms. Asenapine is available in sublingual and transdermal formulations. Sublingually, it is absorbed rapidly, with rapid peak drug levels; therefore, it can be used as a rapid-acting oral PRN (as needed) drug for psychosis to "top up" patients without resorting to an injection (Stahl, 2020; Stahl, 2021).

# Asenapine: Tips and Pearls

## Dosing

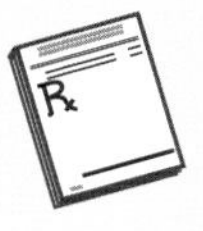

***Formulation:***
2.5, 5, and 10 mg sublingual tablets
3.8, 5.7, and 7.6 mg/24 hours transdermal patches

***Dosage Range:***
10–20 mg/day in 2 divided doses (sublingual)
3.8–7.6 mg/24 hours (transdermal)

***Approved For:***
Schizophrenia in adults (sublingual, transdermal), acute mania/mixed mania monotherapy ages 10–17 and adults (sublingual), acute mania/mixed mania adjunct to lithium or valproate in adults (sublingual), bipolar maintenance in adults (sublingual)

## Side effects I

***Weight Gain***

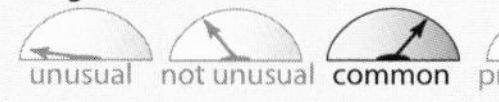


***Sedation***

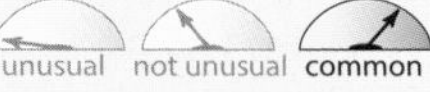

Rare neuroleptic malignant syndrome, seizures; hyperglycemia, ketoacidosis; type 1 hypersensitivity reactions; increased risk of death and cerebrovascular events in elderly patients with dementia; drug-induced movement disorders

## Pearls

Sublingual administration may require prescribing to reliable, adherent patients, or those who have someone who can supervise drug administration

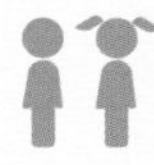

Efficacy of sublingual formulation for schizophrenia has not been demonstrated; transdermal formulation only approved in adults

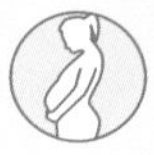

Some animal studies show adverse effects; no controlled studies in pregnant women; recommend either to discontinue drug or bottle feed

## Side effects II

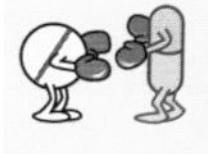

CYP450 1A2 inhibitors increase plasma levels; inhibits CYP450 2D6; may increase effects of antihypertensive agents; may antagonize levodopa, dopamine agonists

Use with caution in patients with cardiac impairments

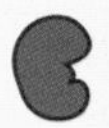

Dose adjustment not generally necessary

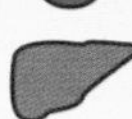

No dose adjustment necessary for mild to moderate impairment; contraindicated in patients with severe hepatic impairment

# The Pines (Peens): Zotepine

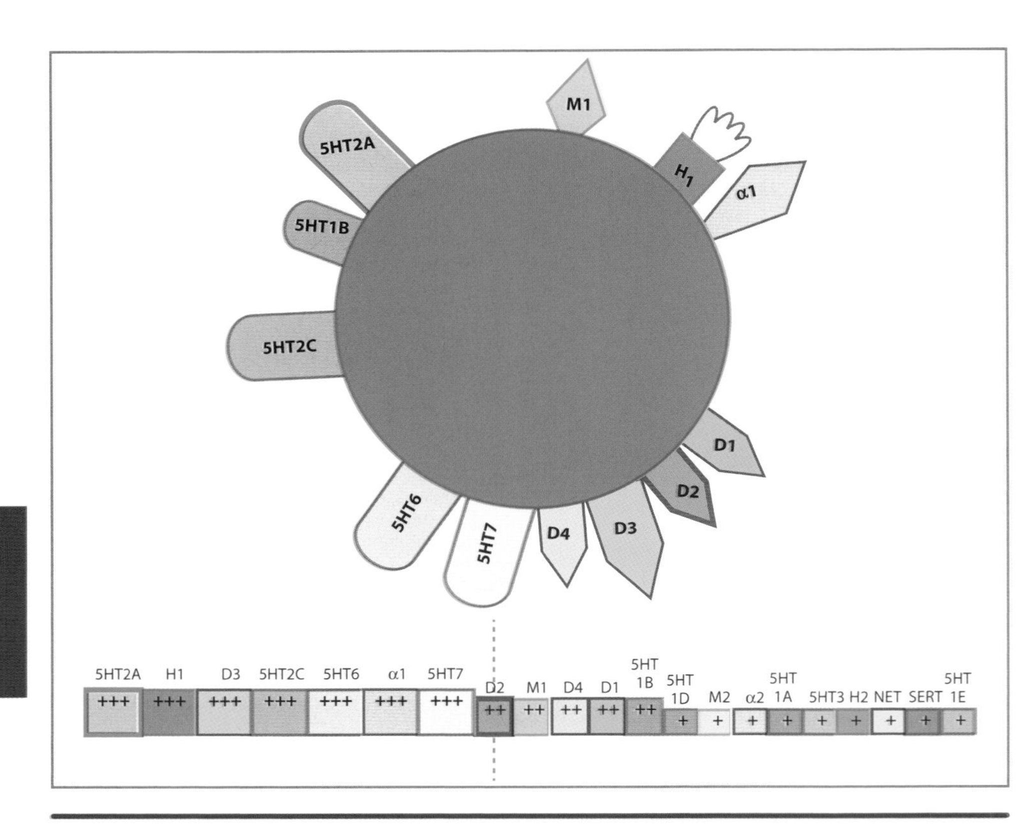


**FIGURE 4.22.** Zotepine has 5HT2A and D2 antagonist properties but is not as popular as other drugs for psychosis because it must be administered three times a day. It is also a 5HT2C antagonist, an α2 antagonist, and a 5HT7 antagonist, suggesting potential antidepressant effects. It is available in Japan and Europe, but not the US (Stahl, 2020; Stahl, 2021).

# Zotepine: Tips and Pearls

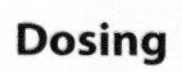

## Dosing

*Formulation:*
25, 50, and 100 mg tablets

*Dosage Range:*
75–300 mg/day in 3 divided doses

*Approved For:*
Not available in the US

## Pearls

Inhibits NE reuptake, thus possibly efficacious for cognitive and mood symptoms

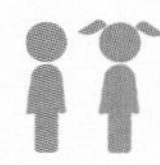

Not recommended for use under age 18

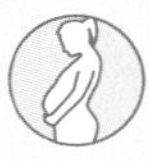

Not recommended during pregnancy or breastfeeding; insufficient data in humans

## Side effects I

*Weight Gain*

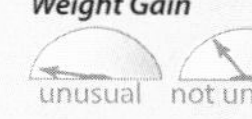


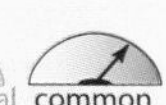


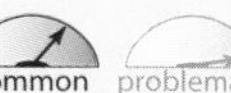


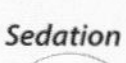

*Sedation*

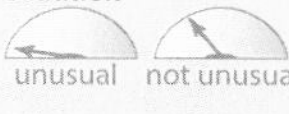


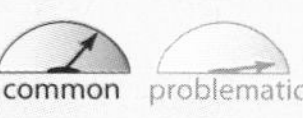


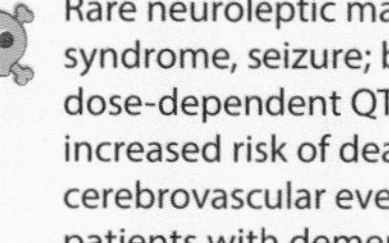

Rare neuroleptic malignant syndrome, seizure; blood dyscrasias; dose-dependent QTc prolongation; increased risk of death and cerebrovascular events in elderly patients with dementia; drug-induced movement disorders

## Side effects II

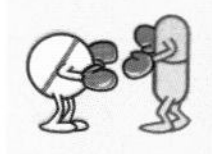

CYP450 1A2 and 3A4 inhibitors increase its plasma levels, CYP 1A2 inducers lower them; combined use with phenothiazines may increase risk of seizures; can decrease the effects of levodopa, dopamine agonists

Use with caution due to dose-dependent increases of QTc prolongation

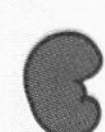

Best to start at 25 mg twice a day, max dose of 75 mg twice a day in patients with renal impairment

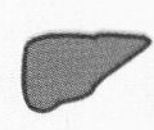

Best to start at 25 mg twice a day, max dose of 75 mg twice a day in patients with hepatic impairment

# The Dones and a Rone: Risperidone

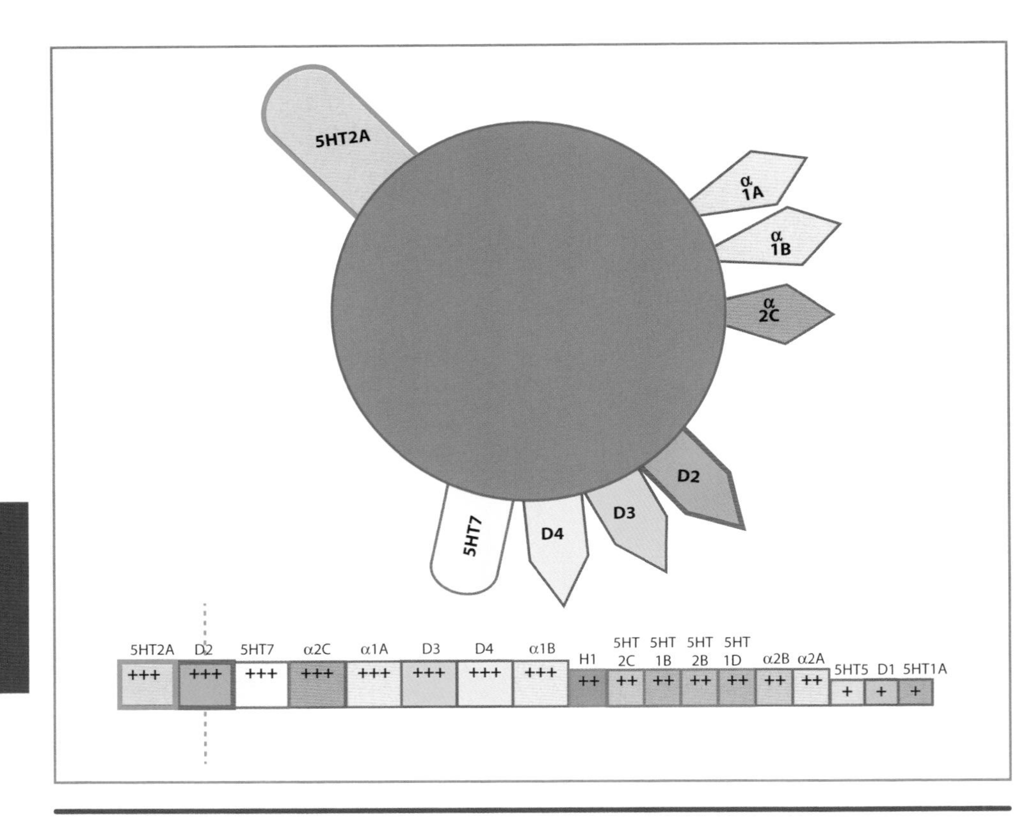


**FIGURE 4.23.** Risperidone is mostly a 5HT2A/D2 antagonist. Alpha-2 antagonist properties may contribute to efficacy for depression, but this can be diminished by simultaneous α1 antagonist properties, which can also contribute to orthostatic hypotension and sedation (Stahl, 2020; Stahl, 2021).

# Risperidone: Tips and Pearls

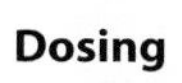

## Dosing

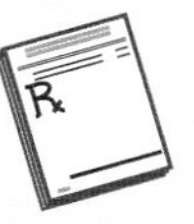

***Formulation:***
0.25, 0.5, 1, 2, 3, 4, and 6 mg tablets
0.5, 1, 2, 3, and 4 mg orally disintegrating tablets
Also available in LAI formulations (IM, SC)

***Dosage Range:***
2–8 mg/day
0.5–2 mg/day for children and elderly

***Approved For:***
Schizophrenia, delaying relapse in schizophrenia, other psychotic disorders, acute mania/mixed mania, autism-related irritability in children ages 5–16, bipolar maintenance

## Pearls

Less may be more; good treatment for agitation/aggression (elderly) and behavioral symptoms (children and adolescents); dose-dependent movement disorder; in women with low estrogen, hyperprolactinemia may accelerate osteoporosis

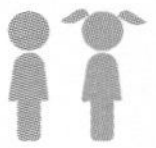

Approved for autism-related irritability (ages 5 to 16), bipolar disorder (ages 10 to 17), and schizophrenia (ages 13 to 17); may need to be monitored more often than adults

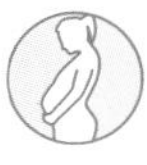

Some animal studies show adverse effects; no controlled studies in pregnant women; recommend either to discontinue drug or bottle feed

## Side effects I

***Weight Gain***

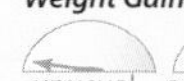
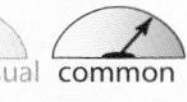
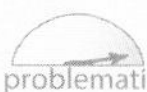


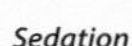

***Sedation***

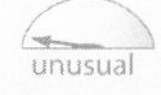
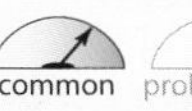
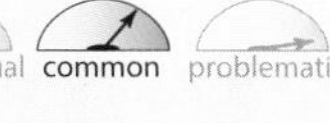


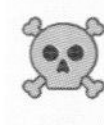

Hyperglycemia, ketoacidosis; rare neuroleptic malignant syndrome, seizure; increased risk of death in elderly; drug-induced movement disorder; hyperprolactinemia

## Side effects II

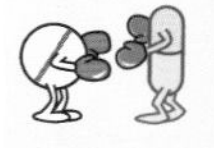

CYP450 2D6 inhibitors can increase its plasma levels; drug increases effects of antihypertensives and decreases DA agonist effects

Use with caution in elderly patients with atrial fibrillation

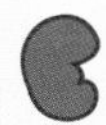

In patients with renal impairments, only use long-acting depot if patient tolerates oral formulation

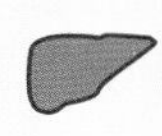

In patients with hepatic impairments, only use long-acting depot if patient tolerates oral formulation

# The Dones and a Rone: Paliperidone

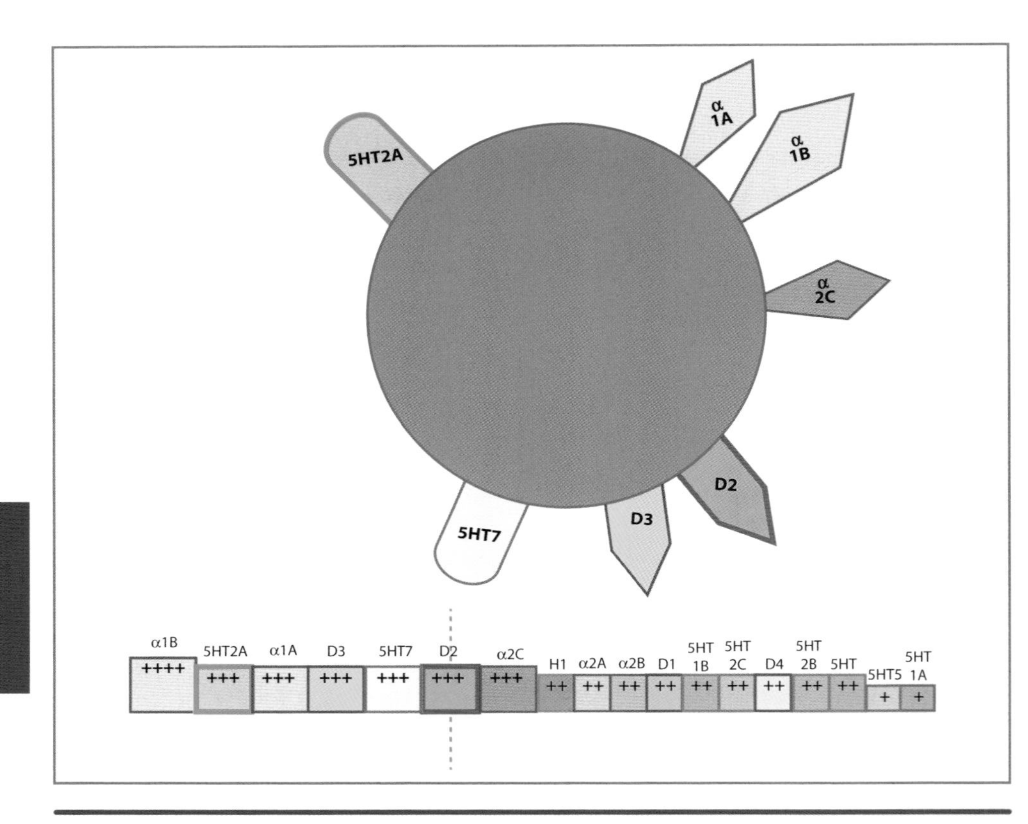


**FIGURE 4.24.** Paliperidone, the active metabolite of risperidone, is also known as 9-hydroxy-risperidone and, like risperidone, has 5HT2A and D2 receptor antagonism. One pharmacokinetic difference, however, between risperidone and paliperidone is that paliperidone, unlike risperidone, is not hepatically metabolized, but its elimination is based upon urinary excretion and thus it has few pharmacokinetic drug interactions. Despite the similar receptor-binding characteristics of paliperidone and risperidone, paliperidone tends to be more tolerable, with less sedation, less orthostasis, and fewer motor side effects, although this is based upon anecdotal clinical experience and not head-to-head clinical studies (Stahl, 2020; Stahl, 2021).

# Paliperidone: Tips and Pearls

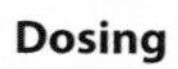
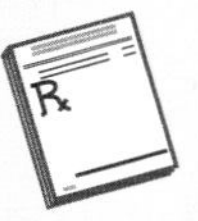

## Dosing

***Formulation:***
1.5, 3, 6, and 9 mg extended-release tablets
Also available in LAI formulations (paliperidone palmitate)

***Dosage Range:***
3–12 mg/day, with 6 mg/day having optimum efficacy
Adolescents <51 kg: initial 3 mg/day; recommended 3–6 mg/day; maximum 6 mg/day
Adolescents >51 kg: initial 3 mg/day; recommended 3–12 mg/day; maximum 12 mg/day

***Approved For:***
Schizophrenia (ages 12 and older), maintaining response in schizophrenia, schizoaffective disorder

## Side effects I

***Weight Gain***

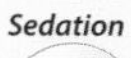

***Sedation***

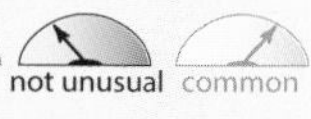
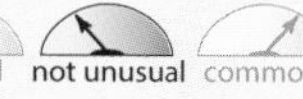

Hyperglycemia, ketoacidosis; rare neuroleptic malignant syndrome, seizure; increased risk of death in elderly; drug-induced movement disorder; hyperprolactinemia

## Pearls

Some patients respond to or tolerate paliperidone better than the parent drug risperidone; dose-dependent increase in some side effects, including drug-induced movement disorders and weight gain; in women with low estrogen, hyperprolactinemia may accelerate osteoporosis

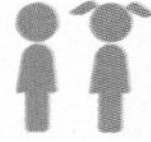
Safety and efficacy have not been established under age 12

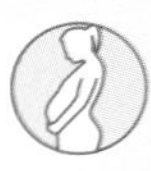
Some animal studies show adverse effects; no controlled studies in pregnant women; recommend either to discontinue drug or bottle feed

## Side effects II

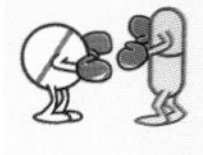
May increase effects of antihypertensive agents; may antagonize levodopa, dopamine agonists; may enhance QTc prolongation of other drugs capable of prolonging QTc interval

Use with caution in patients with cardiac impairments

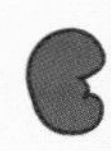
For mild impairment, the maximum recommended dose is 6 mg/day; the initial and maximum dose for moderate impairment is 3 mg/day, the initial dose is 1.5 mg/day, and the maximum dose is 3 mg/day for severe impairment

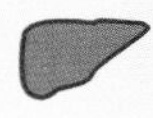
No dose adjustment for mild to moderate impairment; no studies in severe hepatic impairment

# The Dones and a Rone: Ziprasidone

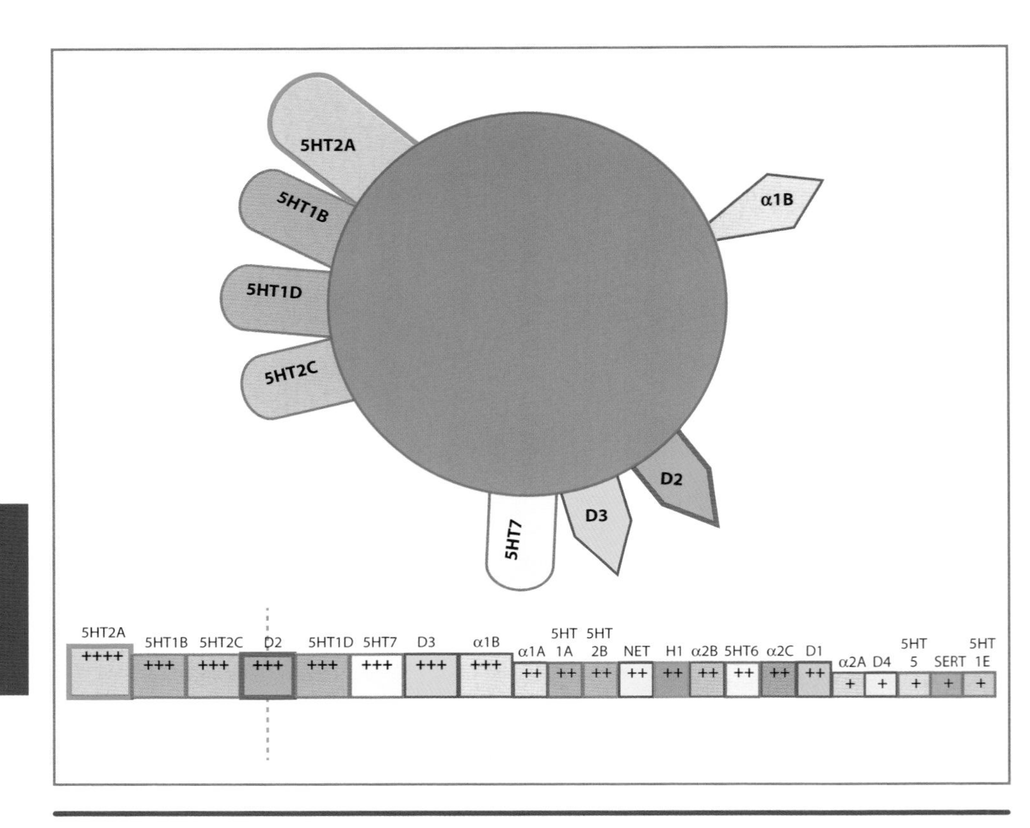


**FIGURE 4.25.** Ziprasidone is a 5HT2A/D2 antagonist that seems to lack the pharmacological actions associated with weight gain and increased cardiometabolic risk, such as increasing fasting plasma triglyceride levels or increasing insulin resistance. Ziprasidone also lacks many of the pharmacological properties associated with significant sedation. However, it is short acting, requires more than once a day dosing, and must be taken with food. Earlier concerns about dangerous QTc prolongation by ziprasidone now appear to be exaggerated (Stahl, 2020; Stahl, 2021).

# Ziprasidone: Tips and Pearls

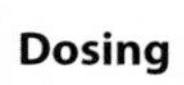

## Dosing

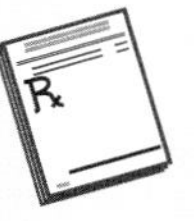

***Formulation:***
20, 40, 60, and 80 mg capsules
20 mg/mL injection

***Dosage Range:***
40–200 mg/day PO in divided doses
10–20 mg IM

***Approved For:***
Schizophrenia, delaying relapse in schizophrenia, acute agitation in schizophrenia (IM), acute mania/mixed mania, bipolar maintenance

## Pearls

It is often underdosed; more activating than some other drugs for psychosis at low doses; food doubles bioavailability; lower metabolic side effects than other drugs for psychosis

Not officially recommended for patients under age 18; clinical experience and early data suggest drug may be safe and effective for behavioral disturbances in children and adolescents

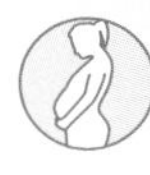

Some animal studies show adverse effects; no controlled studies in pregnant women; recommend either to discontinue drug or bottle feed

## Side effects I

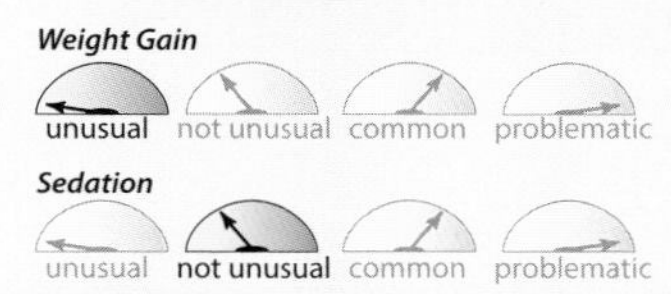


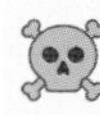

Rare Drug Reaction with Eosinophilia and Systemic Symptoms (DRESS), neuroleptic malignant syndrome, ketoacidosis, seizures; increased risk of death in elderly; drug-induced movement disorder

## Side effects II

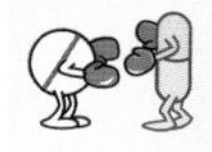

Not affected by CYP450 enzymes; drug increases effects of antihypertensives and decreases DA agonist effects; may enhance QTc prolongation of other drugs that enhance QTc prolongation

Contraindicated in patients with a known history of QTc prolongation, recent acute myocardial infarction, and uncompensated heart failure

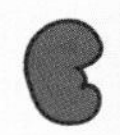

No dose adjustment necessary in patients with renal impairments; use IM formulation with caution

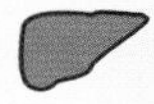

No dose adjustment necessary in patients with hepatic impairments

# The Dones and a Rone: Iloperidone

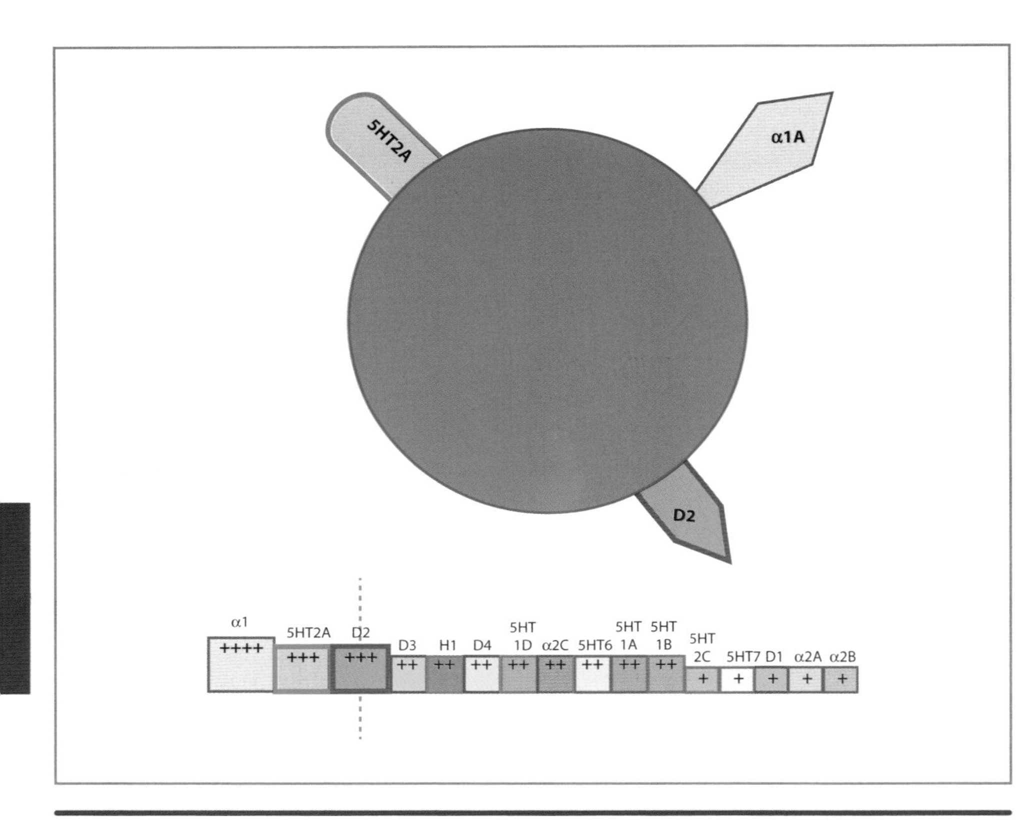


**FIGURE 4.26.** Iloperidone also has 5HT2A/D2 antagonist properties. Among the medications discussed here, iloperidone has one of the simplest pharmacological profiles and comes closest to a serotonin dopamine antagonist (SDA). Its other prominent pharmacological property is potent α1 antagonism, which may be responsible for the risk of orthostatic hypotension but also may contribute to its low risk of drug-induced parkinsonism (DIP). Its most distinguishing clinical properties include a very low level of motor side effects, low level of dyslipidemia, and moderate level of weight gain associated with its use. Iloperidone is generally dosed twice daily and titrated over several days when initiated in order to avoid both orthostasis and sedation. Slow dosing can delay onset of antipsychotic effects, so iloperidone is often used as a switch agent in non-urgent situations (Stahl, 2020; Stahl, 2021).

# Iloperidone: Tips and Pearls

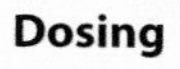

## Dosing

***Formulation:***
1, 2, 4, 6, 8, 10, and 12 mg tablets

***Dosage Range:***
12–24 mg/day in 2 divided doses

***Approved For:***
Schizophrenia and schizophrenia maintenance

## Pearls

Titrate slowly to avoid orthostatic hypotension; low drug-induced parkinsonism and little or no akathisia; QTc warning similar to that for ziprasidone, where this has not materialized into a significant clinical problem

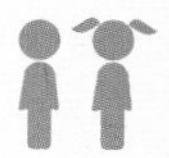

Efficacy and safety not established in children and adolescents

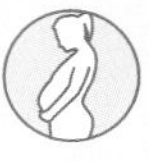

Some animal studies show adverse effects; no controlled studies in pregnant women; recommend either to discontinue drug or bottle feed

## Side effects I

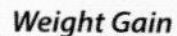

***Weight Gain***

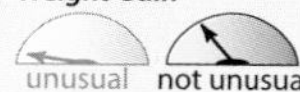

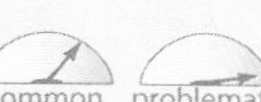

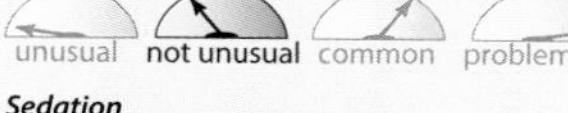


***Sedation***

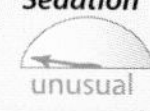

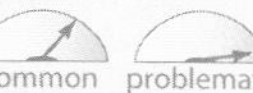

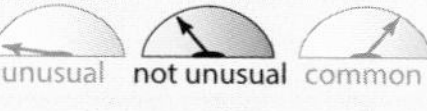


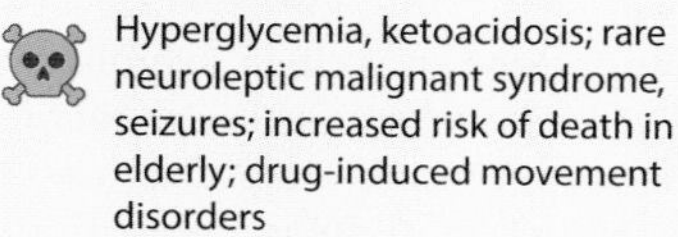

Hyperglycemia, ketoacidosis; rare neuroleptic malignant syndrome, seizures; increased risk of death in elderly; drug-induced movement disorders

## Side effects II

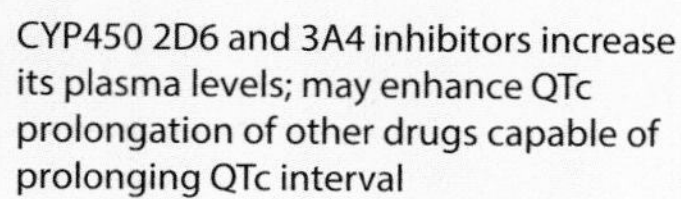

CYP450 2D6 and 3A4 inhibitors increase its plasma levels; may enhance QTc prolongation of other drugs capable of prolonging QTc interval

Not recommended for patients with significant cardiovascular illness

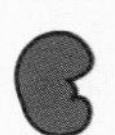

Dose adjustment not necessary for patients with renal impairments

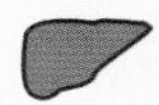

Not recommended for patients with hepatic impairments

# The Dones and a Rone: Lurasidone

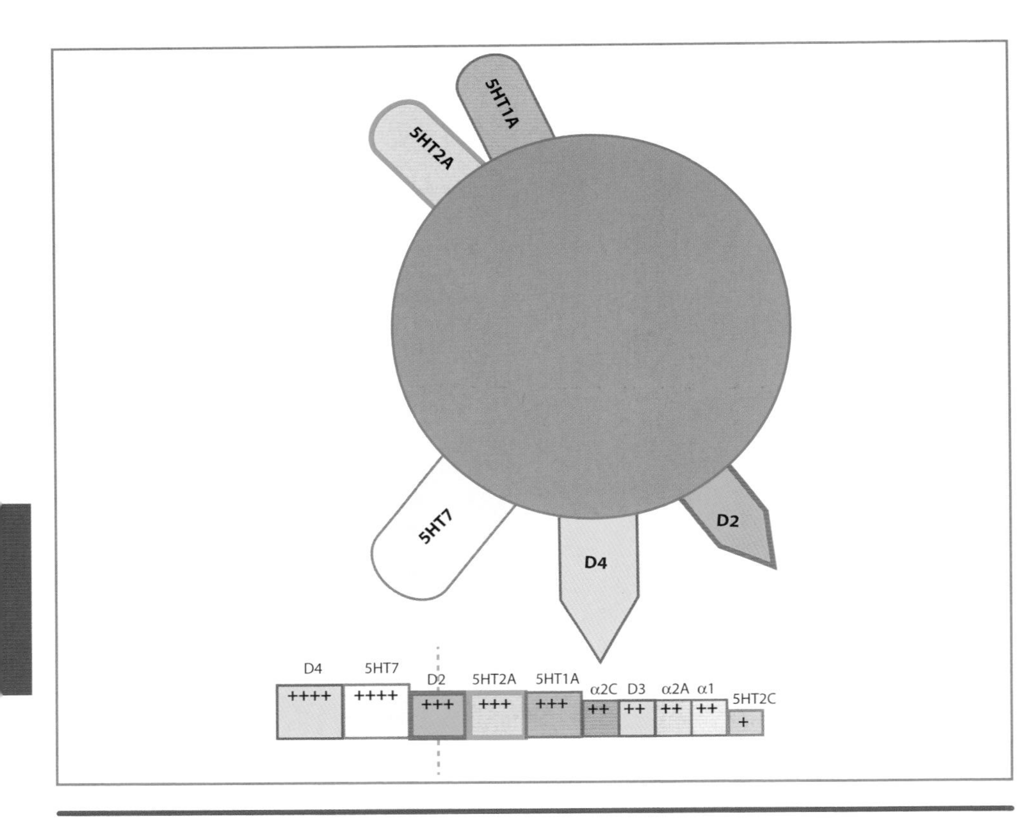


**FIGURE 4.27.** In addition to its 5HT2A/D2 antagonist properties, lurasidone exhibits highest affinity for the D4 and 5HT7 receptors. The effects of D4 are not well understood, but binding at the 5HT7 receptor may contribute to lurasidone's efficacy for mood, cognitive, and sleep symptoms. Indeed, lurasidone is much more popular for use in bipolar depression than schizophrenia (Stahl, 2020; Stahl, 2021).

# Lurasidone: Tips and Pearls

## Dosing

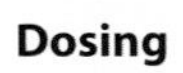

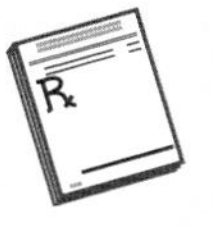

*Formulation:*
20, 40, 50, 80, and 120 mg tablets

*Dosage Range:*
40–80 mg/day for schizophrenia; some patients may benefit from doses up to 160 mg/day

*Approved For:*
Schizophrenia (ages 13 and older), bipolar depression (ages 10 and older, monotherapy), bipolar depression (adults, adjunct)

## Pearls

Dose with food; one of the few "metabolically friendly" drugs for psychosis; low-level drug-induced parkinsonism, especially when dosed at bedtime

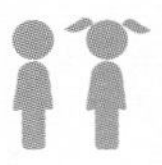

Best to initiate with 20 mg/day dose to test for tolerability; little or no weight gain documented in long-term studies up to 2 years

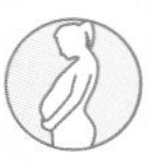

Animal studies have not shown adverse effects; no controlled studies in pregnant women; recommended either to discontinue drug or bottle feed

## Side effects I

*Weight Gain*

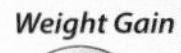

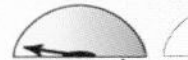

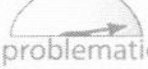

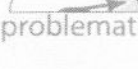



*Sedation*

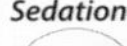

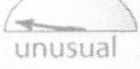

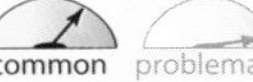

Tachycardia, first-degree atrioventricular block; hyperglycemia, ketoacidosis; rare neuroleptic malignant syndrome, seizures; increased risk of death in elderly; drug-induced movement disorders

## Side effects II

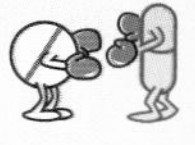

CYP450 3A4 inhibitors may increase drug plasma levels and moderate inducers may decrease drug plasma levels; co-administration with a strong CYP450 3A4 inhibitor or with a strong CYP450 3A4 inducer is contraindicated

Use with caution in patients with cardiac impairments

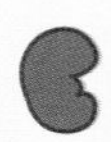

In adults with moderate and severe impairment: initial dose 20 mg/day and maximum dose 80 mg/day

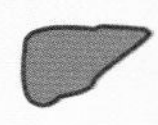

Moderate impairment: initial dose 20 mg/day and maximum dose 80 mg/day; severe impairment: initial dose 20 mg/day and maximum dose 40 mg/day

# The Dones and a Rone: Lumateperone

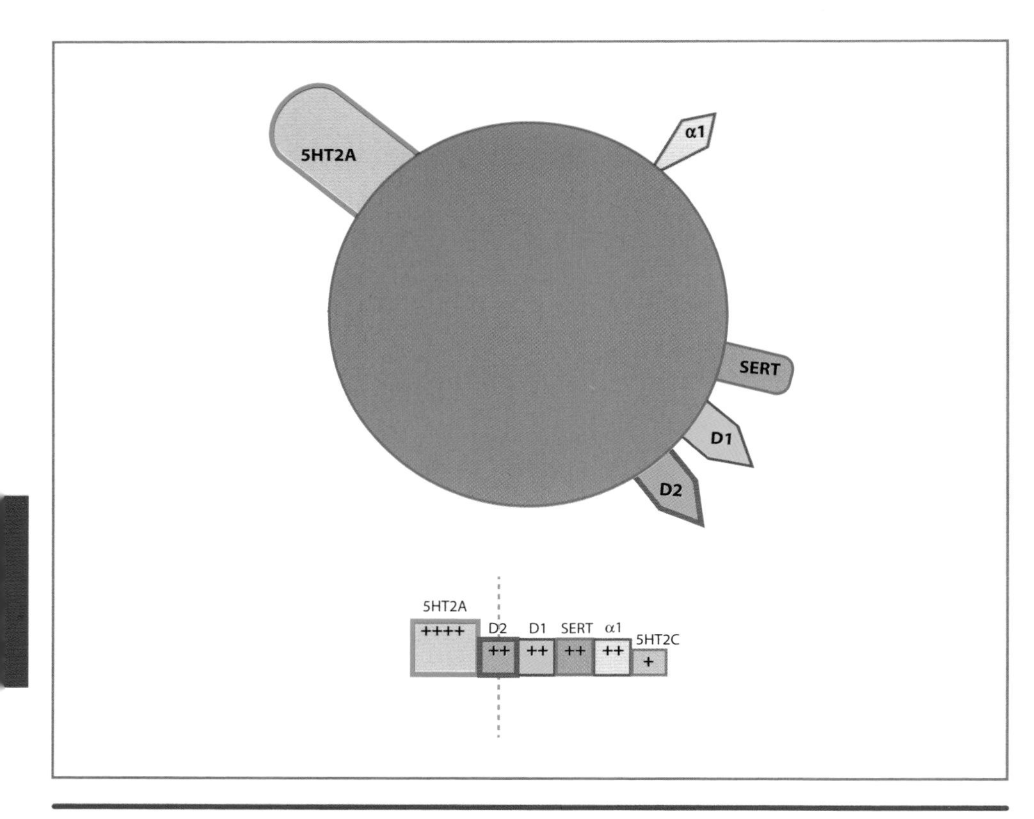


**FIGURE 4.28.** Lumateperone is a 5HT2A/D2 antagonist with very high affinity for the 5HT2A receptor and moderate affinity for the D2, D1, and α1 receptor. It also has moderate affinity for the serotonin transporter. Two key points on its mechanism of action include a wide separation between its 5HT2A antagonist and its D2 antagonist binding, perhaps explaining why it has antipsychotic actions at doses that have relatively low occupancy of D2 receptors, and maybe also why there are low D2-type side effects (e.g., little or no drug-induced parkinsonism or akathisia) (Stahl, 2020; Stahl, 2021).

Although not yet clarified completely, preclinical evidence suggests a novel mechanism of action of lumateperone at D2 receptors. Specifically, lumateperone may have presynaptic agonist actions and postsynaptic antagonist actions, a unique combination of mechanisms that would theoretically turn off dopamine synthesis presynaptically to reduce the oversupply of dopamine present in presynaptic dopamine synapses in psychosis. Further investigations are needed to clarify this possible explanation (Zhang & Hendrick, 2018).

# Lumateperone: Tips and Pearls

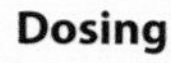

## Dosing

***Formulation:***
42 mg capsule

***Dosage Range:***
42 mg/day

***Approved For:***
Schizophrenia and bipolar depression (monotherapy and adjunct)

## Pearls

Take in the evening to help reduce daytime sedation; favorable metabolic profile; may have prosocial effects; neutral for drug-induced parkinsonism and akathisia

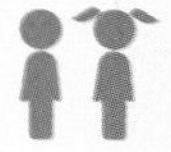

Safety and efficacy have not been established in children and adolescents

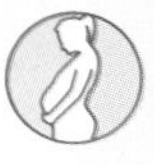

Some animal studies show adverse effects; no controlled studies in pregnant women; recommend either to discontinue drug or bottle feed

## Side effects I

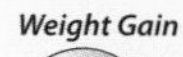



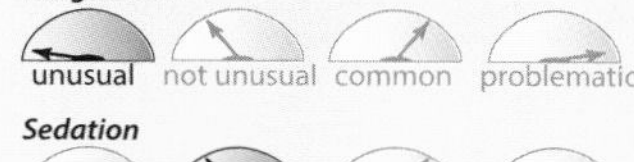



***Sedation***

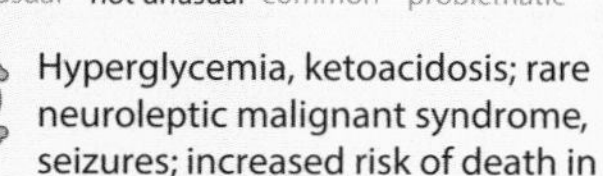



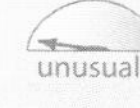

Hyperglycemia, ketoacidosis; rare neuroleptic malignant syndrome, seizures; increased risk of death in elderly; tardive dyskinesia

## Side effects II

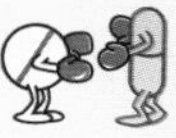

Avoid using with moderate or strong CYP450 3A4 inhibitors and with CYP450 3A4 inducers; avoid using with UGT (uridine 5′-diphospho-glucuronosyltransferase) inhibitors

Use with caution in patients with cardiac impairments

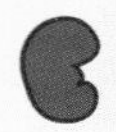

Dose adjustments not necessary in patients with renal impairments

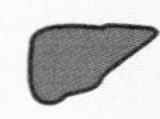

Dose adjustments not necessary in patients with mild hepatic impairments; not recommended for use in patients with moderate to severe impairment

# Other 5HT2A/D2 Antagonists: Sertindole

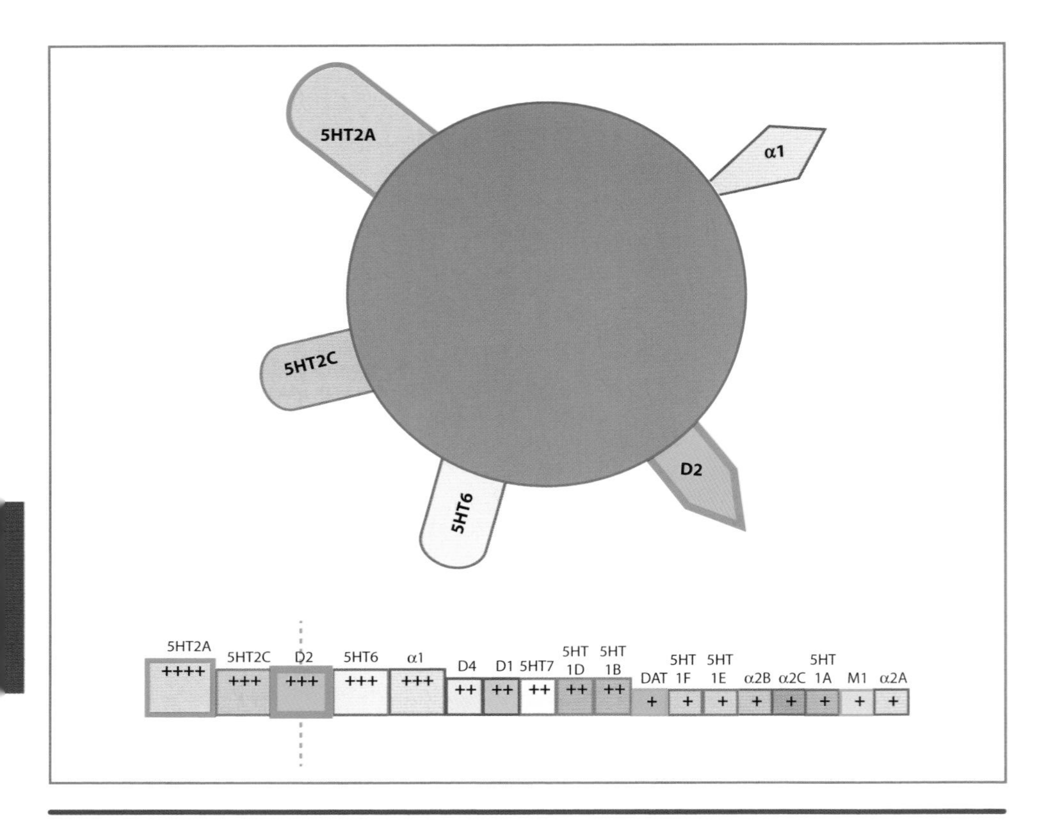


**FIGURE 4.29.** Sertindole is a 5HT2A/D2 receptor antagonist originally approved in some European countries, then withdrawn for further testing of its cardiac safety and QTc-prolonging potential, and then reintroduced into certain countries as a second-line agent. Potent antagonist actions at α1 receptors may account for some of sertindole's side effects. It may be useful for some patients in whom other antipsychotics have failed, and who can have close monitoring of their cardiac status and drug interactions (Stahl, 2020; Stahl, 2021).

# Sertindole: Tips and Pearls

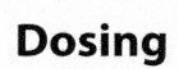

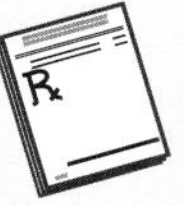

## Dosing

***Formulation:***
4, 12, 16, and 20 mg tablets

***Dosage Range:***
12–20 mg/day

***Approved For:***
Not available in the US

## Side effects I

***Weight Gain***

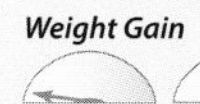
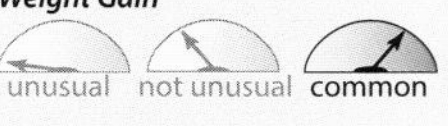


***Sedation***

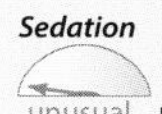
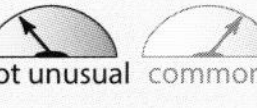
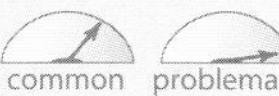


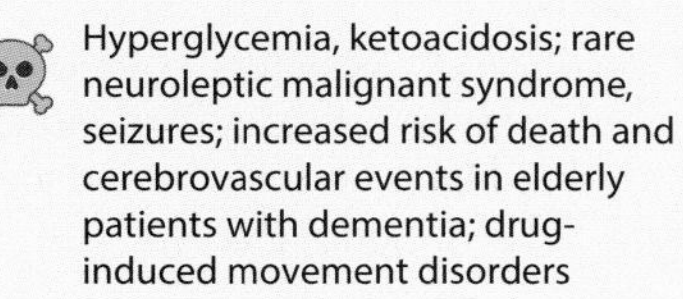

Hyperglycemia, ketoacidosis; rare neuroleptic malignant syndrome, seizures; increased risk of death and cerebrovascular events in elderly patients with dementia; drug-induced movement disorders

## Pearls

Aimed at patients who are intolerant to at least one other antipsychotic and when potential benefits outweigh potential risks

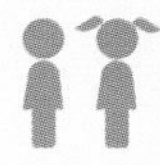

Safety and efficacy unknown in children and adolescents

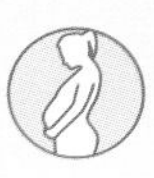

Some animal studies show adverse effects; no controlled studies in pregnant women; recommend either to discontinue drug or bottle feed

## Side effects II

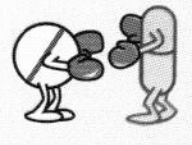

CYP450 2D6 and 3A4 inhibitors increase its plasma levels, and inducers decrease its plasma levels; may enhance QTc prolongation of other drugs capable of prolonging QTc interval

Do not use in patients with significant cardiovascular disease, congestive heart failure, cardiac hypertrophy, arrythmia, bradycardia, personal or family history of congenital prolonged QTc syndrome

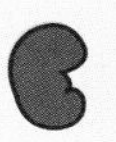

Dose adjustments not necessary in patients with renal impairments

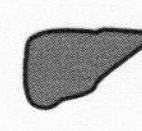

For mild to moderate impairment, use slower titration and lower maintenance dose; contraindicated in patients with severe hepatic impairment

# Other 5HT2A/D2 Antagonists: Perospirone

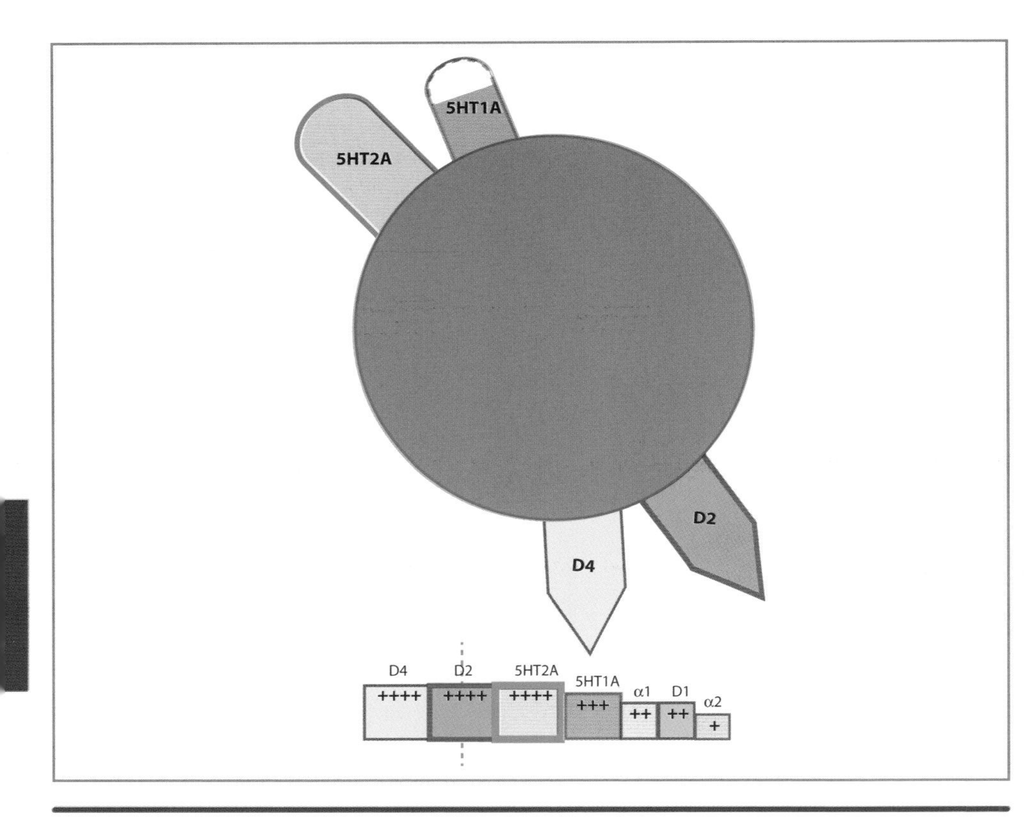


**FIGURE 4.30.** Perospirone is another 5HT2A and D2 antagonist available in Asia to treat schizophrenia. 5HT1A partial agonist actions may contribute to efficacy for mood and cognitive symptoms. Its ability to cause weight gain, dyslipidemia, insulin resistance, and diabetes is not well investigated (Kishi et al., 2014; Stahl, 2020; Stahl, 2021).

# Perospirone: Tips and Pearls

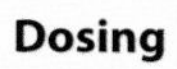
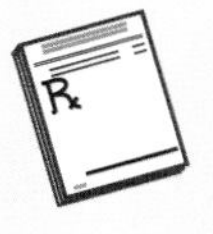

## Dosing

***Formulation:***
4, 8 mg tablets

***Dosage Range:***
8–48 mg/day in 3 divided doses

***Approved For:***
Not available in the US

## Side effects I

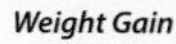

***Weight Gain***

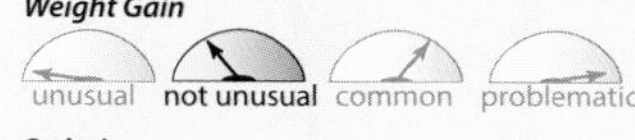


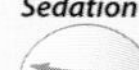

***Sedation***

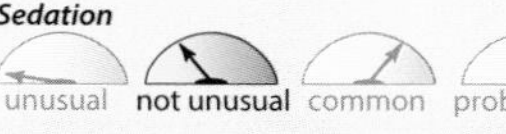

Rare neuroleptic malignant syndrome, seizures; increased risk of death and cerebrovascular events in elderly patients with dementia; drug-induced movement disorders

## Pearls

Drug-induced parkinsonism may be more frequent than with some other second-generation drugs for psychosis; potent 5HT1A binding properties may be helpful for improving cognitive symptoms of schizophrenia in long-term treatment

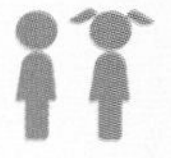

Use with caution in children and adolescents

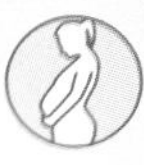

Not recommended during pregnancy or breastfeeding; insufficient data in humans

## Side effects II

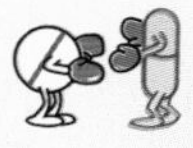

CYP450 3A4 inhibitors increase its plasma levels, CYP450 3A4 inducers decrease its plasma levels

Use with caution in patients with cardiac impairments

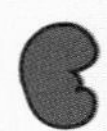

Use with caution in patients with renal impairments

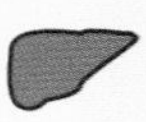

Use with caution in patients with hepatic impairments

# Other 5HT2A/D2 Antagonists: Blonanserin

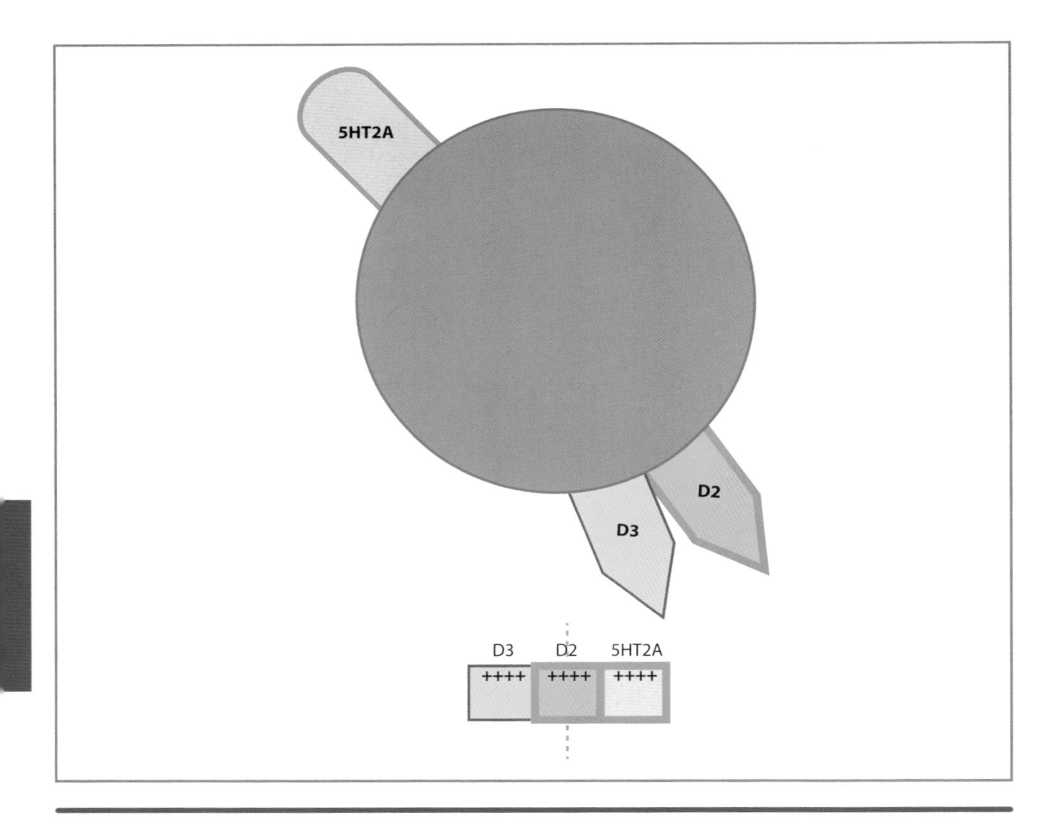


**FIGURE 4.31.** Blonanserin is a 5HT2A/D2 antagonist, available in Asia to treat schizophrenia. It has the unique property of higher affinity for the D3 receptor than DA has for the D3 receptor, suggesting possible utility for the negative symptoms of schizophrenia, but it is not yet well studied for this indication (Stahl, 2020; Stahl, 2021).

# Blonanserin: Tips and Pearls

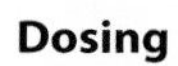

## Dosing

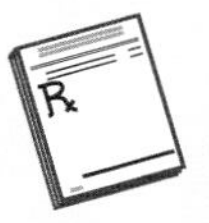

***Formulation:***
2, 4, and 8 mg tablets
20 mg per 1 gram powder

***Dosage Range:***
8–16 mg/day in 2 divided doses

***Approved For:***
Not available in the US

## Side effects I

***Weight Gain***

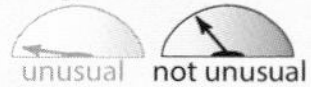


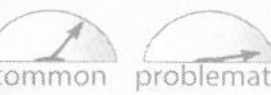


***Sedation***

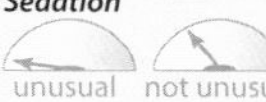

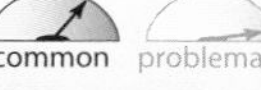


Hyperglycemia, ketoacidosis; rare neuroleptic malignant syndrome, seizures; increased risk of death in elderly patients with dementia; drug-induced movement disorders

## Pearls

D3 antagonist actions have been hypothetically associated with improvement in negative, cognitive, and affective symptoms

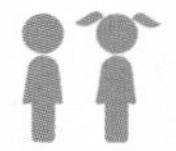

Safety and efficacy have not been established in children or adolescents

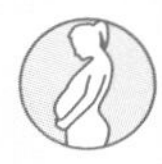

Not recommended during pregnancy or breastfeeding; insufficient data in humans

## Side effects II

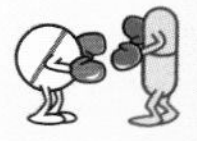

CYP450 3A4 inhibitors increase its plasma levels, CYP450 3A4 inducers decrease its plasma levels

Use with caution in patients with cardiac impairments

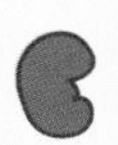

Use with caution in patients with renal impairments

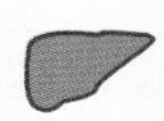

Use with caution in patients with hepatic impairments; may need lower dose

# Two Pips and a Rip: Aripiprazole

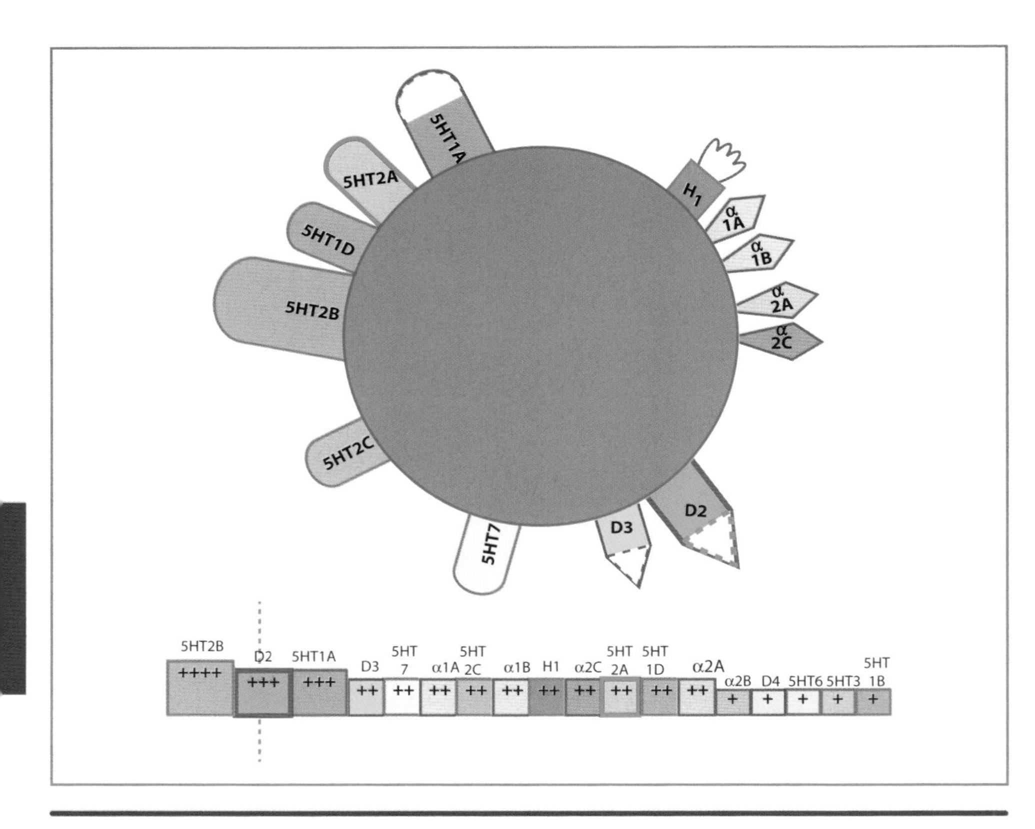


**FIGURE 4.32.** Aripiprazole is a partial agonist at D2 receptors rather than an antagonist. Additional important pharmacological properties that may contribute to its clinical profile include 5HT2A antagonist actions, 5HT1A partial agonist actions, 5HT7 antagonist actions, and 5HT2C antagonist actions. Aripiprazole lacks or has weak binding potency at receptors usually associated with significant sedation. Aripiprazole also seems to lack the pharmacological actions associated with weight gain and increased cardiometabolic risk, such as increasing fasting plasma triglyceride levels or increasing insulin resistance (Stahl, 2020; Stahl, 2021).

# Aripiprazole: Tips and Pearls

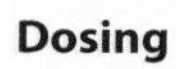

## Dosing

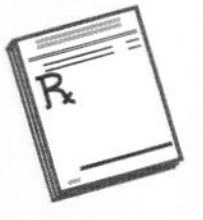

*Formulation:*
2, 5, 10, 15, 20, and 30 mg tablets
10, 15 mg orally disintegrating tablets
1 mg/mL oral solution
9.75 mg/1.3 mL IM injection
Also available in LAI formulations

*Dosage Range:*
15–30 mg/day for schizophrenia

*Approved For:*
Schizophrenia (ages 13 and older); maintaining stability in schizophrenia; acute mania/mixed mania (ages 10 and older); bipolar maintenance; major depressive disorder; autism-related irritability (ages 6 to 17); Tourette's disorder (ages 6 to 18); acute agitation associated with schizophrenia or bipolar disorder

## Side effects I

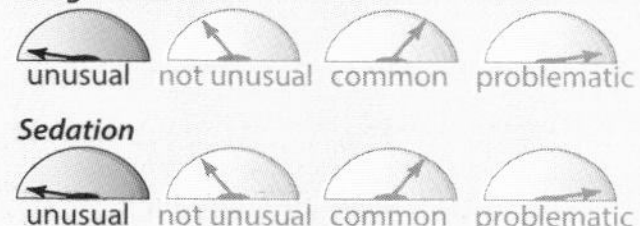

Hyperglycemia; rare impulse control problems, neuroleptic malignant syndrome, seizures; increased risk of death in elderly patients with dementia; drug-induced movement disorders; increased risk of suicide in young people

## Pearls

Can even be activating, which can be reduced by lowering the dose or starting at a lower dose; well accepted in clinical practice when wanting to avoid weight gain or sedation; co-administration (even low doses of 1–5 mg) with another D2 antagonist drug for psychosis can reverse hyperprolactinemia or galactorrhea; anecdotal reports of utility in treatment-resistant cases of psychosis

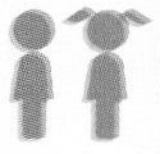

May be more risk of weight gain in children than in adults; children and adolescents may need to be monitored more often than adults and may tolerate lower doses better

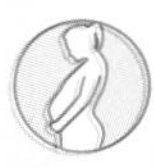

Some animal studies show adverse effects; no controlled studies in pregnant women; recommend either to discontinue drug or bottle feed

## Side effects II

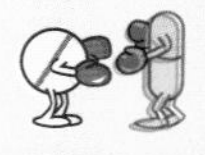

CYP450 3A4 or 2D6 inhibitors increase its plasma levels, and CYP450 3A4 inducers lower them; CYP450 2D6 inhibitors increase its plasma levels; drug increases effects of antihypertensives and decreases DA agonist effects

Use with caution in patients with cardiac impairments due to risk of orthostatic hypotension

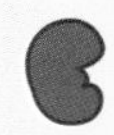

Dose adjustment not necessary in patients with renal impairments

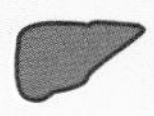

Dose adjustment not necessary in patients with hepatic impairments

# Two Pips and a Rip: Brexpiprazole

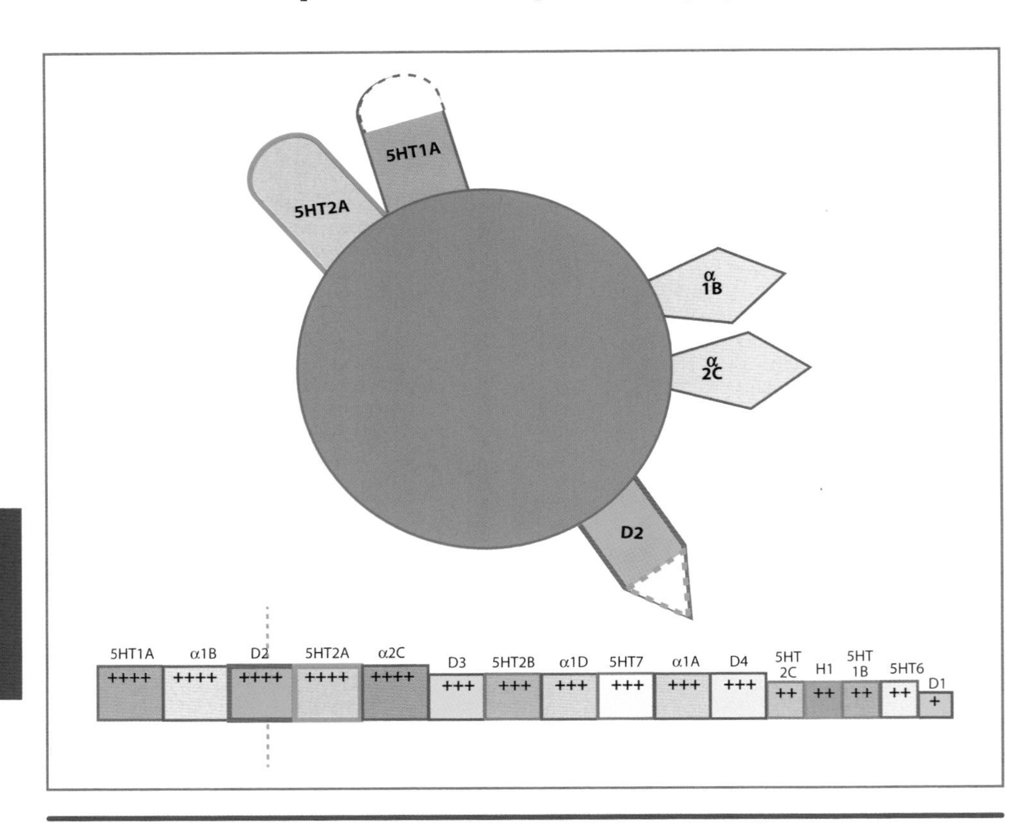


**FIGURE 4.33.** Brexpiprazole is a partial agonist at D2 receptors rather than an antagonist, and binds potently to 5HT2A, 5HT1A, and α1 receptors. Brexpiprazole also seems to lack actions at receptors usually associated with significant sedation, weight gain, and increased cardiometabolic risk, although it is too early to evaluate the clinical profile of this medication (Stahl, 2020; Stahl, 2021).

# Brexpiprazole: Tips and Pearls

## Dosing

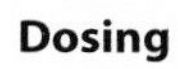

*Formulation:*
0.25, 0.5, 1, 2, 3, and 4 mg tablets

*Dosage Range:*
2–4 mg/day for schizophrenia

*Approved For:*
Schizophrenia (ages 13 and older); major depressive disorder (adjunct); agitation associated with Alzheimer's dementia

## Side effects I

*Weight Gain*

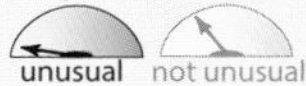
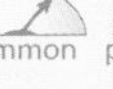


*Sedation*

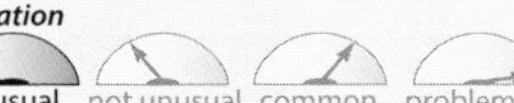

Hyperglycemia, ketoacidosis; rare impulse control problems, neuroleptic malignant syndrome, seizures; increased risk of death in elderly patients with dementia; drug-induced movement disorders; increased risk of suicide in children and young adults

## Pearls

Animal data suggest that drug may improve cognitive impairment in schizophrenia

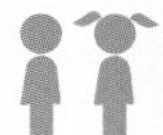
Children and adolescents may need to be monitored more often than adults and may tolerate lower doses better

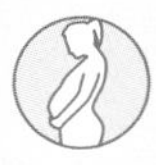
Animal studies have not shown adverse effects; no controlled studies in pregnant women; recommended either to discontinue drug or bottle feed

## Side effects II

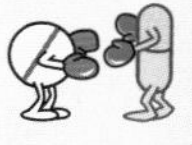
Drug should be administered at half the usual dose when taking with a strong/moderate CYP450 3A4 inhibitor, and at double the dose when taking with a strong inducer; in patients taking strong/moderate CYP450 2D6 inhibitor or who are known poor metabolizer, drug should be administered at half the usual dose (quarter dose if also taking strong/moderate CYP3A4 inhibitor)

Use with caution in patients with cardiac impairments

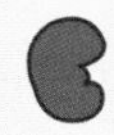
Maximum recommended dose is 3 mg once daily for patients with moderate, severe, or end-stage renal impairment

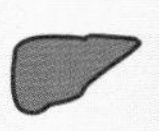
Recommended dose is 3 mg once daily for patients with moderate to severe hepatic impairment

# Two Pips and a Rip: Cariprazine

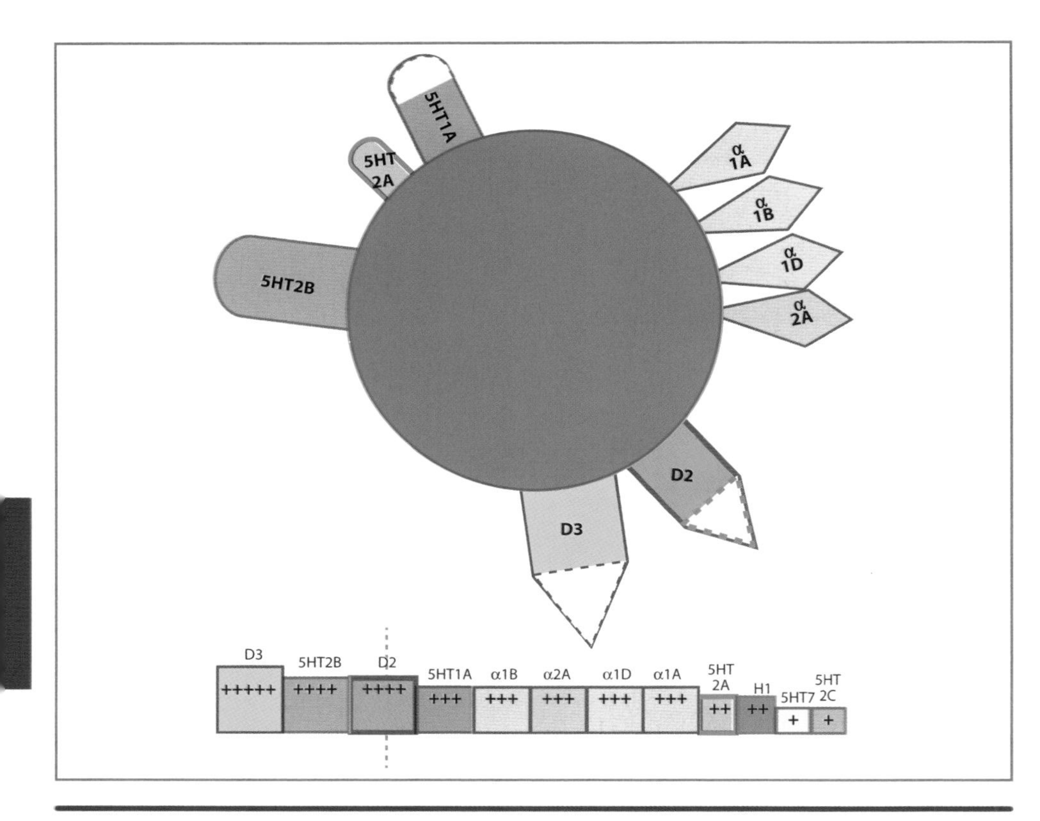


**FIGURE 4.34.** Cariprazine is the "rip" of this group and is another D2/5HT1A partial agonist. It has potent actions at D3, 5HT2B, D2, and 5HT1A receptors, with relatively weaker affinity for 5HT2A and H1 receptors. Cariprazine actually has higher affinity for the D3 receptor than dopamine does. The role of D3 receptors is just now being clarified in humans since preclinical studies suggest therapeutic potential of D3 partial agonism for cognition, mood, emotions, and reward/substance abuse, as well as negative symptoms. In fact, cariprazine has been shown to be superior to D2/5HT2A antagonist treatment for the improvement of negative symptoms in schizophrenia. D3 antagonist/partial agonist action may block key postsynaptic D3 receptors in limbic areas to reduce dopamine overactivity in emotional striatum and key somatodendritic presynaptic D3 receptors in the ventral tegmental area/mesostriatal/integrative hub to increase DA release in the prefrontal cortex and improve negative, affective, and cognitive symptoms (Sokoloff & Le Foll, 2017; Stahl, 2020; Stahl, 2021).

# Cariprazine: Tips and Pearls

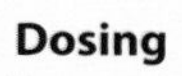

**Dosing**

***Formulation:***
1.5, 3, 4.5, and 6 mg capsules

***Dosage Range:***
1.5–6 mg/day in schizophrenia

***Approved For:***
Schizophrenia (acute and maintenance), acute mania/mixed mania, bipolar depression (bipolar I disorder), major depressive disorder (adjunct)

## Side effects I

***Weight Gain***

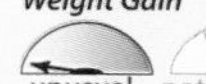
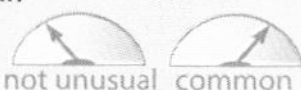
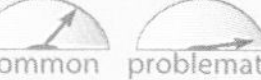

unusual not unusual common problematic

***Sedation***

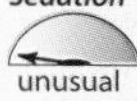
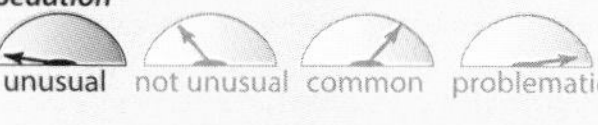

unusual not unusual common problematic

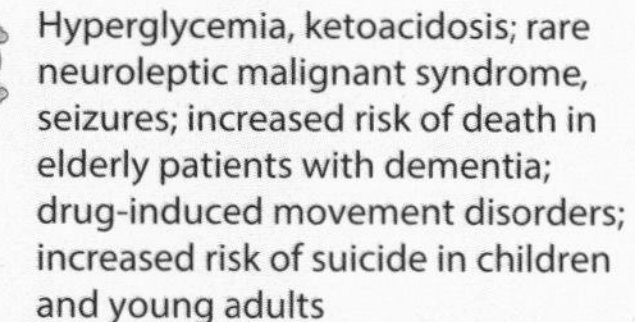

Hyperglycemia, ketoacidosis; rare neuroleptic malignant syndrome, seizures; increased risk of death in elderly patients with dementia; drug-induced movement disorders; increased risk of suicide in children and young adults

## Pearls

Drug is metabolized into a very long-lasting active metabolite; it is thus possible that adverse events could appear several weeks after drug initiation due to accumulation of drug and major metabolites over time; favorable metabolic profile

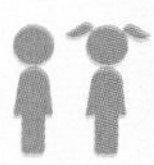

Safety and efficacy have not been established in children or adolescents

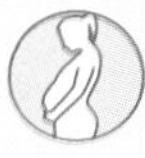

Some animal studies show adverse effects; no controlled studies in pregnant women; recommend either to discontinue drug or bottle feed

## Side effects II

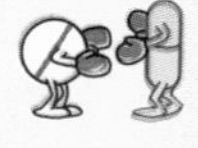

Use of drug with a strong CYP450 3A4 inhibitor requires dose adjustments; concomitant use of drug and a CYP450 3A4 inducer is not recommended; drug increases effects of antihypertensives and decreases DA agonist effects

Use with caution in patients with cardiac impairments

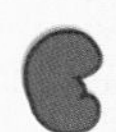

Dose adjustment is not necessary for patients with mild-to-moderate renal impairment; drug is not recommended for patients with severe renal impairment or end-stage renal disease

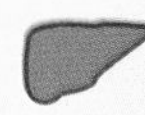

Dose adjustment is not necessary for patients with mild-to-moderate hepatic impairment; drug is not recommended for patients with severe hepatic impairment

# Selective 5HT2A Antagonist: Pimavanserin

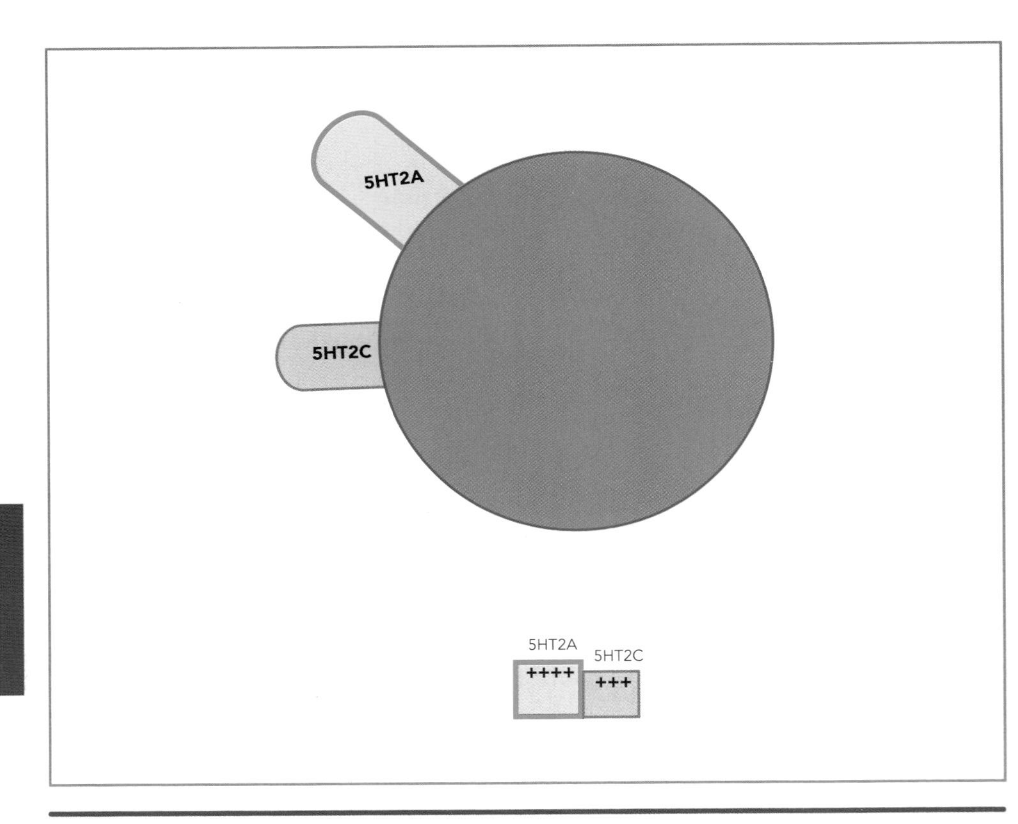


**FIGURE 4.35.** Pimavanserin is the only known drug with proven antipsychotic efficacy that does not bind to D2 receptors. Instead, it has potent 5HT2A antagonism (sometimes called inverse agonism) with lesser 5HT2C antagonist actions. The role, if any, of 5HT2C antagonism in the treatment of psychosis is not clear but 5HT2C antagonist actions would theoretically improve dopamine release in both depression and in the negative symptoms of schizophrenia.
It is only indicated for Parkinson's disease psychosis, but results from a recent phase 2 randomized clinical trial show that pimavanserin improves negative symptoms of schizophrenia (Bugarski-Kirola et al., 2022; Darwish et al., 2022; Stahl, 2020; Stahl, 2021). A phase 3 study evaluating the efficacy of pimavanserin in patients with predominant negative symptoms of schizophrenia is ongoing.

# Pimavanserin: Tips and Pearls

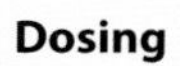

## Dosing

***Formulation:***
34 mg capsule
10 mg tablet

***Dosage Range:***
34 mg/day

***Approved For:***
Hallucinations and delusions associated with Parkinson's disease psychosis

## Side effects I

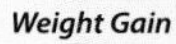

***Weight Gain***

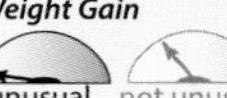

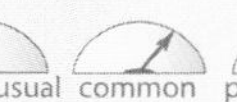


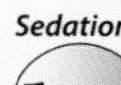

***Sedation***

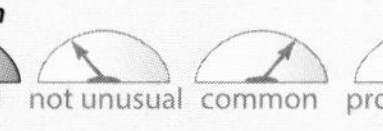

QTc prolongation; increased risk of death in elderly patients with dementia

## Pearls

Does not worsen motor symptoms of Parkinson's disease; is not associated with metabolic side effects or sedation; enhances slow wave sleep and may have hypnotic properties

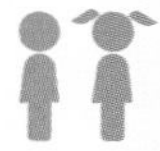

Safety and efficacy have not been established in children or adolescents

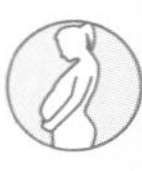

Some animal studies show adverse effects; no controlled studies in pregnant women; recommend either to discontinue drug or bottle feed

## Side effects II

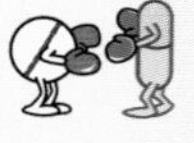

Recommended dose of drug is 10 mg/day when taking moderate or strong CYP450 3A4 inhibitors; avoid use with moderate or strong CYP450 3A4 inducers

Avoid in patients with known QTc prolongation or who are taking drugs that are known to prolong QTc interval; avoid in patients with a history of cardiac arrhythmias, symptomatic bradycardia, hypokalemia or hypomagnesemia, or presence of congenital prolongation of the QT interval

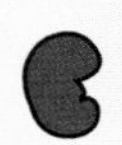

Use with caution in patients with severe impairment or end-stage renal disease

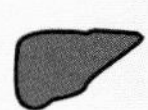

Dose adjustment not necessary in patients with hepatic impairment

Stahl's Illustrated | Chapter 5

# Switching Strategies and Converting to Long-Acting Injectables

Figuring out how to treat psychosis in different patients can be challenging, particularly when recovery necessitates switching to different second-generation drugs for psychosis. Practical switching strategies are presented that will aid in properly changing medications in patients when different treatments are required. Additionally, key information for converting patients from oral to long-acting injectable (LAI) formulations is provided. The use of LAIs can be instrumental for treating patients with psychosis, particularly those who struggle with adherence (Citrome, 2021). Non-adherence and even partial adherence can increase the risk of relapse in patients with schizophrenia (Goff et al., 2017). Several formulations are now available, each with a unique profile in terms of pharmacokinetics, administration factors, initiation strategy, and maintenance dosing schedule.

| Abbreviations Used in This Chapter | |
|---|---|
| 5HT2A | Serotonin 2A receptor |
| ALND | Aripiprazole lauroxil nanocrystal dispersion |
| CYP | Cytochrome P450 |
| D2 | Dopamine 2 receptor |
| DPA | D2 partial agonist |
| LAI | Long-acting injectable |
| q1M | Every month |
| q2M | Every 2 months |
| SDA | 5HT2A/D2 antagonist |

# How NOT to Switch between Second-Generation Drugs for Psychosis

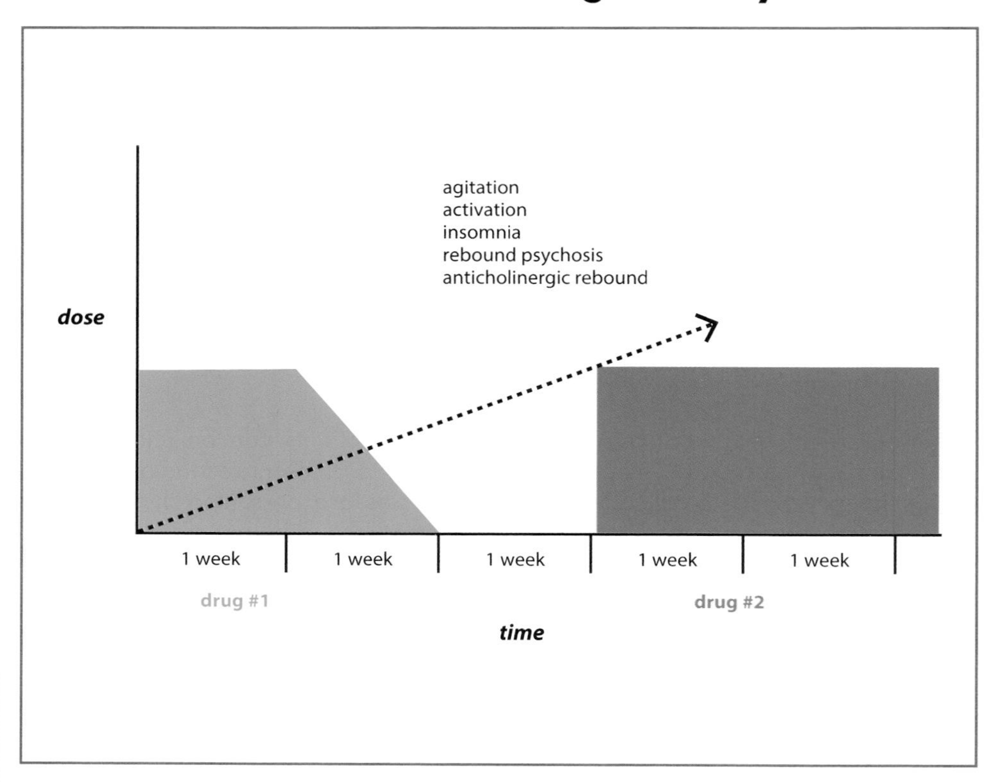


**FIGURE 5.1.** There are strategies for switching between second-generation drugs for psychosis and strategies to avoid in order to prevent rebound psychosis, aggravation of side effects, or withdrawal symptoms. Generally, it is preferable to (1) not rush the discontinuation of the first treatment, (2) not allow gaps between two treatments, and (3) not start the second treatment at full dose (Stahl, 2013; Takeuchi & Remington, 2020).

# Switching from One Second-Generation Drug for Psychosis to Another

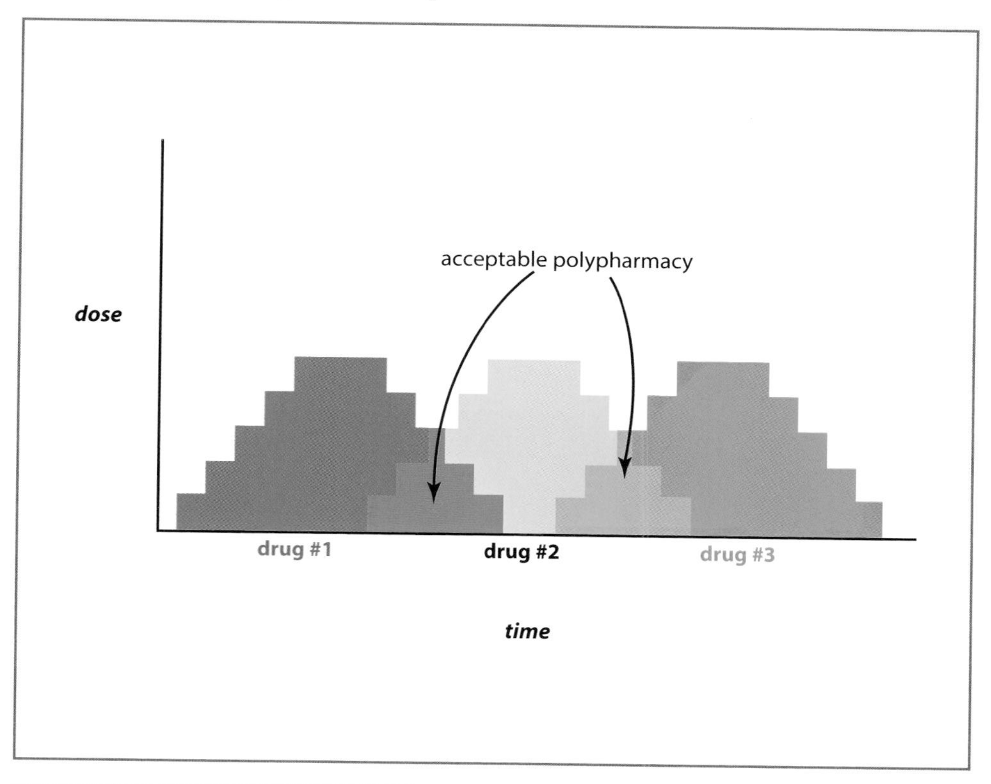


**FIGURE 5.2.** When switching from one drug to another, it is frequently prudent to "cross-titrate"—that is, to build down the dose of the first drug while building up the dose of the other over a few days to a few weeks. This leads to transient administration of two drugs but is justified in order to reduce side effects and the risk of rebound symptoms, and to accelerate the successful transition to the second drug (Stahl, 2013).

# Getting Trapped in Cross-Titration

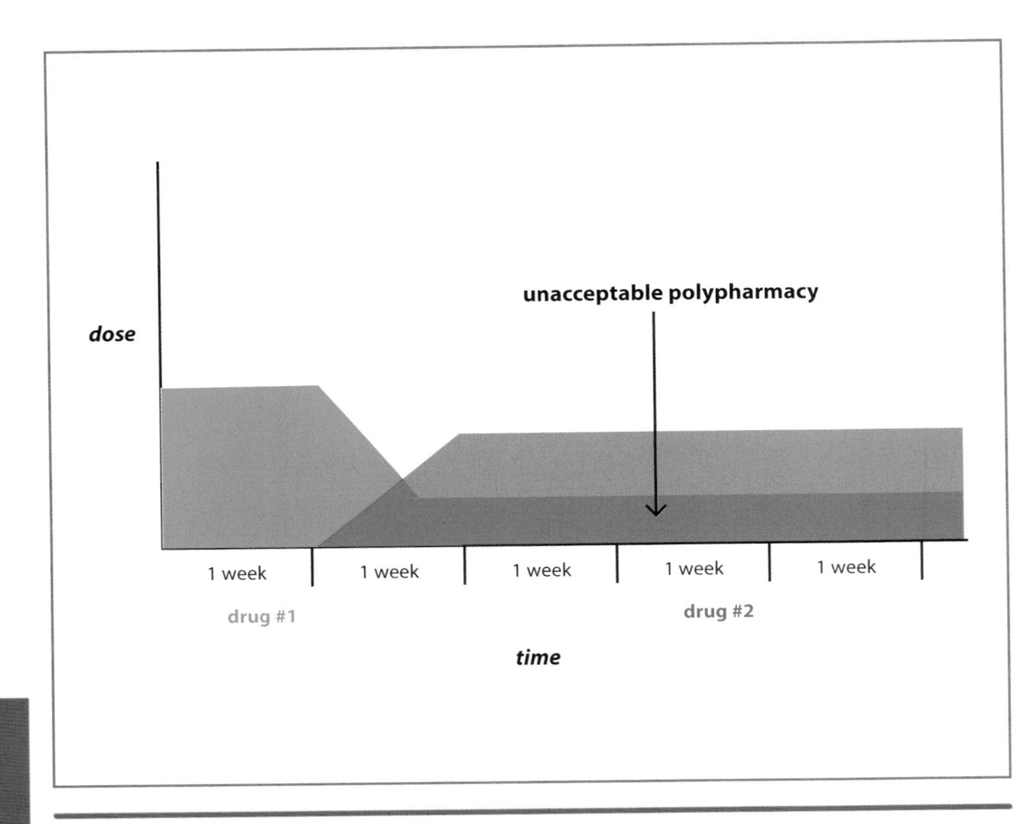


**FIGURE 5.3.** When initiating cross-titration, it is imperative to not forget to taper the first drug. Patients may improve in the middle of a cross-titration, but this should not be the reason to stop the process. An unfinished cross-titration will lead to polypharmacy where the patient takes two drugs indefinitely. While polypharmacy is sometimes a necessity in hard-to-treat cases, an adequate monotherapy trial of a second drug should be the first option (Stahl, 2013).

# Switching from Pines to Pines or Dones to Dones

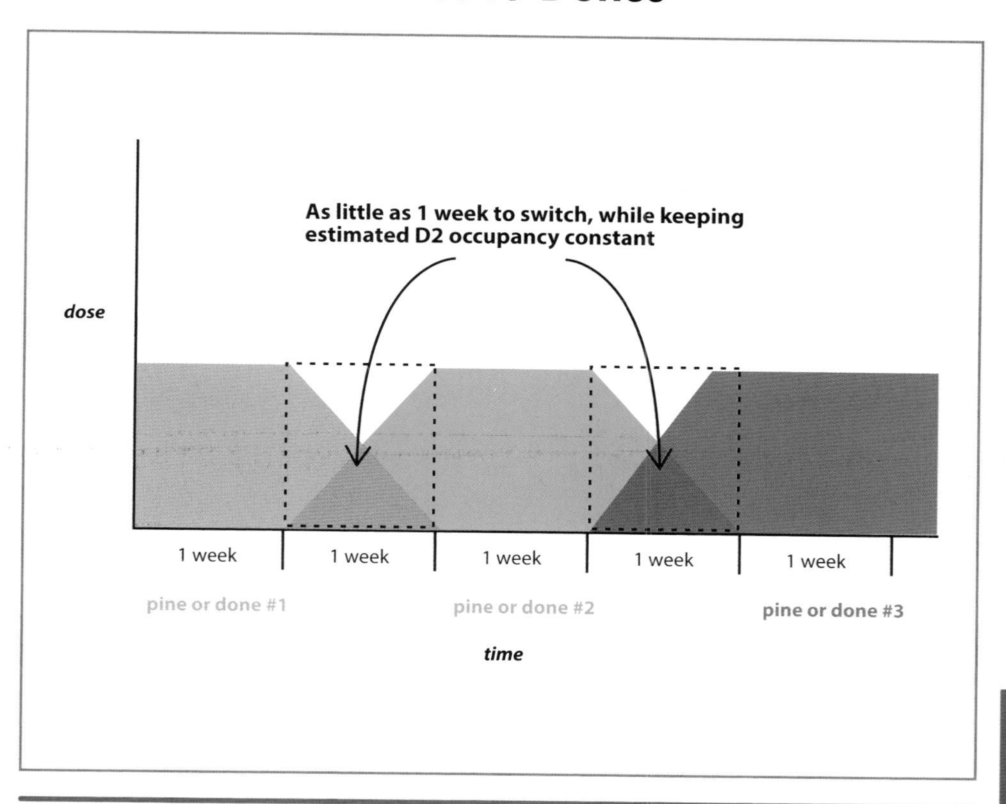


**FIGURE 5.4.** When switching from one "pine" (clozapine, olanzapine, quetiapine, asenapine) to another, it is prudent to make the switch in as little as 1 week, while keeping estimated D2 receptor occupancy constant. Likewise, when switching from one "done" (risperidone, paliperidone, ziprasidone, iloperidone, lurasidone) to another, it is prudent to make the switch in as little as 1 week, while keeping estimated D2 receptor occupancy constant (Keks et al., 2019; Stahl, 2013).

# Switching from a Pine to a Done: Stop the Pine Slowly

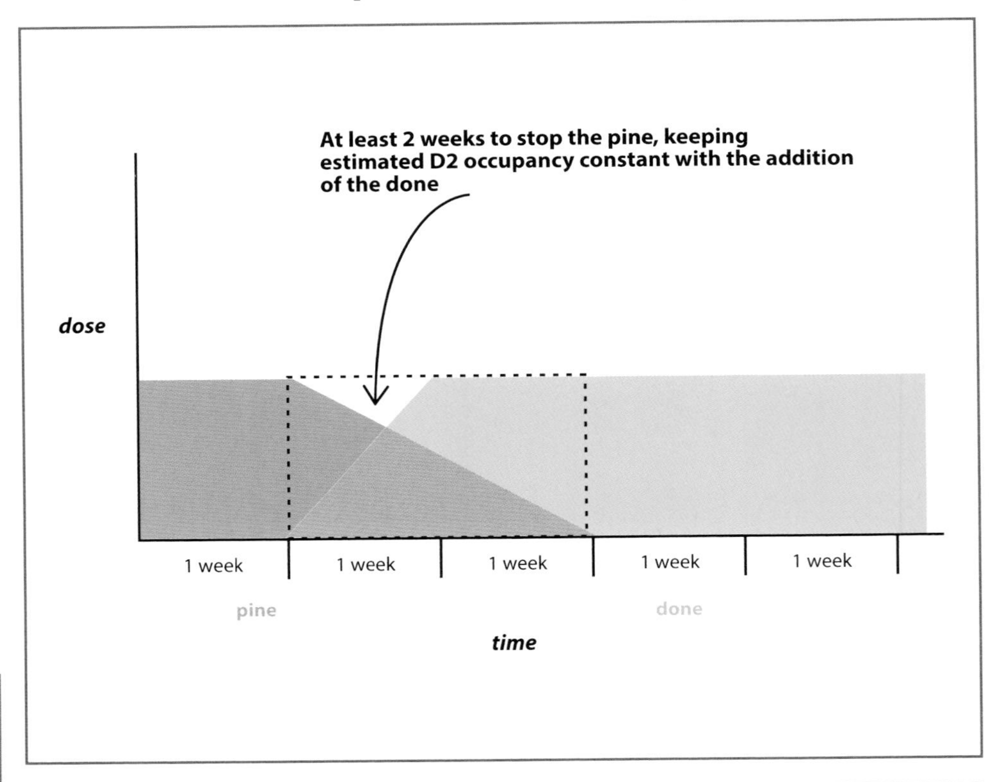


**FIGURE 5.5.** When switching from a "pine" (clozapine, olanzapine, quetiapine, asenapine) to a done (risperidone, paliperidone, ziprasidone, iloperidone, lurasidone), it is prudent to take at least 2 weeks to stop the pine, while keeping the estimated D2 receptor occupancy constant during the addition of the done (Keks et al., 2019; Stahl, 2013).

# Always Stop Clozapine Slowly

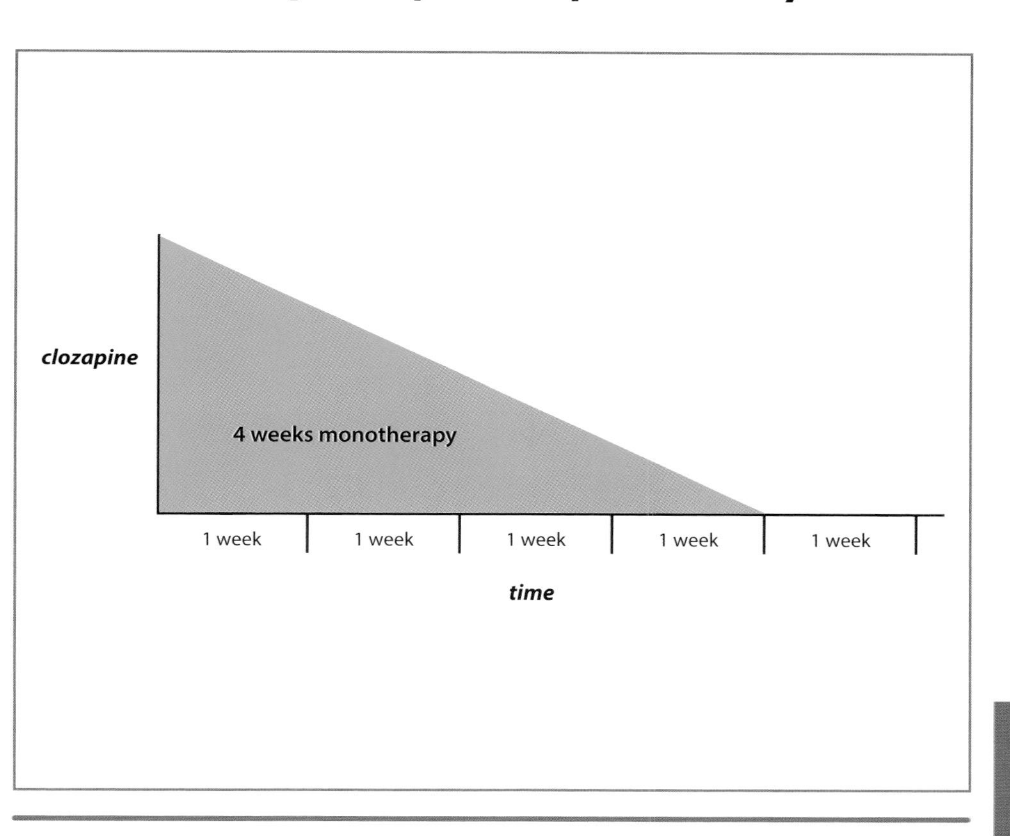


**FIGURE 5.6.** When stopping clozapine, it is always necessary to do so slowly, with 4 weeks of down-titration prior to starting another antipsychotic (Meyer & Stahl, 2019; Stahl, 2013).

# Switching from a Done to a Pine: Start the Pine Slowly

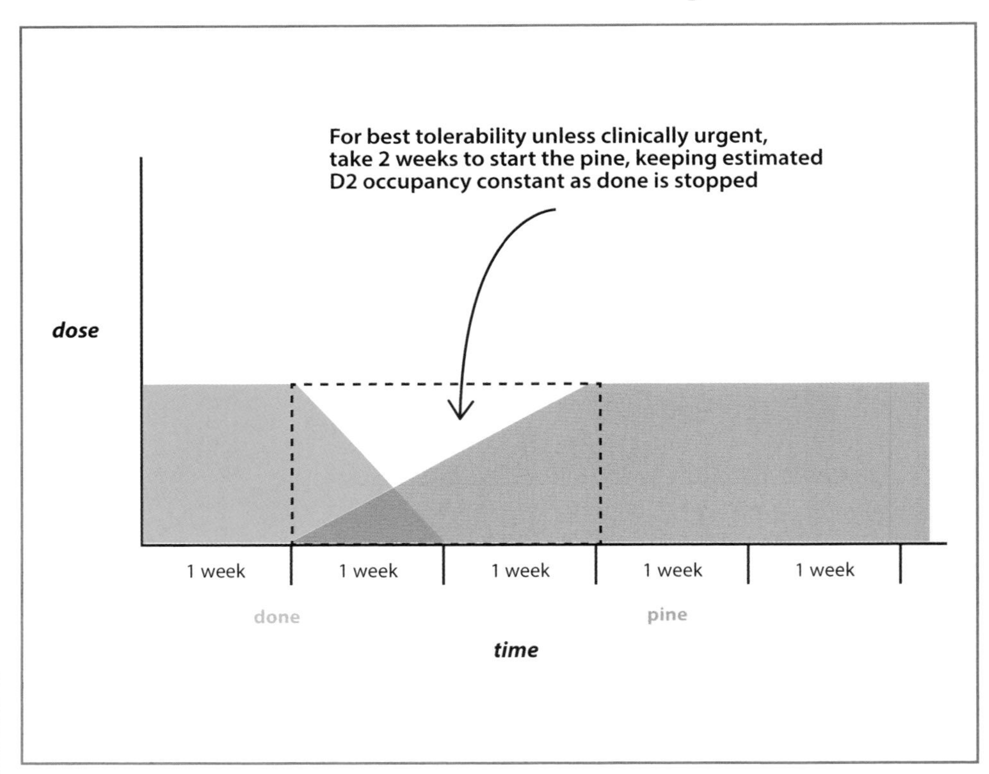


**FIGURE 5.7.** When switching from a "done" (risperidone, paliperidone, ziprasidone, iloperidone, lurasidone) to a "pine" (clozapine, olanzapine, quetiapine, asenapine), tolerability may be best if the pine can be titrated up over the course of 2 weeks, while keeping the estimated D2 receptor occupancy constant as the done is stopped (Keks et al., 2019; Stahl, 2013).

# Switching to Aripiprazole from a Pine

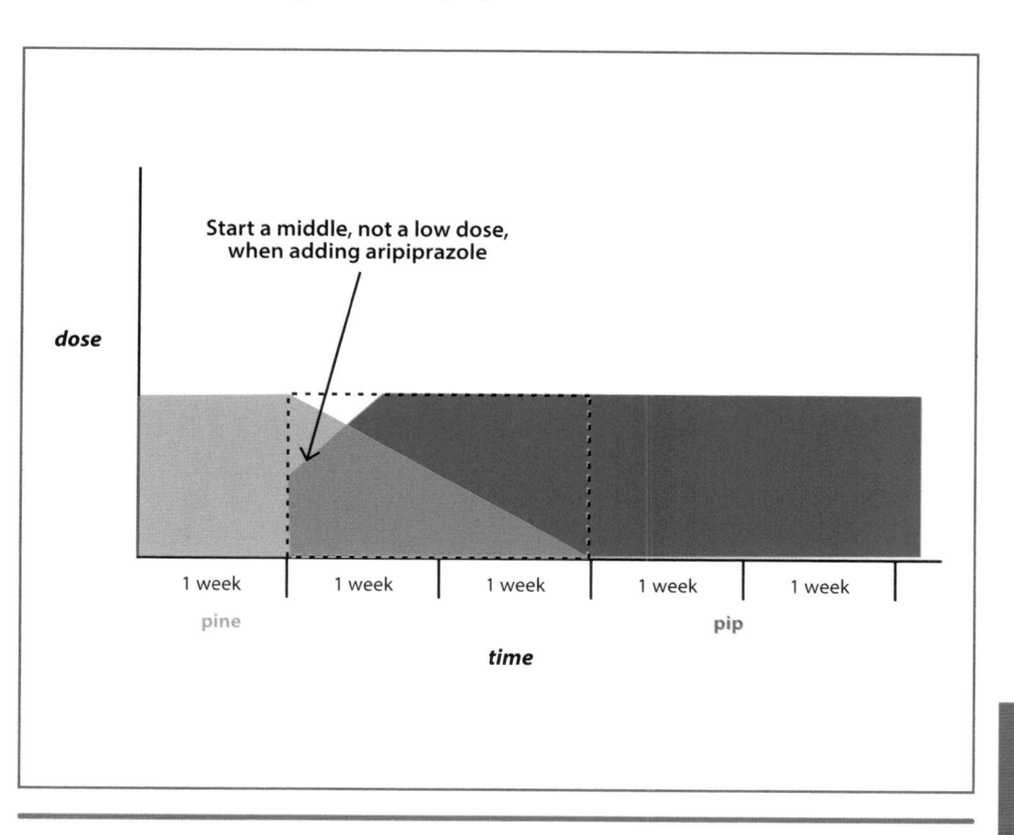


**FIGURE 5.8.** Aripiprazole has higher affinity for D2 receptors than most "pines" (clozapine, olanzapine, quetiapine, asenapine); thus, breakthrough symptoms may be more likely when switching from a pine to aripiprazole. A prudent approach, therefore, is to start aripiprazole at a middle dose, rather than a low dose, while down-titrating the pine slowly over 2 weeks (Keks et al., 2019; Stahl, 2013).

# Switching to Aripiprazole from a Done

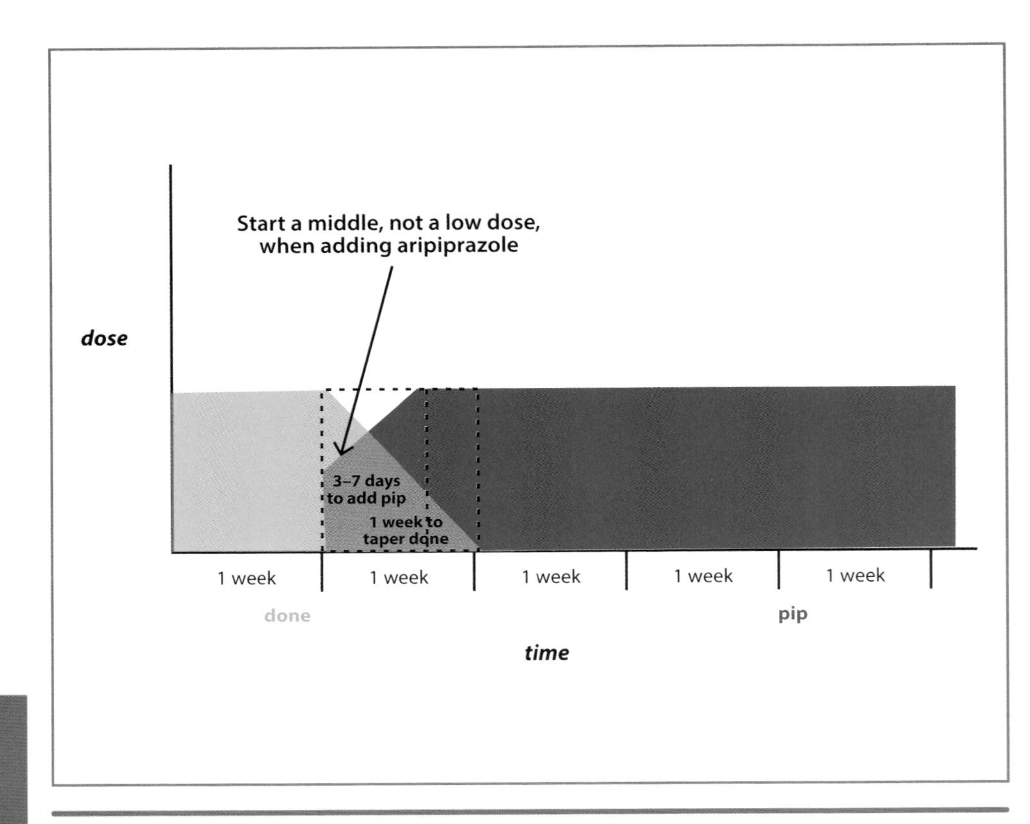


**FIGURE 5.9.** When switching to aripiprazole from a "done" (risperidone, paliperidone, ziprasidone, iloperidone, lurasidone), it is recommended to start aripiprazole at a middle dose, rather than a low dose, while down-titrating the done over 1 week (Keks et al., 2019; Stahl, 2013).

# Switching from Aripiprazole to a Pine

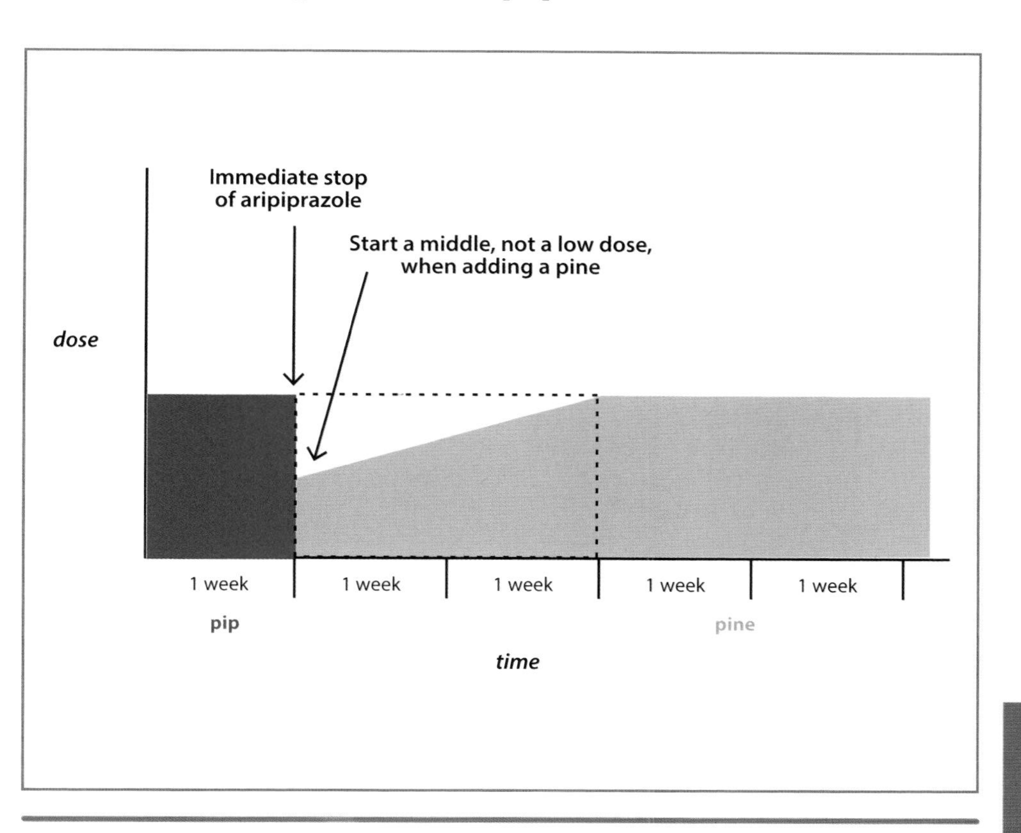


**FIGURE 5.10.** When switching from aripiprazole to a "pine" (clozapine, olanzapine, quetiapine, asenapine), it is recommended to stop aripiprazole immediately and start the pine at a middle, rather than a low, dose. The pine can be up-titrated over a period of 2 weeks (Keks et al., 2019; Stahl, 2013).

# Switching from Aripiprazole to a Done

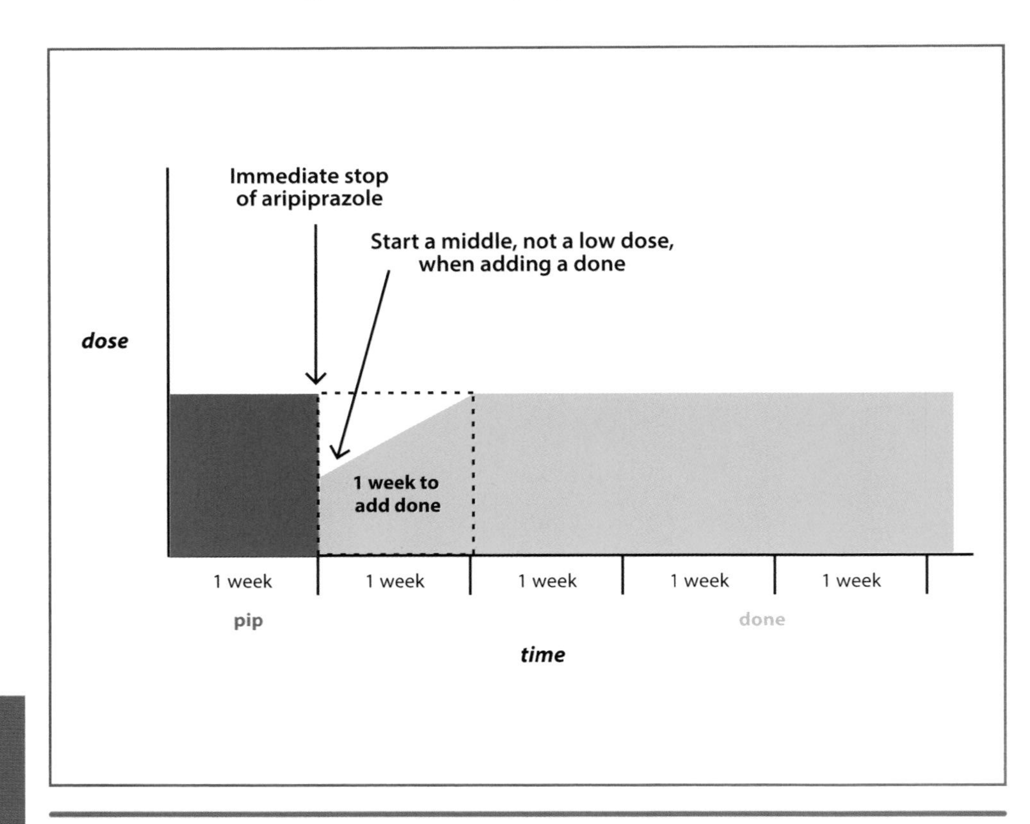


**FIGURE 5.11.** When switching from aripiprazole to a "done" (risperidone, paliperidone, ziprasidone, iloperidone, lurasidone), it is recommended to stop aripiprazole immediately and start the done at a middle, rather than a low, dose. The done can be up-titrated over a period of 1 week (Keks et al., 2019; Stahl, 2013).

# Converting from Oral to LAI: Haloperidol Decanoate

| Brand name | Haldol Decanoate |
|---|---|
| Starting dose | 10–20 times the previous oral dose |
| Maintenance dose | 10–15 times the previous oral dose |
| Apparent half-life | 21 days |
| Injection interval | 4 weeks |
| Injection site | Intramuscular (deltoid or gluteal) |
| Dosage forms | 50 mg, 100 mg ampules |
| Injection volume | 50 or 100 mg/mL; not to exceed 3 mL |

**FIGURE 5.12.** Haloperidol decanoate can be loaded; the loading dose is 10 times the oral daily dose, given weekly for the first 3 weeks. Discontinuation of oral antipsychotic can begin immediately if adequate loading is pursued; however, the time to maximum concentration ranges from 3 to 9 days, and oral coverage may still be necessary for the first week for some patients. Steady state is reached after 4 weeks with loading. The terminal half-life with multiple dosing is 21 days; therefore, the maintenance dosing schedule for haloperidol decanoate is every 4 weeks. The maintenance dose is 20 times the oral daily dose and should start 2 weeks after the last loading injection. Depending on the appropriate maintenance dose, some patients may require a different dosing schedule. Single injection volumes greater than 300 mg are not tolerated, so patients who require higher doses typically receive the monthly dose as split injections every 2 weeks (Citrome, 2021; Correll et al., 2021; Meyer, 2017).

# Converting from Oral to LAI: Fluphenazine Decanoate

| Brand name | Prolixin Decanoate |
|---|---|
| Starting dose | 12.5–25 mg |
| Maintenance dose | 25–100 mg |
| Apparent half-life | 7–10 days |
| Injection interval | 2 weeks |
| Injection site | Subcutaneous or intramuscular (deltoid or gluteal) |
| Dosage forms | 25 mg, 100 mg ampules, syringes, and vial kits |
| Injection volume | 25 or 100 mg/mL |

**FIGURE 5.13.** For fluphenazine decanoate, the response threshold is 0.8 ng/mL. Plasma levels greater than 2 to 3 ng/mL are generally not well tolerated. With a single dose, the time to maximum concentration is only 0.3 to 1.5 days, after which the concentration drops steeply. This early peak relative to other LAIs may make fluphenazine decanoate preferable in acute situations, but it also carries the risk of drug-induced parkinsonism or akathisia in the first 48 hours. In addition, the steep drop in levels can lead to relapse, which is why one must provide either weekly loading injections or oral coverage at half dose when converting to fluphenazine decanoate. The formula for converting patients from oral to long-acting fluphenazine is not as well established as for some other LAIs, and the best way to determine the loading schedule is by obtaining a plasma level. After steady state is achieved, one should convert to a 2-week dosing schedule, based on the terminal half-life of 14 days. The usual maintenance dose is 12.5 to 100 mg every 2 weeks (Citrome, 2021; Correll et al., 2021; Meyer, 2017).

# Converting from Oral to LAI: Risperidone Microspheres

| Brand name | Risperdal Consta, Rykindo |
|---|---|
| Starting dose | 25 mg |
| Maintenance dose | 25 mg, maximum 50 mg/2 weeks |
| Apparent half-life | 3–6 days |
| Injection interval | 2 weeks |
| Injection site | Intramuscular (deltoid or gluteal [Rykindo only gluteal]) |
| Dosage forms | 12.5 mg, 25 mg, 37.5 mg, 50 mg vial kits or injectable suspension |
| Injection volume | ~2 mL |
| Oral supplementation | 7 (Rykindo) or 21 (Risperdal Consta) days after the initial injection and after any change in dose |

**FIGURE 5.14.** For Risperdal Consta, there is a lag time to active release, such that maximum concentration is not achieved until 21 days. For Rykindo, a single injection leads to an initial release of risperidone followed by a stable release phase of 2 to 4 weeks; the median time to peak concentration is 14 and 17 days for a 25 and 50 mg dose, respectively. However, the terminal half-life with multiple doses for risperidone microspheres is 3 to 6 days, which is why it needs to be dosed every 2 weeks. Risperidone microspheres cannot be loaded, and so requires oral supplementation for 7 days for Rykindo and 21 days for Risperdal Consta in order to maintain therapeutic plasma levels, which are generally 20 to 60 ng/mL. Plasma concentrations can be estimated as 7 times the oral dose, which can in turn be used to predict the appropriate long-acting dose. However, this is an average and can vary by individual patient, so obtaining plasma levels is ideal when deciding on the maintenance dose of the LAI formulation. If dose adjustments are needed after a patient has started risperidone microspheres, titration should occur at intervals of no less than 4 weeks. If a dose is missed by 2 or more weeks, then oral coverage while reinitiating injections may be necessary. The usual maintenance dose range is 12.5–50 mg every 2 weeks, with 50 mg per vial as the highest available dosing option. This means that patients who are taking 8 mg per day or higher of oral risperidone may not be good candidates for the long-acting formulation, since more than one injection would be required (Citrome, 2021; Correll et al., 2021; Luye Pharma Group, 2023; Meyer, 2017).

# Converting from Oral to LAI: Risperidone Monthly

| Brand name | Perseris |
|---|---|
| Starting dose | 90 or 120 mg |
| Maintenance dose | Same as above |
| Apparent half-life | 9–11 days |
| Injection interval | 4 weeks |
| Injection site | Subcutaneous (abdomen) |
| Dosage forms | 90 mg, 120 mg syringe kits |
| Injection volume | 0.6 mL (90 mg), 0.8 mL (120 mg) |

**FIGURE 5.15.** The 1-month long-acting formulation of risperidone is administered subcutaneously. The delivery system hardens upon contact with bodily fluids, subsequently releasing the active drug at a controlled rate and for an extended period. There are two absorption peaks: the first occurs 4 to 6 hours after injection due to an initial release of the active drug during the depot formation process. The second occurs 10 to 14 days after the injection, with similar magnitude and at levels that approach steady state; thus, no oral supplementation or loading is necessary. The 1-month formulation of risperidone is available in a 90 mg dose and a 120 mg dose, which correspond to 3 and 4 mg doses of oral risperidone, respectively (Citrome, 2021; Correll et al., 2021; Meyer, 2017).

# Converting from Oral to LAI: Risperidone Every 1 or 2 Months

| Brand name | Uzedy |
|---|---|
| Starting dose | q1M: 25 times the previous oral dose<br>q2M: 50 times the previous oral dose |
| Maintenance dose | Same as above |
| Apparent half-life | 14–22 days |
| Injection interval | 4 or 8 weeks |
| Injection site | Subcutaneous (abdomen or deltoid) |
| Dosage forms | 50 mg, 75 mg, 100 mg, 125 mg, 150 mg, 200 mg, and 250 mg single-dose prefilled syringes |
| Injection volume | 50.14 mL (50 mg), 0.21 mL (75 mg),<br>0.28 mL (100 mg), 0.35 mL (125 mg),<br>0.42 mL (150 mg), 0.56 mL (200 mg),<br>and 0.7 mL (250 mg) |

**FIGURE 5.16.** A monthly or bi-monthly injectable suspension of risperidone was approved by the Food and Drug Administration in April 2023 for the treatment of schizophrenia in adults. It is administered subcutaneously every month (q1M) or 2 months (q2M) and does not require a loading dose or oral supplementation. This formulation utilizes SteadyTeq™, a proprietary copolymer technology that controls the steady release of risperidone. Tolerability with oral risperidone must be established prior to initiating this treatment. Monthly doses are 25 times the previous oral dose, while bi-monthly doses are 50 times the previous oral dose. Therapeutic blood concentrations are reached within 6–24 hours of a single dose (Teva Pharmaceuticals, 2023).

# Converting from Oral to LAI: Paliperidone Palmitate Monthly

| Brand name | Invega Sustenna |
|---|---|
| Starting dose | 234 mg day 1 and 156 mg day 8 (deltoid) |
| Maintenance dose | 117 mg, range 39–234 mg/4 weeks |
| Apparent half-life | 25–49 days |
| Injection interval | 4 weeks |
| Injection site | Intramuscular (deltoid at initiation, then either deltoid or gluteal) |
| Dosage forms | 39 mg, 78 mg, 117 mg, 156 mg, 234 mg injectable suspension |
| Injection volume | 156 mg/mL; range 0.25–1.5 mL |

**FIGURE 5.17.** For patients switching from oral medication, or who are not on active medication, the 1-month formulation of paliperidone palmitate can be loaded, with a standard loading schedule of 234 mg on day 1 and 156 mg on day 8, plus or minus 2 days. The initiation doses must be administered in the deltoid muscle. The maintenance dose should start 4 weeks after the second loading injection, but the dosing window is flexible and can vary by plus or minus 1 week. The maintenance dose of 1-month paliperidone palmitate is determined based on the oral dose, although ideally plasma levels would be obtained (recommended therapeutic plasma levels for paliperidone are 20 to 60 ng/mL) (Citrome, 2021; Correll et al., 2021; Meyer, 2017).

# Converting from Oral to LAI: Paliperidone Palmitate Every 3 Months

| Brand name | Invega Trinza |
|---|---|
| Starting dose | 273 mg, 410 mg, 546 mg, 819 mg (3.5 times the last dose of the once monthly formulation) |
| Maintenance dose | Same as above |
| Apparent half-life | 84–95 days (deltoid), 118–139 (gluteal) |
| Injection interval | 12 weeks |
| Injection site | Intramuscular (deltoid or gluteal) |
| Dosage forms | 273 mg, 410 mg, 546 mg, 819 mg injectable suspension |
| Injection volume | 312 mg/mL; range 0.9–2.6 mL |

**FIGURE 5.18.** The injection of the 3-month formulation of paliperidone palmitate is given in place of the next scheduled 1-month injection, with dosing based on the previous 1-month injection dose. The dosing window is also flexible for the 3-month formulation, and it can be given up to 2 weeks before or after the 3-month time period (Citrome, 2021; Correll et al., 2021; Meyer, 2017).

# Converting from Oral to LAI: Paliperidone Palmitate Every 6 Months

| Brand name | Invega Hafyera |
|---|---|
| Starting dose | Option A: After treatment with 1-month paliperidone palmitate for at least 4 months: 1092 mg if the last dose was 156 mg, or 1560 mg if the last dose was 234 mg<br>Option B: After treatment with 3-month paliperidone palmitate for at least one 3-month cycle: 1092 mg if the last dose was 546 mg, or 1560 mg if the last dose was 819 mg |
| Maintenance dose | Same as above |
| Apparent half-life | 148–159 days |
| Injection interval | 6 months |
| Injection site | Intramuscular (gluteal) |
| Dosage forms | 1092 mg, 1560 mg injectable suspension |
| Injection volume | 3.5 mL (1092 mg), 5 mL (1560 mL) |

**FIGURE 5.19.** The injection of the 6-month formulation of paliperidone palmitate is given in place of the next scheduled 1-month or 3-month injection, with dosing based on the previous 1-month or 3-month product. When switching from the 1-month LAI, the last two doses of the 1-month formulation should be the same dosage strength so that a consistent maintenance dose is established prior to starting the 6-month formulation. When switching from the 3-month LAI, the 6-month injection can be given up to 2 weeks before or after the next scheduled 3-month dose (Peters et al., 2023).

# Converting from Oral to LAI: Aripiprazole Monohydrate

| Brand name | Abilify Maintena |
|---|---|
| Starting dose | 400 mg |
| Maintenance dose | 300 or 400 mg (adjust for CYP2D6 or CYP3A4 inhibitors; cannot give with CYP3A4 inducers) |
| Apparent half-life | 29.9–46.5 days |
| Injection interval | 4 weeks |
| Injection site | Intramuscular (deltoid or gluteal) |
| Dosage forms | 300 mg, 400 mg vial kits and dual-chambered prefilled syringes |
| Injection volume | 200 mg/mL; range 0.8–2 mL |
| Oral supplementation | 14 days after the initial injection |

**FIGURE 5.20.** Aripiprazole monohydrate is poorly soluble, resulting in slow and prolonged dissolution and absorption, with maximum concentration achieved after about a week. It requires an initial injection of 400 mg and, because it cannot be loaded, oral coverage is necessary for the first 14 days. The maintenance dosing schedule is typically 300 to 400 mg every 4 weeks. The maximum dose of aripiprazole monohydrate, 400 mg, is equivalent to 20 mg of oral aripiprazole, which generally corresponds to a plasma level in the 200s. Aripiprazole monohydrate cannot be used with strong CYP3A4 inducers and requires dose adjustment in the presence of CYP2D6 and CYP3A4 inhibitors, as well as in patients who are poor CYP2D6 metabolizers (Citrome, 2021; Correll et al., 2021; Meyer, 2017).

# Converting from Oral to LAI: Aripiprazole Lauroxil

| Brand name | Aristada |
|---|---|
| Starting dose | 441 mg/4 weeks, 662 mg/4 weeks, 882 mg/ 4 weeks, 882 mg/6 weeks, 1064 mg/8 weeks |
| Maintenance dose | Same as above (adjust for CYP2D6 or CYP3A4 modulators) |
| Apparent half-life | 53.9–57.2 days |
| Injection interval | 4, 6, or 8 weeks |
| Injection site | Intramuscular (deltoid [441 mg only] or gluteal) |
| Dosage forms | 441 mg, 662 mg, 882 mg, 1064 mg injectable suspension |
| Injection volume | 276 mg/mL: range 1.6–3.9 mL |
| Oral supplementation | 21 days after the initial injection or 1 day when used with the nanocrystal dispersion formulation |

**FIGURE 5.21.** Aripiprazole lauroxil dissolves slowly, reaching maximum concentration after 44 to 50 days, with four monthly injections required to reach steady state. There are two options for how to initiate treatment: (1) oral coverage for the first 21 days, or (2) use of the 675 mg single-dose initiation injection in combination with a 30 mg dose of oral aripiprazole. The first maintenance aripiprazole lauroxil injection can be administered on the same day as the single-dose injection or up to 10 days later. One should avoid injecting both the single-dose injection and maintenance-dose injection into the same deltoid or gluteal muscle. Dose adjustments are needed in the presence of CYP2D6 inhibitors, CYP3A4 inhibitors, and CYP3A4 inducers. However, dose adjustments are not possible for the single-dose injection, so this treatment initiation option should be avoided in patients who are known CYP2D6 poor metabolizers or who are taking strong CYP3A4 inhibitors, strong CYP2D6 inhibitors, or strong CYP3A4 inducers (Citrome, 2021; Correll et al., 2021 Meyer, 2017).

# Converting from Oral to LAI: Aripiprazole Lauroxil Nanocrystal Dispersion

| Brand name | Aristada Initio |
|---|---|
| Starting dose | NA |
| Maintenance dose | NA |
| Apparent half-life | 15–18 days |
| Injection interval | NA |
| Injection site | Intramuscular (deltoid or gluteal) |
| Dosage forms | 675 mg injectable suspension |
| Injection volume | 2.4 mL |
| Oral supplementation | One day of aripiprazole 30 mg |

**FIGURE 5.22.** When initiating aripiprazole lauroxil (see **FIGURE 5.21**), one injection of aripiprazole lauroxil nanocrystal dispersion (ALNCD) formulation, plus administration of oral aripiprazole 30 mg that same day, can substitute for 21 days of supplementation with oral aripiprazole. The first injection of aripiprazole lauroxil may be administered the same day or within 10 days. The ALNCD formulation may also be used instead of oral supplementation in cases where the regularly scheduled aripiprazole lauroxil injection is delayed. The ALNCD formulation should not be used in the presence of strong CYP2D6 or CYP3A4 inhibitors or strong CYP3A4 inducers, since there is only one dose of ALNCD that cannot be adjusted (Citrome, 2021; Correll et al., 2021).

# Converting from Oral to LAI: Aripiprazole Every 2 Months

| Brand name | Abilify Asimtufii |
|---|---|
| Starting dose | 960 mg or 720 mg |
| Maintenance dose | Same as above |
| Apparent half-life | Not determined |
| Injection interval | 8 weeks |
| Injection site | Intramuscular (gluteal) |
| Dosage forms | 960 mg, 720 mg single-dose prefilled syringes |
| Injection volume | 3.2 mL (960 mg), 2.4 mL (720 mg) |
| Oral supplementation | 14 days (10–20 mg) after the initial injection |

**FIGURE 5.23.** A bi-monthly injectable suspension of aripiprazole was approved by the Food and Drug Administration in April 2023 for the treatment of schizophrenia and bipolar I disorder in adults. It is administered intramuscularly every 2 months and requires oral supplementation when converting from oral aripiprazole. The recommended dose is 960 mg, but the dose may be reduced to 720 mg in case of adverse reactions. A dose of 720 mg should also be used in patients who are CYP2D6 poor metabolizers or in patients with concomitant use of a strong CYP2D6 or CYP3A4 inhibitor (Otsuka Pharmaceutical, 2023).

# Converting from Oral to LAI: Olanzapine Pamoate

| Brand name | Zyprexa Relprevv |
|---|---|
| Starting dose | 210 mg/2 weeks, 405 mg/4 weeks, 300 mg/2 weeks |
| Maintenance dose | 150 mg/2 weeks, 300 mg/4 weeks, 210 mg/2 weeks, 405 mg/4 weeks, 300 mg/2 weeks |
| Apparent half-life | ~30 days |
| Injection interval | 2 weeks or 4 weeks |
| Injection site | Intramuscular (gluteal) |
| Dosage forms | 210 mg, 300 mg, 405 mg vial kit |
| Injection volume | 150 mg/mL (range 1.0–2.7 mL) |

**FIGURE 5.24.** For olanzapine pamoate, the response threshold is generally 20 ng/mL, and the recommended therapeutic range is 20 to 80 ng/mL, although the tolerability threshold is higher, perhaps up to 180 ng/mL. The time to maximum concentration is 3 to 4 days, and time to steady state is 3 months. The dose should be loaded for the first 8 weeks, with the specific dosage determined based on the previous oral dose. The main limitation to using olanzapine pamoate is that it requires 3-hour post-injection monitoring due to the rare risk of post-injection delirium/sedation syndrome from vascular breach (Citrome, 2021; Correll et al., 2021, Meyer, 2017).

# Future Treatments

In this chapter, we discuss novel treatments for psychosis that act through mechanisms that are not traditional for current drugs with antipsychotic properties. This includes the unique receptor targets muscarinic M1 and M4 acetylcholine receptors and TAAR1 receptors. Upstream binding at these receptors appears to modify dopamine release presynaptically, and postsynaptic mechanisms may also contribute to antipsychotic efficacy (Paul et al., 2022; Stahl, 2021; Yohn et al., 2023). The muscarinic treatments that are farthest along in development for the treatment of schizophrenia are xanomeline-trospium (submitted for FDA approval November 2023), emraclidine (phase 2), and NBI-1117568 (phase 2). Xanomeline-trospium and emraclidine are also being investigated for the treatment of Alzheimer's disease psychosis. The TAAR1 treatment that is farthest along in development for the treatment of schizophrenia is ulotaront (phase 3). Ulotaront is also being investigated for the treatment of Parkinson's disease psychosis (phase 2).

# Upstream M1 Binding Decreases DA Release in Striatum

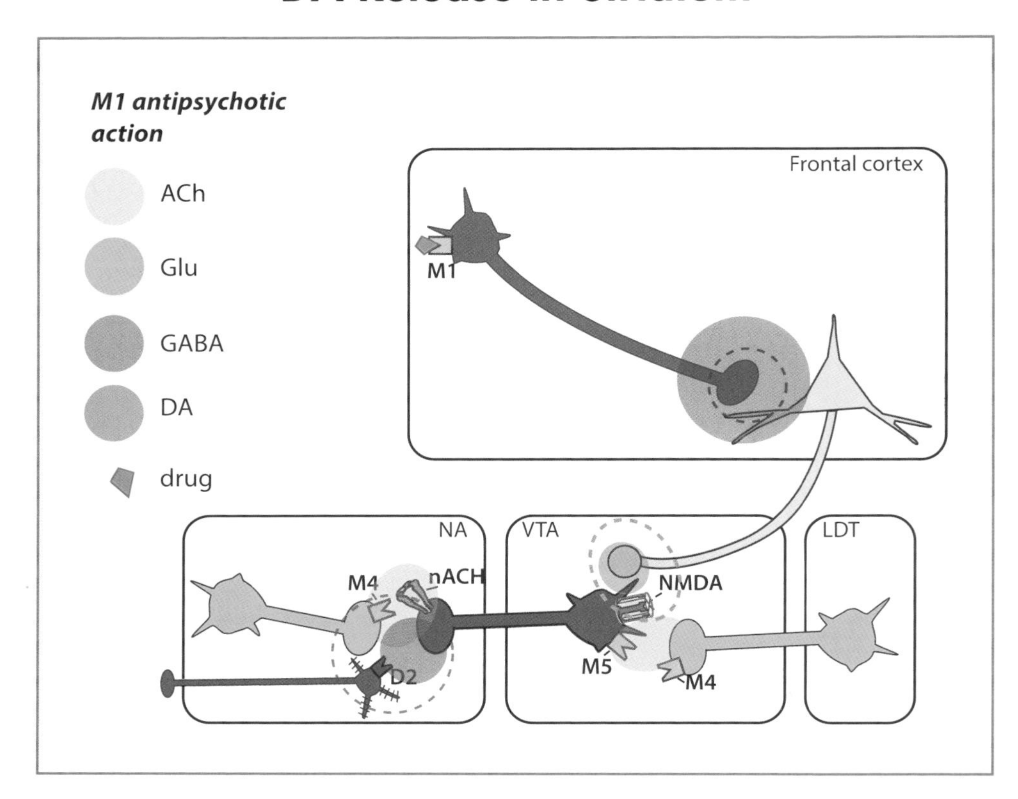

# Upstream M1 Binding Decreases DA Release in Striatum

**FIGURE 6.1.** In the frontal cortex, activation of muscarinic M1 receptors on inhibitory γ-aminobutyric acid (GABA) interneurons by an M1 agonist leads to a reduction of excitatory glutamate (Glu) release in the ventral tegmental area (VTA). This reduction in Glu decreases the activity of dopamine (DA) neurons via N-methyl-D-aspartate (NMDA) receptors, hypothetically resulting in a decrease in DA release and positive symptoms of psychosis (Paul et al., 2022; Yohn et al., 2022).

# Upstream M1 Binding Decreases DA Release in Prefrontal Cortex

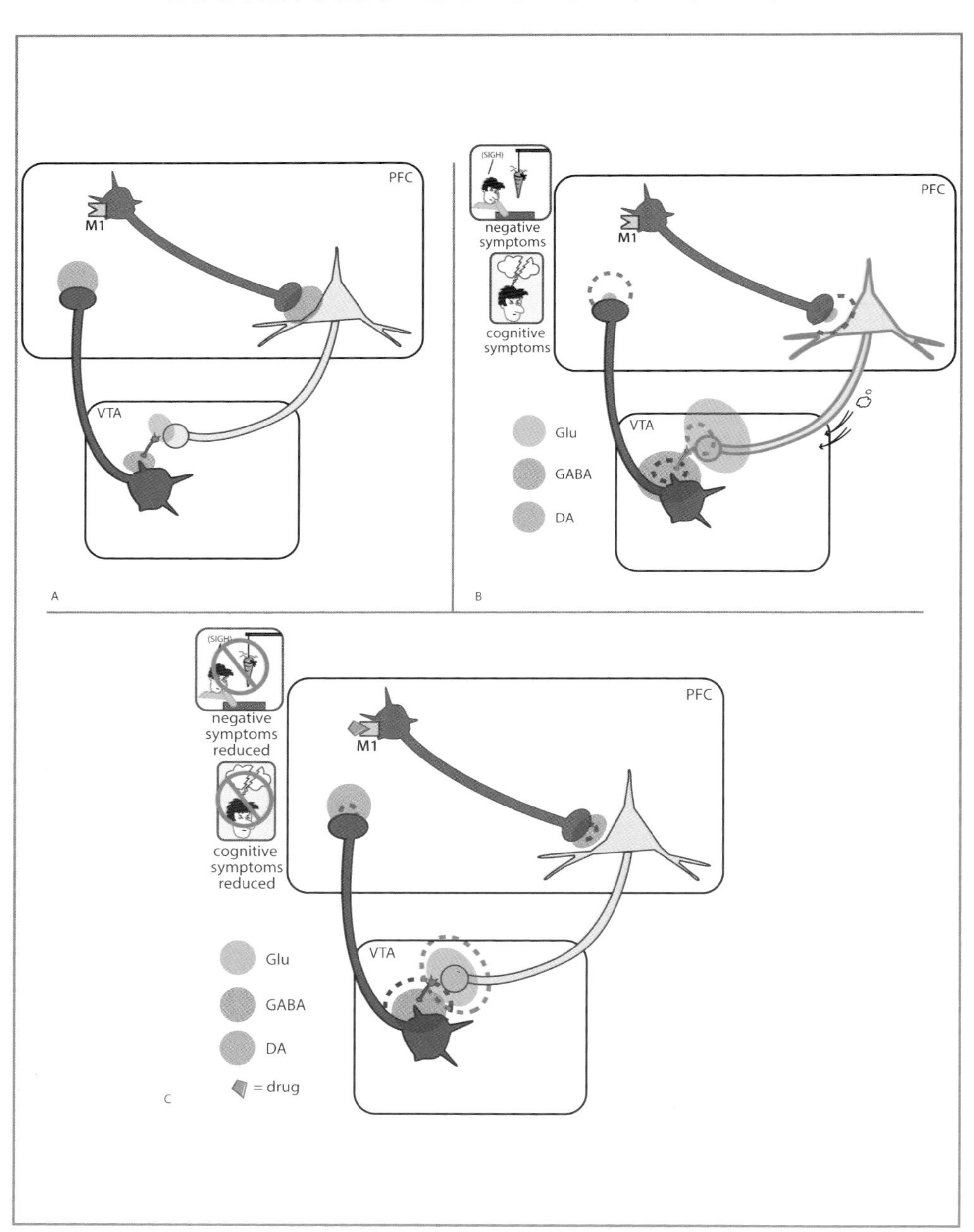

# Upstream M1 Binding Decreases DA Release in Prefrontal Cortex

**FIGURE 6.2.** (A) At baseline, cortical acetylcholine regulates dopamine (DA) projecting back to the prefrontal cortex (PFC). (B) In the context of psychosis, hypofunctional GABA interneurons in the PFC result in disinhibition of glutamate (Glu) and subsequent activation of GABA in the ventral tegmental area (VTA). In turn, the increase in GABA inhibits DA release in the PFC, hypothetically causing negative and cognitive symptoms of psychosis. (C) When muscarinic M1 receptors on hypofunctional GABA interneurons in the PFC are activated by an M1 agonist, this decreases release of Glu and subsequent release of GABA in the VTA. This disinhibition leads to an increase in DA release in the PFC and the hypothetical reduction of negative and cognitive symptoms of psychosis.

# Upstream M4 Binding Decreases Presynaptic DA Release

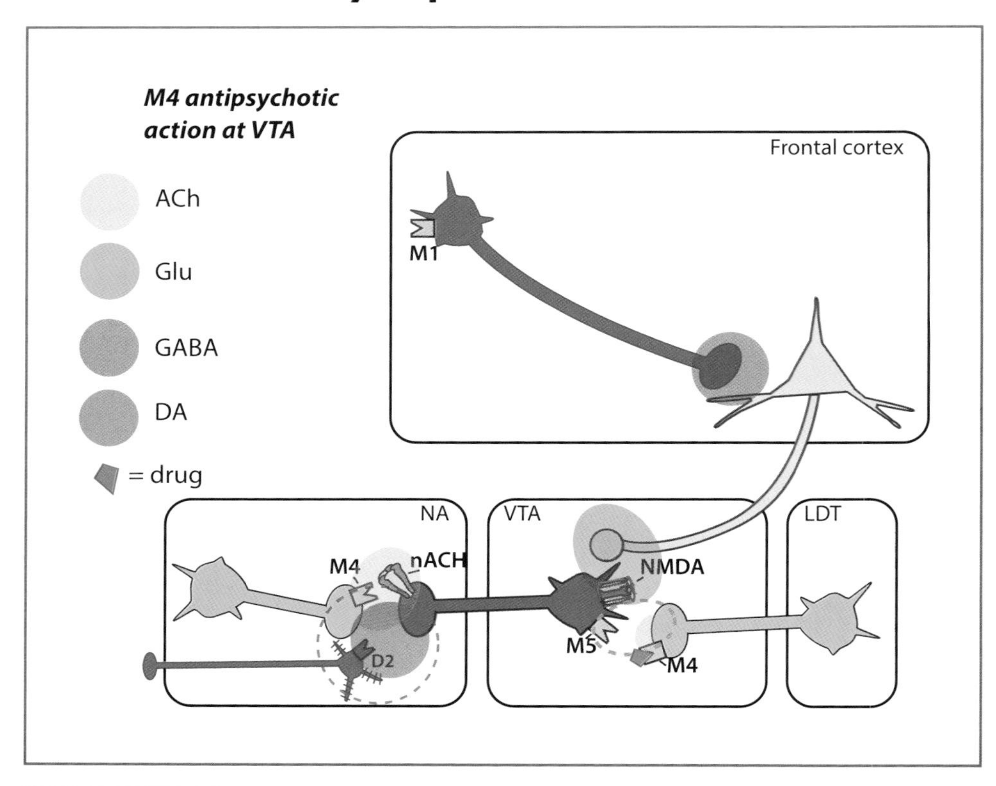


**FIGURE 6.3.** Muscarinic M4 receptors on cholinergic projections from the laterodorsal tegmental nucleus (LDT) in the hindbrain act as autoreceptors and turn off acetylcholine (ACh) release from these projections when activated by an M4 agonist or positive allosteric modulator. This reduction in ACh leads to decreased activation of muscarinic M5 receptors located on DA cell bodies, decreased neuronal excitability in the VTA, and reduced DA release in the nucleus accumbens (NA), thereby hypothetically decreasing positive symptoms of psychosis (Paul et al., 2022; Yohn et al., 2022).

# Local M4 Binding Decreases Presynaptic DA Release

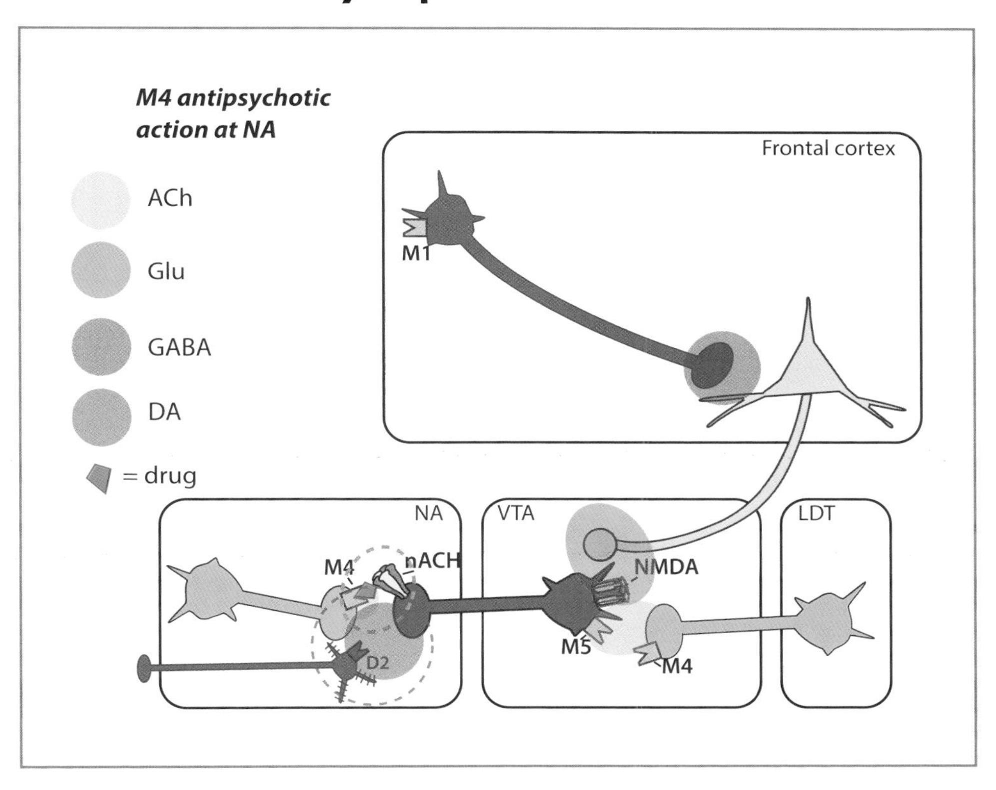


**FIGURE 6.4.** Muscarinic M4 receptors that reside locally in the nucleus accumbens (NA) act as autoreceptors on cholinergic interneurons. Like their actions in the hindbrain, activation of M4 receptors by an M4 agonist or positive allosteric modulator turns off ACh release from cholinergic neurons. Reduced ACh release causes decreased activation of nicotinic ACh (nACh) receptors found on DA terminals, resulting in decreased DA release and hypothetically decreased positive symptoms of psychosis (Paul et al., 2022; Yohn et al., 2022).

# M1/M4 Agonist: Xanomeline-Trospium

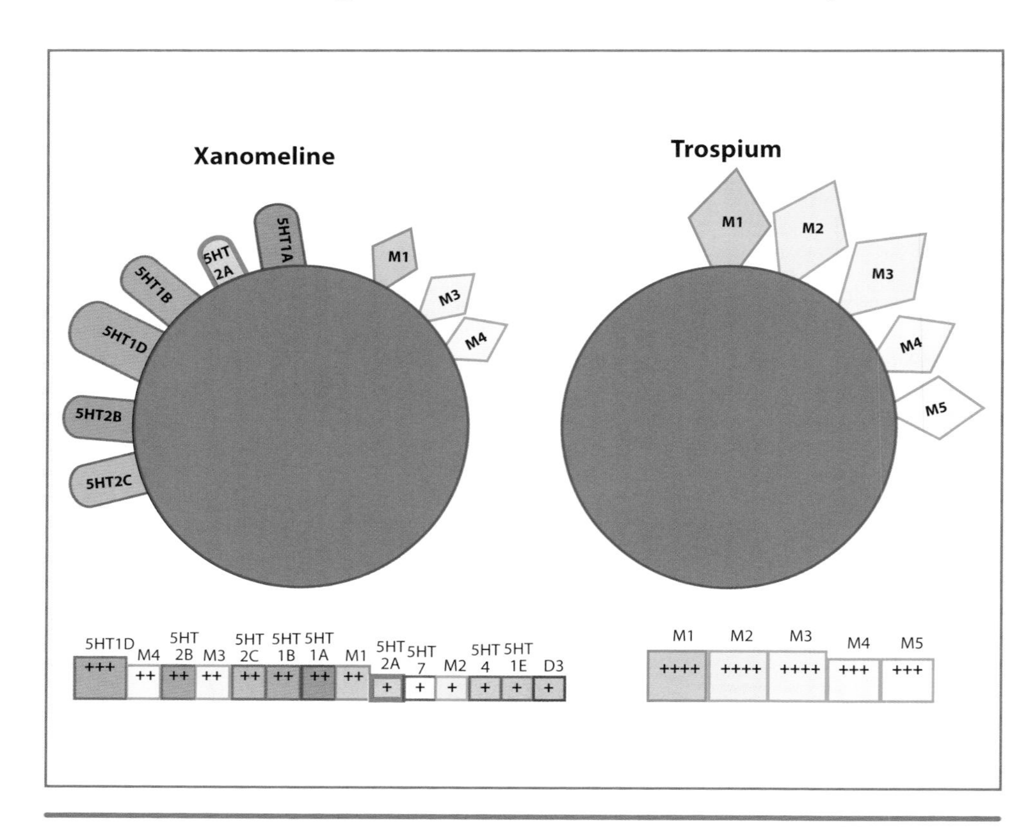


**FIGURE 6.5.** Xanomeline is a relatively selective muscarinic M1/M4 agonist that was previously studied for its antipsychotic properties (Shekhar et al., 2008). Its clinical development was hindered due to gastrointestinal side effects, primarily related to M1 agonism (Dean & Scarr, 2020). The addition of trospium has allowed further investigation. Trospium is a non-selective muscarinic receptor antagonist that has minimal, if any, penetration of the blood–brain barrier, blocking unwanted peripheral cholinergic side effects of xanomeline (Abrams & Andersson, 2007; Pak et al., 2003). Indeed, clinical trial data show that discontinuations of treatment due to adverse effects in xanomeline-trospium and placebo study arms are comparable. Critically, data from clinical trials also show that xanomeline-trospium effectively reduces psychosis symptoms in adults with schizophrenia, compared to placebo (Brannan et al., 2021). To date, results on the effects of xanomeline-trospium on Alzheimer's disease psychosis have not been published.

# M4 Positive Allosteric Modulator: Emraclidine

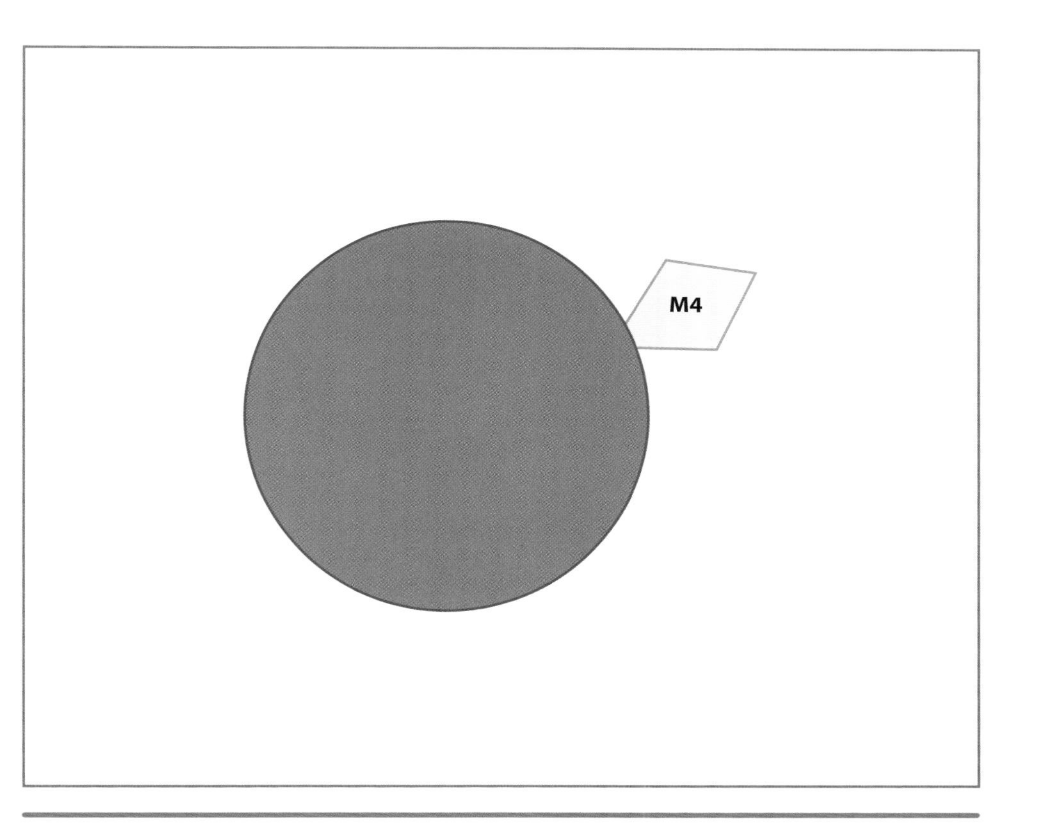


**FIGURE 6.6.** Emraclidine is a brain-penetrant selective muscarinic M4 positive allosteric modulator (PAM) being developed for schizophrenia and Alzheimer's disease psychosis. Allosteric modulators bind to a different receptor site than the endogenous agonist, in this case acetylcholine. Allosteric binding changes the receptor's overall response to stimulation. Positive allosteric binders increase the response of the receptor by increasing the probability that an agonist will bind to a receptor (i.e., affinity), increasing its ability to activate the receptor (i.e., efficacy), or both (Stahl, 2021). The muscarinic M4 receptor is differentially expressed in the striatum; therefore, emraclidine's selective M4 receptor binding may avoid side effects associated with other pan-muscarinic agonists. Results from an early phase clinical trial showed that compared to placebo, emraclidine reduced symptoms of psychosis in adults with schizophrenia. Additionally, the incidence of adverse events was similar across groups (Krystal et al., 2022). To date, results on the effects of emraclidine on Alzheimer's disease psychosis have not been published.

# M4 Agonist: NBI-1117568

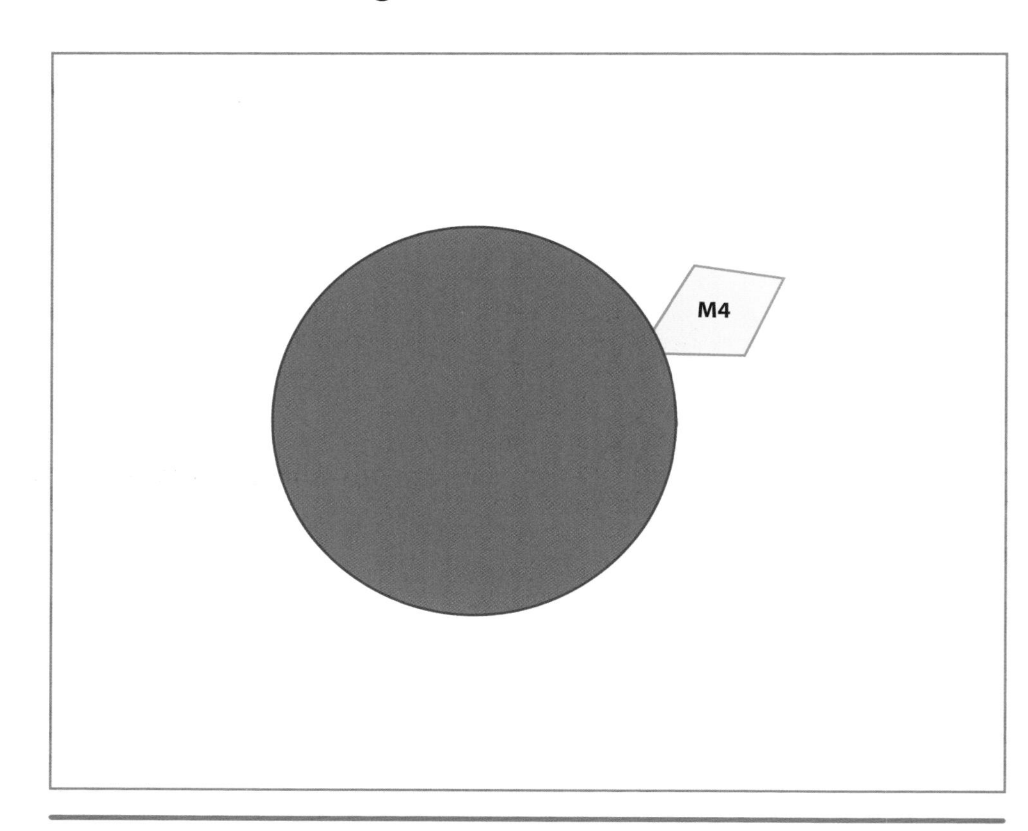


**FIGURE 6.7.** NBI-1117568 is an investigational drug that selectively agonizes the muscarinic M4 receptor. This binding selectivity offers the potential for an improved safety profile without the need for combination therapy to minimize adverse effects. An early phase clinical trial investigating its efficacy in schizophrenia is underway (Kantrowitz et al., 2023).

# Pre- and Postsynaptic Agonism of TAAR1

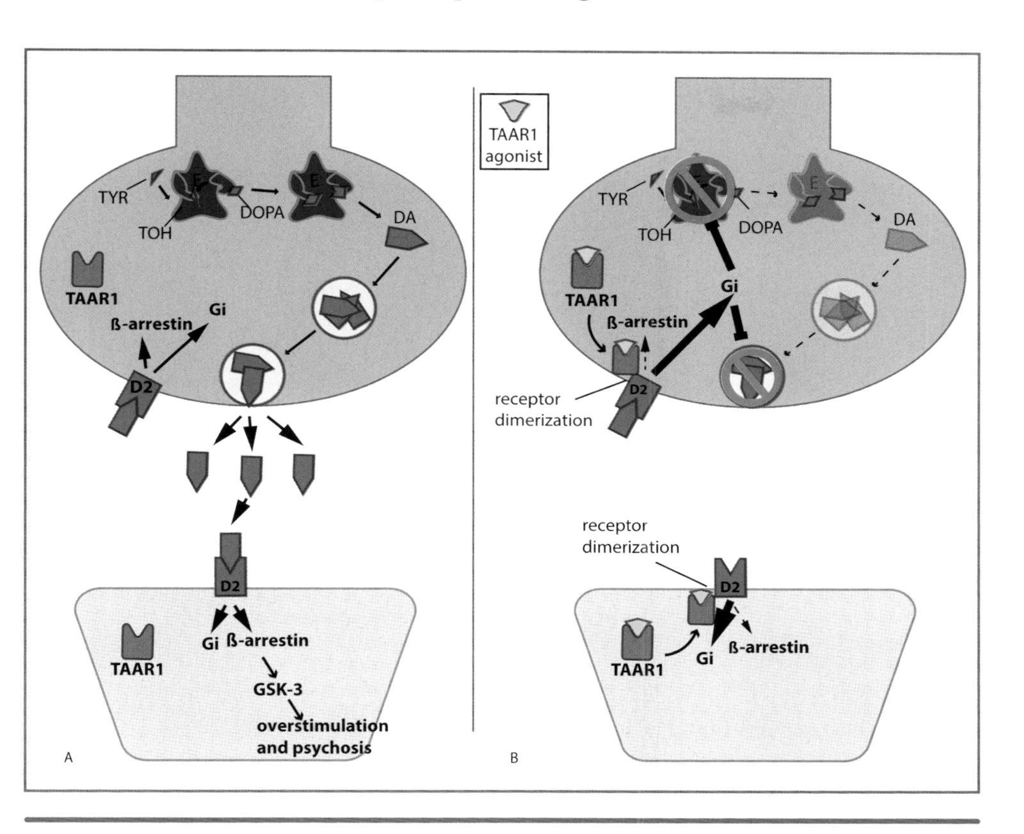


**FIGURE 6.8.** Trace amines are formed from amino acids when either the tyrosine hydroxylase (TYR) step or the tryptophan hydroxylase (TOH) step is omitted during production of dopamine or serotonin, respectively. (A) Dopamine is produced and packaged into synaptic vesicles, then released into the synapse. Dopamine binding at both pre- and postsynaptic D2 receptors can either trigger the inhibitory G (Gi) protein signal transduction cascade or the β-arrestin 2 signal transduction cascade. The β-arrestin 2 cascade leads to production of glycogen synthase kinase 3 (GSK-3); too much GSK-3 activation may be associated with mania or psychosis. (B) When TAAR1 receptors are bound by an agonist, they translocate to the synaptic membrane and couple with D2 receptors (heterodimerization). This biases the D2 receptor toward activating the Gi signal transduction cascade instead of the β-arrestin cascade. Presynaptically, amplification of the Gi pathway leads to inhibition of the synthesis and release of dopamine, which would be beneficial in cases of psychosis. Postsynaptically, amplification of the Gi pathway can lead to reduced production of GSK-3 (Pei et al., 2016; Stahl et al., 2020).

# TAAR1 Agonist: Ulotaront

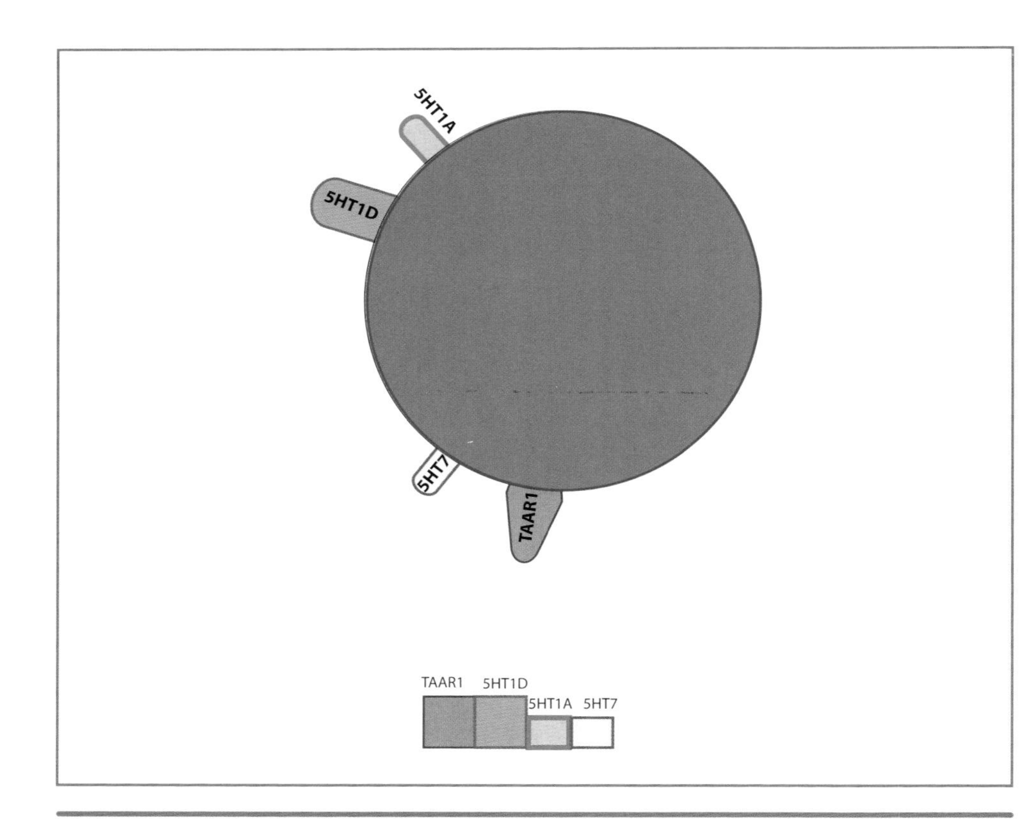


**FIGURE 6.9.** Ulotaront is an agonist at TAAR1 receptors; it also has 5HT1D, 5HT1A, and 5HT7 receptor binding properties (Stahl, 2021). Results from a phase 2 randomized clinical trial show that ulotaront decreases psychotic and negative symptoms in patients with schizophrenia. The data also indicate an absence of motor, metabolic, or endocrine adverse effects, compared to placebo (Koblan et al., 2020). A 6-month open-label extension study indicates that ulotaront improves positive and negative symptoms over the long term, and that the same may apply to cognitive symptoms (Correll et al., 2021). Results from phase 3 clinical trials are pending publication. To date, results on the effects of ulotaront on Parkinson's disease psychosis have not been published.

Stahl's Illustrated | Summary

Our understanding of the underlying pathophysiology of psychosis and schizophrenia continues to evolve and inform the development of novel treatments. Dopamine, glutamate, and serotonin are three of the most important neurotransmitter systems involved in schizophrenia and in the mechanism of action of currently available drugs for psychosis. Emerging research strongly indicates that muscarinic M1 and M4 acetylcholine receptors and TAAR1 receptors also play an important role in the pathophysiology and treatment of psychosis. Each drug for psychosis has a unique receptor profile that influences both the amelioration of symptoms and the induction of side effects. A savvy psychopharmacologist must consider these profiles when selecting and switching treatments in order to maximize patient outcomes.

Optional Posttest and CME/CE Credit: The optional posttest with CME/CE credits is available online for a fee (waived for NEI Members). A posttest score of 70% or higher is required to receive credit. To purchase and/or open the posttest, go to **https://nei.global/24-Stahl-illus-psychosis3**.

# References

Abrams P, Andersson KE. Muscarinic receptor antagonists for overactive bladder. BJU Int 2007;100(5):987–1006.

Alex KD, Pehak EA. Pharmacological mechanisms of serotoninergic regulation of dopamine neurotransmission. Pharmacol Ther 2007;113(2):296–320.

Amargós-Bosch M, Bortolozzi A, Puig MV et al. Co-expression and in vivo interaction of serotonin 1A and serotonin 2A receptors in pyramidal neurons of prefrontal cortex. Cereb Cortex 2004;14(3):281–99.

American Psychiatric Association. Schizophrenia spectrum and other psychotic disorders. In: Diagnostic and statistical manual of mental disorders. 5th ed, text rev. Washington, DC: American Psychiatric Association; 2022:101–38.

Arango C, Rapado-Castro M, Reig S et al. Progressive brain changes in children and adolescents with first-episode psychosis. Arch Gen Psychiatry 2012;69(1):16–26.

Beaulieu JM, Gainetdinov RR. The physiology, signaling, and pharmacology of dopamine receptors. Pharmacol Rev 2011;63(1):182–217.

Benjamin KJM, Chen Q, Jaffe AE et al. Analysis of the caudate nucleus transcriptome in individuals with schizophrenia highlights effects of antipsychotics and new risk genes. Nat Neurosci 2022;25(11):1559–68.

Brannan SK, Sawchak S, Miller AC, Lieberman JA, Paul SM, Breier A. Muscarinic cholinergic receptor agonist and peripheral antagonist for schizophrenia. N Engl J Med 2021;384(8):717–26.

Brugger SP, Angelescu I, Abi-Dargham A, Mizrahi R, Shahrezaei V, Howes OD. Heterogeneity of striatal dopamine function in schizophrenia: meta-analysis of variance. Biol Psychiatry 2020;87(3):215–24.

Bubeníková-Valesová V, Horácek J, Vrajová M, Höschl C. Models of schizophrenia in humans and animals based on inhibition of NMDA receptors. Neurosci Biobehav Rev 2008;32(5):1014–23.

Bugarski-Kirola D, Arango C, Fava M et al. Pimavanserin for negative symptoms of schizophrenia: results from the ADVANCE phase 2 randomised, placebo-controlled trial in North America and Europe. Lancet Psychiatry 2022;9(1):46–58.

Calabrese J, Al Khalili Y. Psychosis. [Updated May 1, 2023]. In: StatPearls [Internet]. Treasure Island (FL): StatPearls Publishing; 2023 Jan. Available from https://www.ncbi.nlm.nih.gov/books/NBK546579/. Accessed September 14, 2023.

Calabresi P, Picconi B, Tozzi A, Ghiglieri V, Di Filippo M. Direct and indirect pathways of basal ganglia: a critical reappraisal. Nat Neurosci 2014;17(8):1022–30.

Citrome L. Long-acting injectable antipsychotics: what, when, and how—Addendum. CNS Spectr 2021;26(2):118–29.

Correll CU, Kim E, Sliwa JK et al. Pharmacokinetic characteristics of long-acting injectable antipsychotics for schizophrenia: an overview. CNS Drugs 2021;35(1):39–59.

Correll CU, Koblan KS, Hopkins SC et al. Safety and effectiveness of ulotaront (SEP-363856) in schizophrenia: results of a 6-month, open-label extension study. NPJ Schizophr 2021;7(1):63.

Cummings JL, Devanand DP, Stahl SM. Dementia-related psychosis and the potential role for pimavanserin. CNS Spectr 2022;27(1):7–15.

Darwish M, Bugarski-Kirola D, Passarell J et al. Pimavanserin exposure-response analyses in patients with schizophrenia: results from the phase 2 ADVANCE Study. J Clin Psychopharmacol 2022;42(6):544–51.

de Bartolomeis A, Fiore G, Iasevoli F. Dopamine-glutamate interaction and antipsychotics mechanism of action: implication for new pharmacological strategies in psychosis. Curr Pharm Des 2005;11(27):3561–94.

Dean B, Scarr E. Muscarinic M1 and M4 receptors: hypothesis driven drug development for schizophrenia. Psychiatry Res 2020;288:112989.

DeLong MR, Wichmann T. Circuits and circuit disorders of the basal ganglia. Arch Neurol 2007;64(1):20–4.

Fink KB, Göthert M. 5-HT receptor regulation of neurotransmitter release. Pharmacol Rev 2007;59(4):360–417.

Gellings Lowe N, Rapagnani MP, Mattei C, Stahl SM. The psychopharmacology of hallucinations: ironic insights into mechanisms of action. In: The neuroscience of hallucinations; Jardri R, Thomas P, Cachia A and Pins D (eds.). Berlin: Springer; 2012:471–92.

Goff DC, Falkai P, Fleischhacker WW et al. The long-term effects of antipsychotic medication on clinical course in schizophrenia. Am J Psychiatry 2017;174(9):840–9.

Goff DC, Zeng B, Ardekani BA et al. Association of hippocampal atrophy with duration of untreated psychosis and molecular biomarkers during initial antipsychotic treatment of first-episode psychosis. JAMA Psychiatry 2018;75(4):370–8.

Grajales D, Ferreira V, Valverde ÁM. Second-generation antipsychotics and dysregulation of glucose metabolism: beyond weight gain. Cells 2019;8(11):1336.

Hansen KB, Yi F, Perszyk RE et al. Structure, function, and allosteric modulation of NMDA receptors. J Gen Physiol 2018;150(8):1081–105.

Homayoun H, Moghaddam B. NMDA receptor hypofunction produces opposite effects on prefrontal cortex interneurons and pyramidal neurons. J Neurosci 2007;27(43):11496–500.

Howes OD, Bose SK, Turkheimer F et al. Dopamine synthesis capacity before onset of psychosis: a prospective [18F]-DOPA PET imaging study. Am J Psychiatry 2011;168(12):1311–7.

Jawad MY, Alnefeesi Y, Lui LMW et al. Olanzapine and samidorphan combination treatment: a systematic review. J Affect Disord 2022;301:99–106.

Kahn RS, Kane JM, Correll CU et al. Olanzapine/samidorphan in young adults with schizophrenia, schizophreniform disorder, or bipolar I disorder who are early in their illness: results of the randomized, controlled ENLIGHTEN-Early Study. J Clin Psychiatry 2023;84(3):22m14674.

Kantrowitz JT, Correll CU, Jain R, Cutler AJ. New developments in the treatment of schizophrenia: an expert roundtable. Int J Neuropsychopharmacol 2023;pyad011.

Keks N, Schwartz D, Hope J. Stopping and switching antipsychotic drugs. Aust Prescr 2019;42:152–7.

Kishi T, Matsuda Y, Iwata N. Cardiometabolic risks of blonanserin and perospirone in the management of schizophrenia: a systematic review and meta-analysis of randomized controlled trials. PLoS One 2014;9(2):e88049.

Koblan KS, Kent J, Hopkins SC et al. A non-D2-receptor-binding drug for the treatment of schizophrenia. N Engl J Med 2020;382(16):1497–506.

Kowalchuk C, Teo C, Wilson V et al. In male rats, the ability of central insulin to suppress glucose production is impaired by olanzapine, whereas glucose uptake is left intact. J Psychiatry Neurosci 2017;42(6):424–31.

Krystal JH, Kane JM, Correll CU et al. Emraclidine, a novel positive allosteric modulator of cholinergic M4 receptors, for the treatment of schizophrenia: a two-part, randomised, double-blind, placebo-controlled, phase 1b trial. Lancet 2022;400(10369):2210–20.

Lindström LH, Gefvert O, Hagberg G et al. Increased dopamine synthesis rate in medial prefrontal cortex and striatum in schizophrenia indicated by L-(beta-11C) DOPA and PET. Biol Psychiatry 1999;46(5):681–8.

Luye Pharma Group. Rykindo (risperidone) for extended-release injectable suspension for intramuscular use prescribing information. Rev. January 2023. Available from https://www.accessdata.fda.gov/drugsatfda_docs/label/2023/212849s000lbl.pdf. Accessed July 28, 2023.

McCutcheon RA, Abi-Dargham A, Howes OD. Schizophrenia, dopamine, and the striatum: from biology to symptoms. Trends Neurosci 2019;42(3):205–20.

Meyer JM. Converting oral to long-acting injectable antipsychotics: a guide for the perplexed. CNS Spectr 2017;22(S1):14–28.

Meyer JM, Stahl SM. The clozapine handbook: Stahl's handbooks. New York, NY: Cambridge University Press; 2019.

Niemann N, Jankovic J. Treatment of tardive dyskinesia: a general overview with focus on the vesicular monoamine transporter 2 inhibitors. Drugs 2018;78(5):525–41.

Otsuka Pharmaceutical. Ability Asimtufii (aripiprazole) for extended-release injectable suspension for intramuscular use prescribing information. Rev April 2023. Available from https://www.accessdata.fda.gov/drugsatfda_docs/label/ 2023/217006s000lbl.pdf. Accessed May 2023.

Pak RW, Petrou SP, Staskin DR. Trospium chloride: a quaternary amine with unique pharmacologic properties. Curr Urol Rep 2003;4(6):436–40.

Paoletti P, Neyton J. NMDA receptor subunits: function and pharmacology. Curr Opin Pharmacol 2007;7(1):39–47.

Paul SM, Yohn SE, Popiolek M, Miller AC, Felder CC. Muscarinic acetylcholine receptor agonists as novel treatments for schizophrenia. Am J Psychiatry 2022;179(9):611–27.

Paz RD, Tardito S, Atzori M, Tseng KY. Glutamatergic dysfunction in schizophrenia: from basic neuroscience to clinical psychopharmacology. Eur Neuropsychopharmacol 2008;18(11):773–86.

Pei Y, Asif-Malik A, Canales JJ. Trace amines and the trace amine-associated receptor 1: pharmacology, neurochemistry, and clinical implications. Front Neurosci 2016;10:148.

Peters L, Dyer M, Schroeder E, D'Souza MS. Invega Hafyera (paliperidone palmitate): extended-release injectable suspension for patients with schizophrenia. J Pharm Technol 2023;39(2):88–94.

Reckziegel R, Czepielewski LS, Hasse-Sousa M et al. Heterogeneous trajectories in schizophrenia: insights from neurodevelopment and neuroprogression models. Braz J Psychiatry 2022;44(1):74–80.

Scheefhals N, MacGillavry HD. Functional organization of postsynaptic glutamate receptors. Mol Cell Neurosci 2018;91:82–94.

Shekhar A, Potter WZ, Lightfoot J et al. Selective muscarinic receptor agonist xanomeline as a novel treatment approach for schizophrenia. Am J Psychiatry 2008;165(8):1033–9.

Sokoloff P, Le Foll B. The dopamine D3 receptor, a quarter century later. Eur J Neurosci 2017;45(1):2–19.

St Clair D, Lang B. Schizophrenia: a classic battle ground of nature versus nurture debate. Sci Bull (Beijing) 2021;66(10):1037–46.

Stahl SM. Stahl's essential psychopharmacology: neuroscientific basis and practical applications. 4th ed. New York, NY: Cambridge University Press; 2013.

Stahl SM. Dazzled by the dominions of dopamine: clinical roles of D3, D2, and D1 receptors. CNS Spectr 2017;22(4):305–11.

Stahl SM. Neuronal traffic signals in tardive dyskinesia: not enough "stop" in the motor striatum. CNS Spectr 2017;22(6):427–34.

Stahl SM. Beyond the dopamine hypothesis of schizophrenia to three neural networks of psychosis: dopamine, serotonin, and glutamate. CNS Spectr 2018;23(3):187–91.

Stahl SM. Comparing pharmacologic mechanism of action for the vesicular monoamine transporter 2 (VMAT2) inhibitors valbenazine and deutetrabenazine in treating tardive dyskinesia: does one have advantages over the other? CNS Spectr 2018;23(4):239–47.

Stahl SM. Mechanism of action of vesicular monoamine transporter 2 (VMAT2) inhibitors in tardive dyskinesia: reducing dopamine leads to less "go" and more "stop" from the motor striatum for robust therapeutic effects. CNS Spectr 2018;23(1):1–6.

Stahl SM. Stahl's essential psychopharmacology: the prescriber's guide. 7th ed. New York, NY: Cambridge University Press; 2020.

Stahl SM. Stahl's essential psychopharmacology: neuroscientific basis and practical applications. 5th ed. New York, NY: Cambridge University Press; 2021.

Teva Pharmaceuticals. Uzedy (risperidone) extended-release injectable suspension for subcutaneous use prescribing information. Rev. May 2023. Available from https://www.accessdata.fda.gov/drugsatfda_docs/label/2023/213586s000lbl.pdf. Accessed May 2023.

Wahbeh MH, Avramopoulos D. Gene-environment interactions in schizophrenia: a literature review. Genes (Basel) 2021;12(12):185.

Weinstein JJ, Chohan MO, Slifstein M, Kegeles LS, Moore H, Abi-Dargham A. Pathway-specific dopamine abnormalities in schizophrenia. Biol Psychiatry 2017;81(1):31–42.

Wentland MP, Lu Q, Lou R, Bu Y, Knapp BI, Bidlack JM. Synthesis and opioid receptor binding properties of a highly potent 4-hydroxy analogue of naltrexone. Bioorg Med Chem Lett 2005;15(8):2107–10.

Yohn SE, Weiden PJ, Felder CC, Stahl SM. Muscarinic acetylcholine receptors for psychotic disorders: bench-side to clinic. Trends Pharmacol Sci 2022;43(12):1098–112.

Zhang L, Hendrick JP. The presynaptic D2 partial agonist lumateperone acts as a postsynaptic D2 antagonist. Matters 2018. doi: 10.19185/matters.201712000006.

Stahl's Illustrated | # Index